Management of Infectious Diseases in Stem Cell Transplantation and Hematologic Malignancy

Editor

JO-ANNE H. YOUNG

INFECTIOUS DISEASE CLINICS OF NORTH AMERICA

www.id.theclinics.com

Consulting Editor
HELEN W. BOUCHER

June 2019 • Volume 33 • Number 2

ELSEVIER

1600 John F. Kennedy Boulevard • Suite 1800 • Philadelphia, Pennsylvania, 19103-2899.
http://www.theclinics.com

INFECTIOUS DISEASE CLINICS OF NORTH AMERICA Volume 33, Number 2
June 2019 ISSN 0891–5520, ISBN-13: 978-0-323-67872-8

Editor: Kerry Holland
Developmental Editor: Donald Mumford

Infectious Disease Clinics of North America (ISSN 0891–5520) is published in March, June, September, and December by Elsevier Inc., 360 Park Avenue South, New York, NY 10010-1710. Periodicals postage paid at New York, NY and additional mailing offices. Subscription prices are $330.00 per year for US individuals, $660.00 per year for US institutions, $100.00 per year for US students, $396.00 per year for Canadian individuals, $824.00 per year for Canadian institutions, $432.00 per year for international individuals, $824.00 per year for international institutions, and $200.00 per year for Canadian and international students. To receive student rate, orders must be accompanied by name of affiliated institution, date of term, and the *signature* of program/residency coordinator on institution letterhead. Orders will be billed at individual rate until proof of status is received. Foreign air speed delivery is included in all *Clinics* subscription prices. All prices are subject to change without notice. **POSTMASTER**: Send address changes to *Infectious Disease Clinics of North America*, Elsevier Health Sciences Division, Subcription Customer Service, 3251 Riverport Lane, Maryland Heights, MO 63043. **Customer Service: 1-800-654-2452 (US). From outside of the US and Canada, call 1-314-447-8871. Fax: 1-314-447-8029. E-mail: JournalsCustomerService-usa@elsevier.com (print support) or JournalsOnlineSupport-usa@elsevier.com (online support).**

Infectious Disease Clinics of North America is also published in Spanish by Editorial Inter-Médica, Junin 917, 1er A 1113, Buenos Aires, Argentina.

Reprints. For copies of 100 or more, of articles in this publication, please contact the Commercial Reprints Department, Elsevier Inc., 360 Park Avenue South, New York, New York 10010-1710. Tel. 212-633-3874, Fax: 212-633-3820, E-mail: reprints@elsevier.com.

Infectious Disease Clinics of North America is covered in *MEDLINE/PubMed (Index Medicus), Current Contents/Clinical Medicine, Science Citation Alert, SCISEARCH,* and *Research Alert.*

Printed in the United States of America.

Contributors

CONSULTING EDITOR

HELEN W. BOUCHER, MD, FIDSA, FACP
Director, Infectious Diseases Fellowship Program, Division of Geographic Medicine and Infectious Diseases, Tufts Medical Center, Associate Professor of Medicine, Tufts University School of Medicine, Boston, Massachusetts, USA

EDITOR

JO-ANNE H. YOUNG, MD
Professor, Division of Infectious Disease and International Medicine, Department of Medicine, Executive Medical Director, Program in Adult Transplant Infectious Disease, University of Minnesota, Minneapolis, Minnesota, USA

AUTHORS

DAVID R. ANDES, MD
Department of Medicine, Division of Infectious Disease, University of Wisconsin School of Medicine and Public Health, Madison, Wisconsin, USA

SARAH ATKINS, MD
Department of Internal Medicine, University of Minnesota, Minneapolis, Minnesota, USA

DEREK J. BAYS, MD
Department of Internal Medicine, University of California, Davis Medical Center, Davis, California, USA

SANJEET SINGH DADWAL, MD, FACP
City of Hope National Medical Center, Duarte, California, USA

ERIK R. DUBBERKE, MD, MSPH
Professor, Division of Infectious Disease, Department of Internal Medicine, Washington University School of Medicine, St Louis, Missouri, USA

LAUREN FONTANA, DO
Division of Infectious Disease, Department of Medicine, Oregon Health & Science University, Portland, Oregon, USA

FIONA HE, MD
Division of Hematology, Oncology, and Transplantation, University of Minnesota, Minneapolis, Minnesota, USA

SHERNAN G. HOLTAN, MD
Assistant Professor, Division of Hematology, Oncology, and Transplantation, Department of Medicine, University of Minnesota, Minneapolis, Minnesota, USA

MINI KAMBOJ, MD
Associate Member, Infectious Disease Service, Department of Medicine,
Chief Medical Epidemiologist, Memorial Sloan Kettering Cancer Center, Assistant
Professor of Medicine, Weill Cornell Medical College, New York, New York,
USA

ROY L. KAO, MD
Assistant Professor, Division of Hematology, Oncology, and Transplantation, Department
of Medicine, University of Minnesota, Minneapolis, Minnesota, USA

ELIZABETH ANN MISCH, MD
Department of Medicine, Division of Infectious Disease, University of Wisconsin School of
Medicine and Public Health, Madison, Wisconsin, USA

SUNITA NATHAN, MD
Associate Professor of Medicine, Division of Hematology, Oncology and Cellular Therapy,
Rush University Medical Center, Chicago, Illinois, USA

DIONYSIOS NEOFYTOS, MD, MPH
Division of Infectious Diseases, University Hospital of Geneva, Geneva, Switzerland

KARAM M. OBEID, MD
Division of Infectious Diseases and International Medicine, University of Minnesota,
Minneapolis, Minnesota, USA

ANUPAM PANDE, MD, MPH
Assistant Professor, Division of Infectious Disease, Department of Internal Medicine,
Washington University School of Medicine, St Louis, Missouri, USA

DRIELE PEIXOTO, MD
Sao Paulo State Cancer Institute (ICESP), Hospital das Clínicas, São Paulo, Brazil

DANIEL P. PRESTES, MD
A. C. Camargo Cancer Center, Emilio Ribas Infectious Diseases Institute, São Paulo,
Brazil

NASIA SAFDAR, MD, PhD
Department of Medicine, Division of Infectious Disease, University of Wisconsin School of
Medicine and Public Health, Department of Medicine, William S. Middleton Memorial
Veterans Hospital, Madison, Wisconsin, USA

GOWRI SATYANARAYANA, MD
Assistant Professor, Division of Infectious Diseases, Vanderbilt University Medical Center,
Nashville, Tennessee, USA

MONIKA K. SHAH, MD
Clinical Member, Infectious Disease Service, Department of Medicine, Associate
Professor of Clinical Medicine, Weill Cornell Medical College, New York, New York,
USA

LYNNE STRASFELD, MD
Division of Infectious Disease, Department of Medicine, Oregon Health & Science
University, Portland, Oregon, USA

GEORGE R. THOMPSON III, MD, FIDSA
Associate Professor of Clinical Medicine, Department of Internal Medicine, Division of Infectious Diseases, University of California, Davis Medical Center, Department of Medical Microbiology and Immunology, University of California, Davis, Davis, California, USA

CELALETTIN USTUN, MD
Associate Professor of Medicine, Division of Hematology, Oncology and Cellular Therapy, Rush University Medical Center, Chicago, Illinois, USA

Contents

> Treatment options for hematologic malignancies have been rapidly expanding in the past decade, resulting in better survival outcomes for many patients. Infection is an important cause of morbidity and mortality in this patient population. Cytotoxic chemotherapy has well-studied infectious risks related to the degree and duration of myelosuppression. Targeted therapies and immunotherapies have less clearly predictable infectious risk and diverse effects on immune function. This review discusses contemporary management of hematologic malignancies, followed by special discussion of novel agents, including signaling/small molecule inhibitors, monoclonal antibodies, immunomodulators, and immunotherapies, for treatment of hematologic malignancies with focus on infectious risk.

> Infection contributes significantly to morbidity and mortality in hematopoietic cell transplantation. A complex interplay of host, graft, and technical factors contributes to infectious risk in the recipient. Host factors such as age, underlying disease, and comorbidities; central venous access; and the preparative regimen contribute to mucosal disruption, organ dysfunction, and immunodeficiency before hematopoietic cell transplantation. Graft factors, including donor histocompatibility, cell source, and graft components, along with immunosuppression and graft-versus-host disease, contribute to the speed of immune reconstitution. Evaluation of these factors, plus previous and posttransplant exposure to pathogens, is necessary to best assess an individual recipient's infection risk.

> This article discusses the complications of hematopoietic stem cell transplantion (HSCT) that affect infections in HSCT recipients, with analogies to patients with hematologic malignancies. Mucositis, with mucosal barrier disruption, is common and increases the risk of gram-positive and anaerobic bacterial, and fungal infections, and can evolve to typhlitis. Engraftment syndrome; graft-versus-host disease, hepatic sinusoidal

Clostridioides difficile infection (CDI) is common in the stem cell transplant (SCT) and hematologic malignancy (HM) population and mostly occurs in the early posttransplant period. Treatment of CDI in SCT/HM is the same as for the general population, with the exception that fecal microbiota transplant (FMT) has not been widely adopted because of safety concerns. Several case reports, small series, and retrospective studies have shown that FMT is effective and safe. A randomized controlled trial of FMT for prophylaxis of CDI in SCT patients is underway. In addition, an abundance of novel therapeutics for CDI is currently in development.

This review discusses the epidemiologic and clinical aspects of herpes viruses other than cytomegalovirus in patients who have undergone hematopoietic stem cell transplantation.

Cytomegalovirus (CMV) may no longer be the menace that plagues stem cell transplant outcomes, owing to marked improvements in transplantation techniques and methods of prophylaxis. However, it still remains a common and morbid problem for recipients of stem cell transplant and patients with certain hematologic malignancies. This article discusses the epidemiology and risk factors of CMV infection and disease, associated morbidity and mortality, diagnosis, and clinical features of clinical syndromes associated with CMV and the principles of management of CMV, with special attention to resistant CMV as it pertains to infectious disease specialists.

Infections due to adenovirus, polyomaviruses (BK and JC viruses), and parvovirus B19 may not be as common as infections due to other DNA viruses, such as cytomegalovirus in patients with hematological malignancies and the recipients of hematopoietic stem cell transplantation. However, these infections may result in life-threatening diseases that significantly impact patients' recovery, morbidity, and mortality. Treating physicians should be aware of the diseases associated with these viruses, the patient populations at increased risk for complications due to these infections, and the available diagnostic and therapeutic approaches.

> Respiratory virus infections in hematologic stem cell transplant recipients and patients with hematologic malignancies are increasingly recognized as a cause of significant morbidity and mortality. The often overlapping clinical presentation makes molecular diagnostic strategies imperative for rapid diagnosis and to inform understanding of the changing epidemiology of each of the respiratory viruses. Most respiratory virus infections are managed with supportive therapy, although there is effective antiviral therapy for influenza. The primary focus should remain on primary prevention infection control procedures and isolation precautions, avoidance of ill contacts, and vaccination for influenza.

> Despite advances in chemotherapy and supportive care, morbidity and mortality remain high for patients with hematologic malignances (HMs). Those who require hematopoietic stem cell transplantation (HSCT) often require significant immunosuppression and are subject to a variety of complications. These patients carry multiple risk factors for infectious complications, including the development of invasive fungal infections, compared with the general population. Because antifungal prophylaxis has been widely adopted, there has been a shift away from invasive candidiasis toward invasive mold infections, including breakthrough infections. For patients with HM and HSCT, we outline the epidemiology, manifestations, diagnosis, and treatment of invasive fungal infections.

> Hematopoietic stem cell transplantation (HSCT) recipients may infrequently develop parasitic infections at the time of the procedure via contamination from allograft tissue or blood products, and in the post-transplantation period through the traditional route of infection or as a reactivation caused by immunosuppression related to the transplant. To reduce risk, efforts should be directed at performing a comprehensive history, maintaining a high index of suspicion, and adhering to preventive measures. Additional strategies for the prevention, screening and careful follow-up, identification, and pre-emptive treatment of parasitic infections are required to reduce morbidity and mortality in HSCT patients.

> Patients with hematologic malignancy or those who undergo hematopoietic stem cell transplantation experience variable degrees of immunosuppression, dependent on underlying disease, therapy received, time since

transplant, and complications, such as graft-versus-host disease. Vaccination is an important strategy to mitigate onset and severity of certain vaccine-preventable illnesses, such as influenza, pneumococcal disease, or varicella zoster infection, among others. This article highlights vaccines that should and should not be used in this patient population and includes general guidelines for timing of vaccination administration and special considerations in the context of newer therapies, recent vaccine developments, travel, and considerations for household contacts.

Management of Infectious Diseases in Stem Cell Transplantation and Hematologic Malignancy

INFECTIOUS DISEASE CLINICS
OF NORTH AMERICA

FORTHCOMING ISSUES

September 2019
HIV
Paul Edward Sax, *Editor*

December 2019
Emerging and Re-Emerging Infectious Diseases
Alimuddin Zumla and David SC Hui, *Editors*

March 2020
Collaborative Antimicrobial Stewardship
Elizabeth Dodds-Ashley and S. Shaefer Spires, *Editors*

RECENT ISSUES

March 2019
Updates in Tropical Medicine
Michael Libman and Cédric P. Yansouni, *Editors*

December 2018
Device-Associated Infections
Vivian H. Chu, *Editor*

September 2018
Management of Infections in Solid Organ Transplant Recipients
Sherif Beniameen Mossad, *Editor*

Preface

Management of Infectious Diseases in Stem Cell Transplantation and Hematologic Malignancy

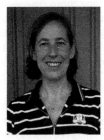

Jo-Anne H. Young, MD
Editor

The approach to treatment of hematologic malignancy started in the 1940s due to failed chemical treatments for malaria. These malaria treatments were destroying white blood cells. The origins of modern bone marrow transplantation followed in short order, with the combining of chemotherapy and radiation treatments following recognition of how to take care of people who were afflicted by radiation accidents. The first human marrow product was infused in 1957, demonstrating that the patient did not die immediately of an infusion reaction and did not get the equivalent of pulmonary embolism from infusing a combination of fat, microparticles of bone, and clumps of marrow cells intravenously.[1] Important breakthroughs in immunology came with HLA description and modern HLA serologic typing in the 1960s. In 1968, the first two successful bone marrow transplants were performed, for immunodeficiency diseases.[2,3]

Clinical bone marrow transplantation took off with steam in the 1970s. In 1977, a landmark article described 100 sibling donor transplants for leukemia, showing engraftment for 94 patients.[4] The original model was myeloablative transplant whereby an intense regimen killed off as many cancer cells as possible. Immunosuppression prevented graft rejection, but complications were frequent and included regimen-related toxicity, graft-versus-host disease, opportunistic infections, and relapse. Anticancer transplantation, regardless of whether the cells come from bone marrow, involves killing all the cancer cells with pretransplant conditioning, managing the aplasia that follows, or expecting the transplant itself will restore immunocompetence. In the process, two outcomes need to be managed: first, prevent infection while restoring a functioning immune system, and second, prevent cancer

Infect Dis Clin N Am 33 (2019) xiii–xv
https://doi.org/10.1016/j.idc.2019.02.013
0891-5520/19/© 2019 Published by Elsevier Inc.

recurrence by graft-versus-leukemia or graft-versus-tumor effects that are associated with any type of a nonsyngeneic donor.

To bring transplants to older patients, the transplant community had to figure out how to limit the toxicity of regimens, to make them more immunosuppressive and less immunotoxic. This led to the development of nonmyeloablative conditioning. As the intensity of the anticancer conditioning decreases, success of the transplant procedure relies more on the immunologic graft-versus-leukemia effect to reduce relapse. The idea is that it is safer overall and less clinically toxic, and indeed, more tolerable for older or sicker people, or people beaten up by previous cancer chemotherapy.

Highlights of changes to the hematology field over subsequent decades include extending indications for chemotherapy and transplantation to many more diseases, extending the donor pool, new drugs, different stem cell sources outside of just bone marrow, changes to conditioning regimens, and new ways of trying to make the whole process work better and safer. In the 2000s, we have seen improved outcomes from safer transplants for all ages, the rise of cord blood and haploidentical products as a stem cell source, and new cellular therapies.[5-8] The current focus is on providing cures and safe transplant.

Nearly 10 years have elapsed since an issue of *Infectious Disease Clinics of North America* included articles dedicated to infections of the hematopoietic stem cell transplant recipient or hematologic malignancy patient. In that time, evolution of diagnostic and therapeutic modalities in the infectious disease world has affected these patients. In addition, there are antimicrobial stewardship initiatives, new vaccines, and a push toward outpatient management whenever possible. The fourteen articles in this issue reflect contemporaneous infectious disease management of patients who are undergoing treatment for hematologic malignancy or who are recipients of hematopoietic cell transplantation.

Jo-Anne H. Young, MD
Division of Infectious Disease and International Medicine
Department of Medicine
University of Minnesota
MMC 250
420 Delaware Street SE
Minneapolis, MN 55455, USA

E-mail address:
vanbu004@umn.edu

REFERENCES

1. Thomas ED, Lochte HL Jr, Lu WC, et al. Intravenous infusion of bone marrow in patients receiving radiation and chemotherapy. N Engl J Med 1957;257(11):491–6.

2. Gatti RA, Meuwissen HJ, Allen HD, et al. Immunological reconstitution of sex-linked lymphopenic immunological deficiency. Lancet 1968;2(7583):1366–9.

3. Bach FH, Albertini RJ, Joo P, et al. Bone-marrow transplantation in a patient with the Wiskott-Aldrich syndrome. Lancet 1968;2(7583):1364–6.

4. Thomas ED, Buckner CD, Banaji M, et al. One hundred patients with acute leukemia treated by chemotherapy, total body irradiation, and allogeneic marrow transplantation. Blood 1977;49(4):511–33.

5. Brunstein CG, Gutman JA, Weisdorf DJ, et al. Allogeneic hematopoietic cell trans-plantation for hematologic malignancy: relative risks and benefits of double umbil-ical cord blood. Blood 2010;116(22):4693–9.
6. Anasetti C, Logan BR, Lee SJ, et al. Peripheral-blood stem cells versus bone marrow from unrelated donors. N Engl J Med 2012;367(16):1487–96.
7. Young JH, Logan BR, Wu J, et al. Infections after transplantation of bone marrow or peripheral blood stem cells from unrelated donors. Biol Blood Marrow Transplant 2016;22(2):359–70.
8. MacMillan ML, DeFor TE, Young JA, et al. Alternative donor hematopoietic cell transplantation for Fanconi anemia. Blood 2015;125(24):3798–804.

Chemotherapy and Beyond

Infections in the Era of Old and New Treatments for Hematologic Malignancies

Sarah Atkins, MD[a], Fiona He, MD[b],*

KEYWORDS

- Infection • Malignant hematology • Chemotherapy • Targeted therapy
- Novel agents

KEY POINTS

- Purine analogues, Alemtuzumab, and multiagent cytotoxic chemotherapy for acute leukemias confer the highest risk for infection due to duration and severity of neutropenia.
- Hepatitis B serostatus for BCR-ABL tyrosine kinase inhibitors, ruxolitinib, and rituximab should be assessed before treatment because reactivation is common.
- Pneumocystis prophylaxis should be given prophylactically with idelalisib, purine analogues, and prednisone to an equivalent of ≥20 mg daily for ≥1 month.
- Cytokine release syndrome is common with chimeric antigen receptor T cells therapy and a mimic of infection.

INTRODUCTION

Infection is a significant cause of morbidity and mortality in the malignant hematology population. In comparison to solid tumors, hematologic malignancies are more likely to have baseline qualitative and quantitative immune deficiencies, and treatment regimens are often more myelosuppressive. Risk of infection with bacterial, fungal, or viral organisms is directly related to severity (absolute neutrophil count [ANC] <100 cells/mm³ highest risk, <500 cells/mm³ high risk) and duration (≥7 days high risk) of neutropenia associated with treatment regimens. Other factors that increase risk of infection in the cancer population include use of indwelling devices, including central venous catheters, Ommaya reservoirs, urinary catheters, and disruption of mucosal barriers from radiation- or chemotherapy-induced mucositis. Susceptibility to

Disclosures: The authors have no relevant conflicts to disclose.
[a] Department of Internal Medicine, University of Minnesota, 420 Delaware Street Southeast, MMC 284, Minneapolis, MN 55455, USA; [b] Division of Hematology, Oncology, and Transplantation, University of Minnesota, 420 Delaware Street Southeast, MMC 480, Minneapolis, MN 55455, USA
* Corresponding author.
E-mail address: fionahe@umn.edu

Infect Dis Clin N Am 33 (2019) 289–309
https://doi.org/10.1016/j.idc.2019.01.001

chemotherapy-induced neutropenia is also conferred by older age due to lower bone marrow reserve, poor performance status, and comorbidities, such as renal and cardiovascular disease.[1] The National Comprehensive Cancer Network recommends the use of prophylactic granulocyte colony-stimulating growth factors (G-CSF) during treatment if febrile neutropenia risk is greater than 20% (high), and consideration based on patient risk factors, such as prior chemotherapy or radiation, persistent neutropenia, bone marrow involvement by tumor, recent surgery, liver dysfunction, renal dysfunction, or age ≥65 for febrile neutropenia risk 10% to 20% (intermediate).[2] In this review, the authors discuss contemporary management by disease type with a focus on infectious risk, followed by special discussion of novel agents, including signaling/small molecule inhibitors, monoclonal antibodies, immunomodulators, and immunotherapies for treatment of hematologic malignancies.

Part 1. Disease-Specific Discussion of Infectious Risk

Acute myeloid leukemia and myelodysplastic syndrome

Patients with acute leukemias undergoing induction or consolidation represent the highest-risk groups for infection among malignancies. Acute myeloid leukemia (AML) patients often present with baseline neutropenia due to hematopoietic stem cell dysfunction and marrow infiltration by leukemic blasts. In AML, the median time of neutrophil recovery to greater than 500 cells/mm^3 after standard induction therapy with anthracycline and antimetabolites (ie, "7 + 3") is 26 days.[3] Risk of neutropenic fever during treatment of AML is estimated at 85% to 95%.[4] During neutropenia, prophylaxis with an antibiotic with gram-negative coverage and a mold-active antifungal agent is recommended to mitigate this risk. Fluoroquinolones, such as levofloxacin, are widely used in practice, although providers should be aware of potential adverse effects of hypoglycemia with concurrent oral hypoglycemic agents or insulin, and QT prolonging effects. In relapsed disease treated with second-line chemotherapy regimens, rates of bacterial and invasive fungal infection further increase, reflecting both myelotoxicity and a susceptible host.[5] Administration of prophylactic myeloid growth factor support with colony-stimulating factors (G-CSF) in AML patients undergoing induction chemotherapy improved time to neutrophil recovery by 4 days, but did not impact infection-related mortality or overall survival in a meta-analysis; therefore, prophylactic G-CSF use is not common practice.[6] CPX-351, a liposomal formulation with a fixed ratio of daunorubicin and cytarabine, is now approved for adults older than 60 years of age with therapy-related AML as frontline therapy. A survival advantage compared with 7 + 3 was reported in a randomized study leading to its approval in this population, but rates of grade 3 to 5 infection were similar at 84% and 86%.[7] Cytotoxic chemotherapy with or without consolidation with allogeneic hematopoietic stem cell transplantation (HCT) remains the standard of care for most AML patients with intermediate or adverse-risk disease.

One subgroup of AML with excellent outcomes in the modern era is acute promyelocytic leukemia, which may be treated with a combination of all-trans retinoic acid (ATRA) and arsenic trioxide in the setting of low- or intermediate-risk disease. This induction and consolidation chemotherapy-free approach was noninferior to ATRA plus chemotherapy and was associated with fewer episodes of neutropenic fever and excellent long-term outcomes.[8]

For treatment of AML patients not fit for intensive therapy or patients with myelodysplastic syndrome (MDS), hypomethylating agents (HMAs), such as azacitidine or decitabine, are commonly used to induce hematologic and morphologic remission. HMAs have low rates of infection requiring treatment with parenteral antibiotics despite higher rates of grade 3 to 4 neutropenia compared with best supportive care.[9] An increase in febrile neutropenia but no difference in infectious mortality was also shown in a meta-analysis.[10] The discordance between febrile neutropenia and infectious mortality highlights the importance of disease control for preventing infections in high-grade myeloid malignancies. Venetoclax, a BCL-2 targeting small molecule inhibitor, may be combined with HMAs in the upfront or relapsed/refractory setting in AML (see section entitled BCL-2 inhibitors).

Acute lymphoblastic leukemia

Treatment of acute lymphoblastic leukemia (ALL) in fit patients consists of intensive multiagent chemotherapy for induction and intensification, including high-dose steroids, anthracycline, vincristine, and peg-asparaginase followed by consolidation, with total duration of therapy usually lasting 1.5 to 2 years (ie, regimens hyper-CVAD ± rituximab, PETHEMA, CALGB 8811).[11] Highest risk of infection is during induction therapy because neutropenia is less frequent during consolidation. In the UKALL 2003 trial of pediatric ALL, infectious mortality accounted for 30% of deaths (2.4% cumulative incidence over 5 years).[12] Of deaths, 68% were secondary to bacteremia (64% gram-negative sepsis) and 20% were due to fungal infection. Down syndrome was the most significant risk factor for infectious mortality (odds ratio [OR] 12.08). In adult patients in the GRAALL 2005 trial, 34% of patients had bacterial infections during induction (82% bacteremia), resulting in 2.8% infectious mortality.[13] Gram-positive cocci (coagulase-negative *Staphylococcus* was most common) and *Escherichia coli* each accounted for greater than 40% of infections. Relapsed ALL also represents a high-risk population for infection when treated with salvage regimens, such as clofarabine or cytarabine.[14] For B-ALL with t(9;22) (Ph positive), targeted therapy with tyrosine kinase inhibitors (TKI) may be added to induction therapy or used with steroids alone (see section entitled Signaling inhibitors: BCR-ABL tyrosine kinase inhibitors). Immunotherapies such as blinatumomab are also an option that is being used more frequently for relapsed/refractory ALL (see section entitled Immunotherapy: Bispecific T-cell engager).

Chronic leukemias and myeloproliferative neoplasms

Cytotoxic chemotherapy remains standard of care as first-line treatment for most adults with chronic lymphocytic leukemia (CLL). CLL is often associated with hypogammaglobulinemia leading to frequent infections; infection may be a primary indication for disease treatment. For fit younger patients, combination chemotherapy with regimens such as fludarabine, cyclophosphamide, and rituximab (FCR) is recommended. FCR was compared with bendamustine and rituximab (BR) in the CLL10 trial for previously untreated CLL and associated with higher rates of grade 4 neutropenia (62% vs 35%) and grade 3 to 5 bacterial infection (40% vs 26%).[15] For CLL in older patients who are not fit for intensive chemotherapy or have high-risk molecular phenotype, such as *TP53* mutation, ibrutinib, a Bruton tyrosine kinase (BTK) inhibitor, is recommended (see section entitled Signaling inhibitors: Bruton tyrosine kinase inhibitors). Other options for relapsed/refractory disease include idelalisib and venetoclax (see sections entitled Signaling inhibitors: Phosphatidylinositol 3-kinase δ inhibitor; B-cell lymphoma 2 inhibitor).

Chronic myeloid leukemia (CML) is largely treated with TKIs targeting the constitutively active BCR-ABL fusion protein (see section entitled Signaling inhibitors: Tyrosine kinase inhibitors).

Classical myeloproliferative neoplasms (MPN), including polycythemia vera, essential thrombocythemia, and primary myelofibrosis, may progress to bone marrow failure or acute leukemia. Treatment with hydroxyurea, an oral chemotherapy agent, causes dose-dependent myelosuppression resulting in reduced platelet counts and improvement in splenomegaly, bone pain, and constitutional symptoms. The infectious risk from hydroxyurea is minimal if the dose is titrated to avoid neutropenia. Targeting the aberrantly overactive JAK/STAT pathway with JAK inhibitors, such as ruxolitinib, may reduce spleen volume and improve symptoms in MPN (see section entitled Signaling inhibitors: JAK inhibitors).[16]

Lymphoma

The backbone of treatment of high-grade non-Hodgkin lymphoma (diffuse large B-cell lymphoma [DLBCL], mantle cell lymphoma, Burkitt lymphoma) and Hodgkin lymphoma is multiagent chemotherapy ± monoclonal antibodies. Typical regimens, such as cyclophosphamide, doxorubicin, vincristine or etoposide, and prednisone with rituximab (R-CHOP), doxorubicin, bleomycin, vinblastine, and dacabazine (ABVD), and BR, are given at 2- to 3-week intervals for 6 to 8 cycles with estimated 15% to 22% incidence of febrile neutropenia.[4,17] Regimens that report higher infectious risk include dose-adjusted (DA) R-EPOCH (double-hit DLBCL, primary mediastinal B-cell lymphoma [PMBCL]), R-HyperCVAD (mantle cell lymphoma, Burkitt lymphoma), and R-CODOX/R-IVAC (Burkitt lymphoma).[18] The increased efficacy of DA-R-EPOCH in high-grade lymphoma with c-myc and bcl-2 or bcl-6 translocation (double hit) is due to dose-intensification postcycle number 1 to goal ANC nadir less than 500 cells/mm³. The dose-intensification is associated with higher rates of grade 3 to 4 febrile neutropenia (37% vs 19% for R-CHOP in all DLBCL) but higher rates of remission and survival for double hit lymphoma in retrospective studies.[19,20] DA-R-EPOCH may also be used as a radiation-sparing approach for PMBCL, a rare subtype of DLBCL, with 13% rate of hospitalization for febrile neutropenia but excellent long-term survival in a typically younger and otherwise healthy population.[21]

T-cell lymphomas are a heterogeneous group but are treated with similar multiagent chemotherapy regimens, such as B-cell NHL, without the addition of rituximab due to lack of CD20 expression. Because cytotoxic chemotherapy has poor efficacy in the relapsed setting, novel treatments for relapsed disease, such as histone deacetylase (HDAC) inhibitors, have been used. Romidepsin, an HDAC inhibitor, induced grade 3 to 4 neutropenia in about one-quarter of patients and infections in 36% (bacteremia and sepsis, upper respiratory bacterial and viral infections, herpes zoster virus [VZV], and hepatitis B virus [HBV] reactivation).[22] Subgroups of T-cell lymphoma, such as anaplastic large cell lymphoma, may be targeted by their CD30 expression (see section entitled Monoclonal antibody: CD30).

Plasma cell myeloma

Patients with plasma cell myeloma also have preexisting risk of infection because of production of antibodies with restricted repertoires. The treatment of myeloma has significantly evolved over the past 10 years since the widespread initiation of proteasome inhibitors (PIs) and immunomodulators ("imides"). Three-drug or 2-drug combinations for primary induction therapy, including PI and/or imide, with dexamethasone have replaced historical approaches of alkylator-based chemotherapy due to improved efficacy and tolerability. A large population-based study from 1988 to 2007 of myeloma patients reported 10% of all deaths within first 60 days of diagnosis related to infection.[23] The impact of prophylactic antibiotics on infection rate in newly diagnosed myeloma patients was assessed in a multicenter trial randomizing patients to levofloxacin or placebo for 12 weeks' duration (n = 977). The investigators reported a decrease in febrile episodes or death (19% vs 27%, P = .002) at 12 weeks, a reduced rate of gram-negative infections, and no change in carriage of resistant organisms.[24] A limited duration of infectious prophylaxis could be considered for this population, but it is currently not standard practice. Disease status and types of prior treatments are an important consideration in myeloma patients, particularly if they have had prior autologous transplantation with high-dose melphalan conditioning, which is associated with immune reconstitution that occurs over at least 2 years.

Part 2. Infectious Risk by Drug Class

Steroids/chemotherapy

High-dose steroid therapy Steroids at high doses ($\geq$20 mg prednisone) affect neutrophil, monocyte, and lymphocyte function. Steroids are commonly used as a backbone in treatment regimens for lymphoid malignancies. Complications directly associated with hematologic malignancies, such as autoimmune manifestations, often require long durations of steroid treatment. Several retrospective studies have shown strong association of higher dose and longer duration of steroid use with bacteremia, sepsis, viral reactivation, and pneumocystis pneumonia (PCP).[25,26] The type of glucocorticoid may also impact infection risk. In a randomized comparison of dexamethasone 10 mg/ m^2/d versus prednisone 60 mg/m^2/d for a 3-week duration in combination with multiagent chemotherapy for pediatric ALL, dexamethasone was associated with reduction in relapse rate, but higher rates of infectious death during induction (2.5 vs 0.9%, $P = .003$).[27]

Purine analogues Purine analogues (fludarabine, clofarabine, nelarabine, cladribine) are used in treatment of a variety of lymphoid malignancies and require special attention because of early and late infectious risk secondary to early neutropenia and prolonged suppression of cell-mediated immunity. For hairy cell leukemia, cladribine monotherapy given over 5 to 7 days has a high disease response rate of greater than 90% and is associated with greater than 70% rates of severe neutropenia (ANC <500 cells/mm^3) and greater than 40% rates of neutropenic fever, but low rates of documented infection (<15%).[28] Prolonged depletion of CD4$^+$ T cells occurs with purine analogues, such as cladribine, with CD4$^+$ nadir less than 200 cells/μL and median recovery time of 40 months.[29] Opportunistic infection has been reported but is relatively rare outside of the immediate neutropenic period. Fludarabine, when given with cyclophosphamide and rituximab (FCR) for frontline treatment of CLL, results in prolonged grade 3 or 4 neutropenia at 1 year in 17% of patients.[30]

Signaling/small molecule inhibitors

BCR-ABL tyrosine kinase inhibitors Inhibitors of BCR-ABL can be very effective for inducing remission in CML and Ph$^+$ B-ALL, due to inhibition of the constitutively active BCR-ABL tyrosine kinase fusion protein associated with t(9;22). The first BCL-ABL TKI, imatinib, preceded newer TKIs dasatinib, nilotinib, bosutinib, and ponatinib, which have varying potencies and off-target effects that may contribute to risk of infection. As a class, myelosuppression resulting in neutropenia is expected and may increase the risk for bacterial infections. Inhibition of T-cell proliferation of both CD4$^+$ and CD8$^+$ subsets also has been demonstrated due to off-target effects.[31] Last, B cells are also affected because humoral responses to pneumococcal vaccine are affected by imatinib, dasatinib, and nilotinib.[32]

Early studies revealed similar rates of neutropenia (14%–25% grade 3–4) but a modest increase in infections, including upper respiratory infections in imatinib compared with interferon/cytarabine.[33] A long-term follow-up (3.5 years) of chronic-phase CML patients treated with first-line imatinib reported infectious complications in 14%, the majority attributed to VZV infections.[34] A larger study reported a lower 2% rate of VZV de novo infection or reactivation among CML patients treated with imatinib that was localized and treatable in all cases.[35] In Ph+ ALL, a 20% rate of febrile neutropenia was reported with a combination of high-dose methotrexate, cytarabine, and imatinib and a 52% rate of grade 3 to 4 infections during induction with a combination of hyper-CVAD and imatinib, similar to historical controls of chemotherapy only.[36,37] Among TKIs, dasatinib may have a higher risk for infection; a retrospective study reported 56% incidence of infection in patients receiving dasatinib, with increased incidence with concurrent high-dose steroid use or ≥3 treatment cycles.[38] In a study of advanced phase CML or Ph+ ALL after failure of imatinib, the incidence of infection with dasatinib monotherapy was 18% (8% grade 3–4 infections).[39] Fewer data exist on infectious risks of nilotinib, bosutinib, and ponatinib, but risk of infection appears similar to that of imatinib, with less than 10% risk of infectious complications.[40–43]

Of infections with BCR-ABL TKIs, viral infections have been well described. HBV reactivation has been repeatedly reported for imatinib,[44,45] nilotinib,[44] and dasatinib.[46] Case reports of cytomegalovirus (CMV) disease have also been reported in nontransplant patients treated with dasatinib (**Table 1**).[47,48]

Overall, BCR-ABL–directed TKI treatment confers a moderate risk of infection due to effects on various immune effector cells, but prophylaxis for bacterial or viral infections is not routinely recommended. HBV serostatus should be determined before initiation of treatment with hepatitis B core antibody (HBc) positivity or hepatitis B surface antigen (HBsAg) positivity indicating higher risk. For +HBsAg or +HBc, prophylaxis with entecavir or regular monitoring of HBV PCR is recommended (**Fig. 1**).

Jak inhibitors (ruxolitinib) Ruxolitinib (Jakafi) is hypothesized to affect immune function via multiple mechanisms, including modulation of dendritic cell priming of T cells, dampening cytokine production (interleukin-1 [IL-1], IL-6, tumor necrosis factor-α, interferon-δ), and impairment of natural killer cells.[49] A meta-analysis of ruxolitinib versus controls reported significantly higher rates of VZV infection (OR 7.39, 95% confidence interval 1.33–41) and similar rates of other infections.[50] However, postmarketing registries have identified isolated reports of opportunistic infections, including toxoplasma retinitis, cryptococcal pneumonia and meningoencephalitis, disseminated tuberculosis (TB), progressive multifocal leukoencephalopathy (PML), Klebsiella liver abscess, and sino-orbital mucormycosis as well as viral reactivation with HBV and Epstein-Barr virus (EBV).[51] Of a series of MPN patients with positive anti-HBc antibody and negative HBsAg and HBV DNA, there was a 40% reactivation rate of HBV at a median of 10 months after ruxolitinib treatment.[52] HBV reactivation prophylaxis or careful monitoring should be considered in HBV carriers (see **Fig. 1**).

Bruton tyrosine kinase inhibitors (ibrutinib) Ibrutinib irreversibly inhibits the BTK pathway involved in B-cell signaling and has activity in multiple B-cell malignancies. High rates of infection have been reported with ibrutinib treatment, with grade 3 to 4 infection rate of up to 56% in patients treated with monotherapy and up to 26% in patients treated with combination therapy in a systematic review.[53] Higher infectious complications have been described in relapsed compared with treatment-naïve CLL patients treated with ibrutinib.[54] In a comparison of a combination with BR with ibrutinib or placebo, similar levels of infection were reported: both overall infections (70% both groups) and in grade 3 to 4 infections (29% in ibrutinib and 25% in placebo).[55] With long-term follow-up for CLL patients on ibrutinib, 42% of patients had a grade 3 to 4 infection over 3 years of treatment, the majority occurring within the first year.[54] BTK is also involved with other immune processes, including innate and adaptive responses that may increase susceptibility to opportunistic infections. The off-target inhibition of the IL-2 inducible T-cell kinase may mediate further immune deficits

Table 1
Infectious risk of treatment regimens by disease

Disease	Treatment Regimen	Infectious Risk[a]			Types of Infection
		Low	Medium	High	
AML	AML induction and consolidation			X	High risk for bacteremia, IFI, HSV, and VZV reactivation
	Azacitidine, decitabine			X	High risk for IFI, HSV, and VZV reactivation
	Venetoclax + azacitidine			X	High risk for IFI, HSV, and VZV reactivation
ALL	ALL induction and consolidation			X	High risk for bacteremia, IFI, HSV, and VZV reactivation
	ALL induction and consolidation + imatinib/dasatinib			X	High risk for bacteremia, IFI, HSV, and VZV reactivation
	Imatinib + steroids		X		High risk for IFI, PCP
	Dasatinib + steroids		X		High risk for IFI, PCP
	Blinatumomab			X	
	CD19 CAR-T			X	High risk for bacteremia, IFI, HSV, and VZV reactivation
MDS	Azacitidine, decitabine		X		
CLL	Purine analogues (FCR)			X	High risk for bacteremia, HSV, and VZV reactivation, HBV reactivation
	Chlorambucil + rituximab		X		HBV reactivation risk
	BR			X	High risk for bacteremia, HBV reactivation risk
	Ibrutinib			X	Rare PCP, aspergillosis
	Venetoclax			X	High risk for respiratory viruses, HSV reactivation, OI, including PCP
	Idelalisib			X	High risk for PCP
	Alemtuzumab			X	High risk for IFI, all viral infections, including CMV reactivation

(continued on next page)

Table 1
(continued)

Disease	Treatment Regimen	Infectious Risk[a]			Types of Infection
		Low	Medium	High	
CML	Imatinib			X	HBV reactivation risk
	Dasatinib			X	HBV reactivation risk
High-grade non-Hodgkin lymphomas	R-CHOP/CHOP		X[b]		HBV reactivation risk
	R-DHAP, R-ICE			X	High risk for bacteremia, HBV reactivation
	DA-R-EPOCH			X	High risk for bacteremia, HBV reactivation
	R-HyperCVAD			X	High risk for bacteremia, HBV reactivation
	CD19 CAR-T			X	High risk for bacteremia, IFI, HSV, and VZV reactivation
	Ibrutinib			X	Rare PCP
Hodgkin	ABVD		X		High risk for bacteremia
	A-AVD (Brentuximab + AVD)			X	High risk for bacteremia
	Escalated BEACOPP			X	Rare CMV reactivation
	Brentuximab			X	
	Nivolumab/pembrolizumab		X		Rare TB reactivation risk
Low-grade non-Hodgkin lymphomas	Rituximab monotherapy		X		HBV reactivation risk
	R-CVP		X		HBV reactivation risk
	BR			X	
Myeloma	RD		X		
	RVD/KRD		X		VZV reactivation risk
	Lenalidomide maintenance		X		
	Bortezomib maintenance		X		VZV reactivation risk
	Daratumumab			X	
	VDT-PACE			X	High risk for bacteremia
MPN	Ruxolitinib	X			VZV reactivation, HBV, and EBV reactivation, rare OI

Abbreviations: IFI, invasive fungal infection; KRD, carfilzomib, lenalidomide, and dexamethasone; OI, opportunistic infections; PCP, *Pneumocystis jirovecii* pneumonia; RVD, lenalidomide, bortezomib, dexamethasone.

[a] Infectious risk defined as low (neutropenic fever <10%), medium (neutropenic fever 10%–20%), or high (neutropenic fever >20%).

[b] Age ≥65 receiving R-CHOP considered high risk.

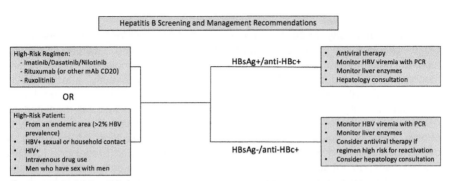

Fig. 1. Screening and management recommendations for HBV before therapy.

predisposing to opportunistic infections with Aspergillus, PCP, and VZV described with ibrutinib (see **Table 1**).[53] Infectious complications from the newer acalabrutinib are limited, although in one prospective study, upper respiratory infections were reported in 23% of relapsed CLL patients.[47,56]

B-cell lymphoma 2 inhibitors (venetoclax) Overexpression of B-cell lymphoma 2 (BCL-2) protein leads to CLL cells resistant to apoptosis. Venetoclax is a BCL-2 inhibitor that promotes apoptosis in Bcl-2 overexpressing cells. Clinical data suggest that venetoclax does not convey increased infection risk, and patients do not require antibacterial, antiviral, or anti-PCP prophylaxis.[47] In a safety analysis of venetoclax derived from 3 phase 1/2 studies, infection of any grade occurred in 72% of patients with 22% of patients having a grade 3 to 4 infection. Cytopenias were most likely to occur during the 5-week dose ramp-up period, with one-third of patients receiving G-CSF support initially, which decreased to 11% beyond 1 year of treatment.[57] Opportunistic infections occurred in 3.1% of patients, including PCP, toxoplasmosis, nocardiosis, herpes pharyngitis, and candida, although no deaths from opportunistic infections occurred.[57] Prior fludarabine exposure was identified as a risk factor for serious infections on venetoclax (33% vs 13%, OR 2.3, $P = .004$). Venetoclax has also been given Food and Drug Administration (FDA) breakthrough designation in combination with low-dose cytarabine or azacitidine with favorable tolerability and ability to induce durable remissions in older adults with AML, who were ineligible for intensive therapy.[58] In an early-phase trial in this population, febrile neutropenia occurred in 31% of patients. Of note, venetoclax dosing should be reduced in patients concurrently receiving azole antifungal therapy due to increased exposure.

Phosphatidylinositol 3-kinase δ inhibitor inhibitors (idelalisib) Idelalisib, an oral phosphatidyl 3-kinase δ inhibitor, is approved for patients with relapsed or refractory CLL or follicular lymphoma. Idelalisib was studied in combination therapy for relapsed CLL in 3 randomized controlled trials and reported increased rates of infection in each.[59] After noticing a significant number of cases of PCP, a retrospective analysis of multiple trials has reported a 2.5% rate of PCP infection, with reduction in risk by greater than 60% with PCP prophylaxis.[60] Based on these data, PCP prophylaxis is recommended for all patients receiving idelalisib. Idelalisib therapy is frequently complicated by serious CMV infection, and routine monitoring with monthly CMV PCR in seropositive patients is recommended. If viremia is encountered, idelalisib should be discontinued and ganciclovir or valganciclovir administered in symptomatic patients (see **Table 1**). Idelalisib is not used as frequently in clinical practice as agents, such as ibrutinib and venetoclax, for treatment of CLL because of tolerability but has activity in refractory disease.

Monoclonal antibodies

Monoclonal antibody CD20 (rituximab) Anti-CD20 monoclonal antibodies target CD20-positive B-cell malignancies and include FDA-approved rituximab, ^{90}Y-ibritumomab, ofatumumab, and obinutuzumab, which vary in molecular structure and mechanisms of inducing cell death. CD20 depletion directly affects CD20-expressing B cells, but also has downstream effects on plasma cells and T cells and can potentially lead to hypogammaglobulinemia and impaired cell-mediated immunity with prolonged treatment.[61–63] Several meta-analyses of rituximab in lymphoma patients, including trials that compared the addition of rituximab to cyclophosphamide, doxorubicin, vincristine or etoposide, and prednisone (CHOP)-like regimens, do not suggest an increase in infections in the early period.[64–68] However, 2 meta-analyses of rituximab given as monotherapy maintenance in lymphoma reported a higher rate of any infection and neutropenia compared with placebo.[69,70] The results of the trials included in these meta-analyses were not uniform, and differences are likely due to prior treatment exposures, such as fludarabine-containing regimens that confer a higher-risk population. Strong evidence exists for increased risk of viral infections with rituximab, particularly HBV reactivation, which occurred in 24% of subjects treated with rituximab compared with 0% with a nonrituximab regimen.[71] Thus, it is recommended that all patients with planned rituximab treatment are checked for HBV serostatus, because preemptive antiviral treatment may be given to prevent acute reactivation (see **Fig. 1**). Opportunistic infections, including PCP, have been reported with rituximab, but are rare and estimated in the 1.3% to 3% range.[72,73] Because of this low incidence, it is not standard practice to use PCP prophylaxis unless other risk factors, such as concurrent steroid use, are present.

Other anti-CD20 monoclonal antibodies are primarily used in combination regimens. Ofatumumab in combination with chlorambucil had similar infectious complications (9%–12%) but higher rate of grade 3 to 4 neutropenia (26% vs 14%) compared with chlorambucil monotherapy for untreated CLL.[74] Obinutuzumab had comparable rates of infection to rituximab with similar overall infections (0% vs 5%) and grade 3 to 4 infections (4% vs 3%).[75] Addition of anti-CD20–directed therapy may confer slightly higher risk of neutropenia, but evidence suggests that overall rate of infection and infection-related mortality are not increased.

Monoclonal antibody CD30 (brentuximab) CD30-expressing T-cell lymphomas, such as anaplastic large cell lymphoma, may be treated with brentuximab vedotin, an antibody-drug conjugate to CD30. Brentuximab vedotin is also frequently used in Hodgkin lymphoma because of its ubiquitous CD30 expression, both in combination with chemotherapy in the frontline setting (brentuximab, doxorubicin, vinblastine, and dacarbazine [A-AVD]) and as monotherapy in relapsed setting and maintenance following autologous HCT. CD30 is a transmembrane glycoprotein that is normally expressed on B, T, and natural killer cells with functions in cytotoxic T-cell expansion and homing. In combination with chemotherapy in previously untreated Hodgkin lymphoma patients, A-AVD–treated patients had a higher rate of grade 3 to 4 infections (18% vs 10%) and febrile neutropenia, which was decreased with addition of G-CSF, compared with patients treated with standard ABVD.[76] Brentuximab may also be given for 2 years after autologous HCT as maintenance therapy and was associated with higher rates of neutropenia, but similar rates of severe infection and febrile neutropenia.[77] Case reports of CMV infection, including retinitis and PML, due to JC virus reactivation have been described.[78]

Monoclonal antibody CD38 (daratumomab) CD38 is a transmembrane glycoprotein expressed predominantly on lymphoid and myeloid cells and is involved in leukocyte activation, differentiation, and proliferation. Because of high expression of CD38 on plasma cells and low expression on normal myeloid and lymphoid cells, it has become a targeted therapy for multiple myeloma.[79] Rates of infection are not significantly increased in patients treated with daratumumab, a monoclonal CD38 antibody. Similar rates of grade 3 to 4 infections and pneumonia occurred in 2 daratumumab-containing regimens, with bortezomib/dexamethasone or with lenalidomide/dexamethasone, compared with the same regimens without daratumumab, although there was a modest increase in febrile neutropenia. Respectively, grade 3 to 4 infections occurred in 21.4% and 28.3% in those randomized to daratumumab regimens therapy compared with 19% and 22.8% in control arms of these 2 studies.[80,81]

Monoclonal antibodyCD52 (alemtuzumab) Alemtuzumab targets CD52, a marker present on mature immune cells, including lymphocytes and neutrophils, and is approved for advanced CLL and some lymphomas. Alemtuzumab can induce profound immunosuppression with reduction in neutrophil, monocyte, T-cell, and B-cell populations for 4 to 9 months after therapy.[82] A Cochrane Review of alemtuzumab for CLL patients reported a significant increase in infections (relative risk [RR] 1.32, $P = .04$) and CMV reactivation (RR 10.52, $P = .02$) in patients treated with alemtuzumab.[83] In patients with CD52[+] lymphoplasmacytic lymphoma, long-term follow-up at 18 months was notable for grade 3 to 4 infection in 17.8% of patients, which was most commonly CMV reactivation.[84] A high rate of viral reactivation was also seen in MDS patients.[85] Overall, patients are at high risk for opportunistic infections, particularly with CMV and herpes simplex virus (HSV) infection (see **Table 1**). Although viral reactivation is high, many cases are subclinical. Thus, the authors recommend monitoring reactivation with CMV PCR during and for at least 2 months following therapy with preemptive treatment of reactivation.

Immunomodulatory drugs/immunotherapy

Imides and proteasome inhibitors (lenalidomide, bortezomib) Immunomodulatory drugs (imides) and PIs are frequently used for treatment of multiple myeloma. Imides target an E3 ubiquitin ligase, causing proteasomal degradation of specific proteins, and ultimately decrease proinflammatory cytokines and increase IL-2 production.[86] The mechanism of PIs is inhibition of the proteasome pathway, leading to apoptosis.

Induction therapy with VRD (bortezomib, lenalidomide, dexamethasone) is the most common induction regimen for standard risk disease and has a similar rate of grade 3 to 4 infection compared with RD (lenalidomide and dexamethasone) at 13% versus 14%.[87] Use of imides appears to confer a modest increase in risk for infection in multiple myeloma patients compared with conventional melphalan-based regimens, with 7% to 20% of patients experiencing severe infection with an imide-based regimen for induction and relapsed disease.[88,89] Lenalidomide is the most common agent used for maintenance following autologous HCT after showing a clear survival benefit over placebo and is associated with slightly higher risk of grade 3 to 4 infection (6% vs 1%) in this patient population.[90] One meta-analysis noted a relative risk of 1.64 ($P<.001$) for grade 3 to 4 infections with maintenance lenalidomide or thalidomide.[91] Pomalidomide, a second-generation imide, has been associated with similar rates of grade 3 to 4 infection (30% for pomalidomide arm vs 24% for comparator arm), with most infections occurring in nonneutropenic patients.[92] Lenalidomide is not clearly associated with increased risk of infection, so prophylactic treatment is not recommended.

In a meta-analysis of PI therapy, there was no difference in risk of severe infection from PI therapy compared with conventional chemotherapy when used for induction in transplant-eligible patients.[88] However, PIs may increase risk of viral infections because of their effects on T cells, particularly VZV infection.[93] VZV reactivation incidence of 13% has been reported in newly diagnosed patients who are treated with a PI (see **Table 1**).[93] Carfilzomib and ixazomib have similar and modest rates of infection.[94,95] Because of increased risk of VZV reactivation with Bortezomib, VZV-seropositive patients should receive acyclovir or valacyclovir prophylaxis during treatment (**Table 2**). Before starting bortezomib, VZV-seronegative patients should receive the live-attenuated vaccination; patients older than 50 can be considered for adjuvant subunit zoster vaccination. Influenza is also more prevalent in patients treated with a PI, so immunization before initiation is recommended if seasonally appropriate.[93]

Bispecific T-cell engager (blinatumomab) Blinatumomab, a bispecific CD19-directed CD3[+] T-cell engager, is approved for relapsed or refractory B-cell ALL. Blinatumomab has binding sites for both CD3[+] T cells and CD19[+] target cells, to induce cell-mediated death. Blinatumomab, compared with salvage chemotherapy for B-ALL, was associated with lower rates of grade 3 to 4 neutropenia (38% vs 58%) and infection (34% vs 52%).[96] Fungal pneumonia has been reported with Blinatumomab, with risk factors of lower ANC at time of initiation and longer duration of neutropenia.[97] Fevers and cytokine release syndrome (CRS) are common with blinatumomab, but a thorough infectious workup is warranted due to the impaired immunity of the ALL patient, especially in relapsed and refractory disease.

Programmed cell death protein 1 blockade (pembrolizumab) Inhibitors of the programmed cell death protein 1 (PD-1)/programmed death-ligand 1 pathway (immune checkpoint blockers) are approved for relapsed or refractory Hodgkin lymphoma and under investigation for other hematologic malignancies. PD-1 blockade with nivolumab or pembrolizumab does not cause immune suppression leading to infections, but has been reported to reactivate latent TB in case reports.[98] TB reactivation is hypothesized to be secondary to reactivation of suppressed TB-specific CD4[+] and CD8[+] T cells expressing PD-1, inducing a proinflammatory state similar to immune reactivation inflammatory syndrome in patients with human immunodeficiency virus. In patients with known risk factors for TB (exposure to endemic areas, prisons, homeless shelters, health care workers, or prior positive testing), an interferon-gamma release assay (IGRA) or Mantoux test should be checked before initiation of immune checkpoint therapies. Notably, IGRA and Mantoux both may be uninterpretable in the setting of an immunocompromised host because they measure T-cell immune response. There is currently insufficient evidence to recommend systematic TB screening without risk factors in patients with cancer receiving immunotherapy.

During treatment with immune checkpoint blockers, immune-mediated adverse events are more common than infection. Fever is frequent, and although may be attributed to the drug, infection should remain on the differential diagnosis for Hodgkin lymphoma patients who have been heavily pretreated, particularly if they are postautologous transplantation.

Chimeric antigen receptor T cells Chimeric antigen receptor (CAR) T cells are genetically modified autologous T cells that are engineered to express CARs, fusion proteins containing antigen-binding, and costimulatory domains. CD19-directed CAR T cells are approved for pediatric and young adults with relapsed or refractory B-ALL and adults with relapsed or refractory DLBCL. Multiple other CAR-T products with other

Table 2
Suggested prophylaxis by treatment regimen

Disease	Treatment Regimen	Prophylaxis Recommended?				
		Bacterial	CMV	HSV/VZV	IFI	PCP
AML	AML induction and consolidation					
	Azacitidine, Decitabine					
	Venetoclax + Azacitidine					
ALL	ALL induction and consolidation					
	ALL induction and consolidation + TKI					
	Imatinib + steroids					
	Dasatinib + steroids					
	Blinatumomab					
	CD19 CAR-T					
MDS	Azacitidine, Decitabine					
CLL	Purine analogues (FCR)					
	Chlorambucil + Rituximab					
	Bendamustine + Rituximab					
	Ibrutinib					
	Venetoclax					
	Idelalisib		b			
	Alemtuzumab		b			
CML	Imatinib					
	Dasatinib					
High Grade Non-Hodgkin Lymphomas	R-CHOP/CHOP					
	R-DHAP, R-ICE					
	DA-R-EPOCH					
	R-HyperCVAD					
	CD19 CAR-T					
	Ibrutinib					
Hodgkin	ABVD					
	A-AVD (Brentuximab + AVD)					
	Escalated BEACOPP					
	Brentuximab		a			a
	Nivolumab/Pembrolizumab					
Low Grade Non-Hodgkin Lymphomas	Rituximab monotherapy					
	R-CVP					
	BR					
Myeloma	RD					
	RVD/KRD					
	Lenalidomide maintenance		a			a
	Bortezomib maintenance		a			a
	Daratumumab					
	VDT-PACE					
MPN	Ruxolitinib					

Recommended	Consider for multiply relapsed disease or susceptible host[c] during periods of neutropenia	Not recommended

[a] Prophylaxis recommended for maintenance post–auto-HCT in seropositive patients.
[b] Monitoring recommended.
[c] Susceptible host includes older age, poor nutrition, indwelling catheters or mucositis, prior chemotherapy-induced febrile neutropenia.

antigen targets are currently in clinical trials. There has been widespread enthusiasm for CAR-T therapy high-response rates in these 2 highly refractory populations leading to approval of 2 cellular products targeting CD19, Kymriah, and Yescarta. CAR-T therapy is usually given with lymphodepleting chemotherapy (cyclophosphamide and fludarabine), which improves proliferation and persistence. Grade 3 to 4 neutropenia is frequently observed in trials with and without lymphodepletion and may persist for weeks, particularly with concurrent CRS.[99]

CRS is a systemic inflammatory syndrome mediated by cytokines, such as IL-6, IL-2, and interferon-δ, that presents with clinical symptoms of fever, hypotension, depressed cardiac ejection fraction, pulmonary edema, neurotoxicity, renal injury, coagulopathy, and cytopenias. CRS of any grade occurs in 3 of 4 patients treated with CAR-T therapy and mimics sepsis. Infections in CAR-T patients occurred in 23% of patients in 1 study of 133 adult patients with relapsed B-ALL, CLL, or NHL and were most frequent within the first 28 days.[100] Seventeen percent of patients had bacterial infections, 9% had viral infections, 4% had invasive fungal infection, and 4% had fatal infections. CRS severity (0 vs 1–3 vs 4) was associated with risk for infection within 28 days (hazard ratio 3.38, $P<.001$). Other studies show similar rates of infection at 24% to 29%, with most patients recovering.[101–103]

Because of the high risk of infection with this treatment, G-CSF may be given if ANC level is less than 500 cells/mm^3 after lymphodepletion, and prophylactic antibiotics, antifungals, and antiviral therapy are standard (see **Table 2**). Because of healthy B cells also being targeted by CD19 CAR-T, hypogammaglobulinemia is frequent after CAR-T, and immunoglobulin therapy is considered if serum immunoglobulin G concentration is less than 400 mg/dL.

SUMMARY

The infectious risk and suggested prophylaxis of various treatment regimens for hematologic malignancies based on the available literature are summarized in **Tables 1** and **2**. Because of heterogeneity of patient populations regarding performance status, comorbidities, and disease status at time of treatment, this should serve as a guideline for providing context for infectious risk. The underlying disease and prior cytotoxic treatments have paramount importance in judging the overall infectious risk with each agent.

Significant advances in the treatment landscape for hematologic malignancies have been made in the past decade with a greater understanding of underlying pathophysiology of each disease. There are now options beyond cytotoxic chemotherapy, which carries predictable immediate and cumulative infectious risk due to induction of neutropenia. Long-term safety data on monoclonal antibodies, TKIs, B-cell signaling inhibitors, JAK inhibitors, immunomodulators, PIs, immune checkpoint inhibitors, and CAR-T cell therapies will inform us of their specific infectious risks that require close monitoring and management.

REFERENCES

1. Lyman GH. Risk models for predicting chemotherapy-induced neutropenia. Oncologist 2005;10(6):427–37.
2. National Comprehensive Cancer Network. Myeloid Growth Factors (Version 2.2018). Available at: https://www.nccn.org/professionals/physician_gls/pdf/myeloid_growth.pdf. Accessed February 27, 2019.
3. Mandelli F, Vignetti M, Suciu S, et al. Daunorubicin versus mitoxantrone versus idarubicin as induction and consolidation chemotherapy for adults with acute myeloid leukemia: the EORTC and GIMEMA groups study AML-10. J Clin Oncol 2009;27(32):5397–403.
4. Taplitz RA, Kennedy EB, Bow EJ, et al. Antimicrobial prophylaxis for adult patients with cancer-related immunosuppression: ASCO and IDSA clinical practice guideline update. J Clin Oncol 2018;18:00374.

5. He F, Sapkota S, Parker S, et al. A real-world study of clofarabine and cytarabine combination therapy for patients with acute myeloid leukemia. Leuk Lymphoma 2018;(612):2–3.

6. Heuser M, Zapf A, Morgan M, et al. Myeloid growth factors in acute myeloid leukemia: systematic review of randomized controlled trials. Ann Hematol 2011; 90(3):273–81.

7. Lancet JE, Uy GL, Cortes JE, et al. CPX-351 (cytarabine and daunorubicin) liposome for injection versus conventional cytarabine plus daunorubicin in older patients with newly diagnosed secondary acute myeloid leukemia. J Clin Oncol 2018;36(26):2684–92.

8. Platzbecker U, Avvisati G, Cicconi L, et al. Improved outcomes with retinoic acid and arsenic trioxide compared with retinoic acid and chemotherapy in non–high-risk acute promyelocytic leukemia: final results of the randomized Italian-German APL0406 trial. J Clin Oncol 2017;35(6):605–12.

9. Fenaux P, Mufti GJ, Hellstrom-Lindberg E, et al. Efficacy of azacitidine compared with that of conventional care regimens in the treatment of higher-risk myelodysplastic syndromes: a randomised, open-label, phase III study. Lancet Oncol 2009;10(3):223–32.

10. Shargian-Alon L, Gurion R, Raanani P, et al. Hypomethylating agents-associated infections—systematic review and meta-analysis of randomized controlled trials. Clin Lymphoma Myeloma Leuk 2018;18(9):603–10.e1.

11. National Comprehensive Cancer Network Guidelines. Acute Lymphoblastic Leukemia (Version 1.2018). Available at: https://www.nccn.org/professionals/physician_gls/pdf/all.pdf. Accessed February 27, 2019.

12. O'Connor D, Bate J, Wade R, et al. Infection-related mortality in children with acute lymphoblastic leukemia: an analysis of infectious deaths on UKALL2003. Blood 2014;124(7):1056–61.

13. Honeyman F, Tavernier E, Richez V, et al. Epidemiology of bacterial infections during induction chemotherapy in adult patients with acute lymphoblastic leukemia (ALL): analysis of the Graall-2005 Study. Blood 2016;128(22):2777.

14. Barba P, Sampol A, Calbacho M, et al. Clofarabine-based chemotherapy for relapsed/refractory adult acute lymphoblastic leukemia and lymphoblastic lymphoma. The Spanish experience. Am J Hematol 2012;87(6):631–4.

15. Eichhorst B, Fink AM, Bahlo J, et al. First-line chemoimmunotherapy with bendamustine and rituximab versus fludarabine, cyclophosphamide, and rituximab in patients with advanced chronic lymphocytic leukaemia (CLL10): an international, open-label, randomised, phase 3, non-inferiority trial. Lancet Oncol 2016;17(7):928–42.

16. Cervantes F, Vannucchi AM, Kiladjian J-J, et al. Three-year efficacy, safety, and survival findings from COMFORT-II, a phase 3 study comparing ruxolitinib with best available therapy for myelofibrosis. Blood 2013;122(25):4047–53.

17. Pettengell R, Schwenkglenks M, Leonard R, et al. Neutropenia occurrence and predictors of reduced chemotherapy delivery: results from the INC-EU prospective observational European neutropenia study. Support Care Cancer 2008; 16(11):1299–309.

18. Maruyama D, Watanabe T, Maeshima AM, et al. Modified cyclophosphamide, vincristine, doxorubicin, and methotrexate (CODOX-M)/ifosfamide, etoposide, and cytarabine (IVAC) therapy with or without rituximab in Japanese adult patients with Burkitt lymphoma (BL) and B cell lymphoma, unclassifiable, with. Int J Hematol 2010;92(5):732–43.

19. Wilson WH, Grossbard ML, Pittaluga S, et al. Dose-adjusted EPOCH chemotherapy for untreated large B-cell lymphomas : a pharmacodynamic approach with high efficacy Plenary paper Dose-adjusted EPOCH chemotherapy for untreated large B-cell lymphomas : a pharmacodynamic approach with high efficacy. Blood 2013;99(8):2685–93.

20. Petrich AM, Gandhi M, Jovanovic B, et al. Impact of induction regimen and stem cell transplantation on outcomes in double-hit lymphoma: a multicenter retrospective analysis. Blood 2014;124(15):2354–61.

21. Dunleavy K, Pittaluga S, Maeda LS, et al. Dose-adjusted EPOCH-rituximab therapy in primary mediastinal B-cell lymphoma. N Engl J Med 2013;368(15):1408–16.

22. Piekarz RL, Frye R, Prince HM, et al. Phase 2 trial of romidepsin in patients with peripheral T-cell lymphoma. Blood 2011;117(22):5827–34.

23. Blimark C, Holmberg E, Mellqvist UH, et al. Multiple myeloma and infections: a population-based study on 9253 multiple myeloma patients. Haematologica 2015;100(1):107–13.

24. Drayson MT, Bowcock S, Planche T, et al. Tackling early morbidity and mortality in myeloma (TEAMM): assessing the benefit of antibiotic prophylaxis and its effect on healthcare associated infections in 977 patients. Blood 2017;130(Suppl 1):903.

25. Teh BW, Harrison SJ, Worth LJ, et al. Risks, severity and timing of infections in patients with multiple myeloma: a longitudinal cohort study in the era of immunomodulatory drug therapy. Br J Haematol 2015;171(1):100–8.

26. Maeda T, Babazono A, Nishi T, et al. Quantification of the effect of chemotherapy and steroids on risk of Pneumocystis jiroveci among hospitalized patients with adult T-cell leukaemia. Br J Haematol 2015;168(4):501–6.

27. Möricke A, Zimmermann M, Valsecchi MG, et al. Dexamethasone vs. prednisone in induction treatment of pediatric ALL: results of the randomized trial AIEOP-BFM ALL 2000. Blood 2016;127(17):2101–12.

28. Saven A, Burian C, Koziol JA, et al. Long-term follow-up of patients with hairy cell leukemia after cladribine treatment. Blood 1998;92(6):1918–26.

29. Tadmor T. Purine analog toxicity in patients with hairy cell leukemia. Leuk Lymphoma 2011;52(sup2):38–42.

30. Fischer K, Bahlo J, Fink AM, et al. Long-term remissions after FCR chemoimmunotherapy in previously untreated patients with CLL: updated results of the CLL8 trial. Blood 2016;127(2):208–15.

31. Reinwald M, Boch T, Hofmann W-K, et al. Risk of infectious complications in hemato-oncological patients treated with kinase inhibitors. Biomark Insights 2015;10(Suppl 3):55–68.

32. de Lavallade H, Khoder A, Hart M, et al. Tyrosine kinase inhibitors impair B-cell immune responses in CML through off-target inhibition of kinases important for cell signaling. Blood 2013;122(2):227–38.

33. O'Brien SG, Guilhot F, Larson RA, et al. Imatinib compared with interferon and low-dose cytarabine for newly diagnosed chronic-phase chronic myeloid leukemia. N Engl J Med 2003;348(11):994–1004.

34. Breccia M, Girmenia C, Latagliata R, et al. Low incidence rate of opportunistic and viral infections during imatinib treatment in chronic myeloid leukemia patients in early and late chronic phase. Mediterr J Hematol Infect Dis 2011;3(1):e2011021.

35. Mattiuzzi GN, Cortes JE, Talpaz M, et al. Development of Varicella-Zoster virus infection in patients with chronic myelogenous leukemia treated with imatinib mesylate. Clin Cancer Res 2003;9(3):976–80.

36. Yanada M, Takeuchi J, Sugiura I, et al. High complete remission rate and promising outcome by combination of imatinib and chemotherapy for newly diagnosed BCR-ABL-positive acute lymphoblastic leukemia: a phase II study by the Japan adult leukemia study group. J Clin Oncol 2006;24:460–6.

37. Daver N, Thomas D, Ravandi F, et al. Final report of a phase II study of imatinib mesylate with hyper-CVAD for the front-line treatment of adult patients with Philadelphia chromosome-positive acute lymphoblastic leukemia. Haematologica 2015;100(5):653–61.

38. Rodriguez GH, Ahmed SI, Al-akhrass F, et al. Characteristics of, and risk factors for, infections in patients with cancer treated with dasatinib and a brief review of other complications. Leuk Lymphoma 2012;53(8):1530–5.

39. Lilly MB, Ottmann OG, Shah NP, et al. Dasatinib 140 mg once daily versus 70 mg twice daily in patients with Ph-positive acute lymphoblastic leukemia who failed imatinib: results from a phase 3 study. Am J Hematol 2010;85(3):164–70.

40. Koren-Michowitz M, le Coutre P, Duyster J, et al. Activity and tolerability of nilotinib. Cancer 2010;116(19):4564–72.

41. Gambacorti-Passerini C, Cortes JE, Lipton JH, et al. Safety of bosutinib versus imatinib in the phase 3 BELA trial in newly diagnosed chronic phase chronic myeloid leukemia. Am J Hematol 2014;89(10):947–53.

42. Brümmendorf TH, Cortes JE, de Souza CA, et al. Bosutinib *versus* imatinib in newly diagnosed chronic-phase chronic myeloid leukaemia: results from the 24-month follow-up of the BELA trial. Br J Haematol 2015;168(1):69–81.

43. Cortes JE, Kim D-W, Pinilla-Ibarz J, et al. A phase 2 trial of ponatinib in philadelphia chromosome-positive leukemias. N Engl J Med 2013;369(19):1783–96.

44. Lai G-M, Yan S-L, Chang C-S, et al. Hepatitis B reactivation in chronic myeloid leukemia patients receiving tyrosine kinase inhibitor. World J Gastroenterol 2013;19(8):1318.

45. Ikeda K, Shiga Y, Takahashi A, et al. Leukemia & Lymphoma Fatal hepatitis B virus reactivation in a chronic myeloid leukemia patient during imatinib mesylate treatment. Leuk Lymphoma 2006;47(1):155–7.

46. Ando T, Kojima K, Isoda H, et al. Reactivation of resolved infection with the hepatitis B virus immune escape mutant G145R during dasatinib treatment for chronic myeloid leukemia. Int J Hematol 2015;102(3):379–82.

47. Reinwald M, Silva JT, Mueller NJ, et al. ESCMID study group for infections in compromised hosts (ESGICH) consensus document on the safety of targeted and biological therapies: an infectious diseases perspective (Intracellular signaling pathways: tyrosine kinase and mTOR inhibitors). Clin Microbiol Infect 2018;24:S53–70.

48. Yassin MA, Nashwan AJ, Soliman AT, et al. Cytomegalovirus-induced hemorrhagic colitis in a patient with chronic myeloid leukemia (chronic phase) on dasatinib as an upfront therapy. Clin Med Insights Case Rep 2015;8:77–81.

49. Manduzio P. Ruxolitinib in myelofibrosis: to be or not to be an immune disruptor. Ther Clin Risk Manag 2017;13:169–77.

50. Lussana F, Cattaneo M, Rambaldi A, et al. Ruxolitinib-associated infections: a systematic review and meta-analysis. Am J Hematol 2018;93(3):339–47.

51. Sylvine P, Thomas S, Pirayeh E. Infections associated with ruxolitinib: study in the French Pharmacovigilance database. Ann Hematol 2018;97(5):913–4.

52. Gill H, Leung GMK, Seto WK, et al. Risk of viral reactivation in patients with occult hepatitis B virus infection during ruxolitinib treatment. Ann Hematol 2019;98(1):215–8.

53. Tillman BF, Pauff JM, Satyanarayana G, et al. Systematic review of infectious events with the Bruton tyrosine kinase inhibitor ibrutinib in the treatment of hematologic malignancies. Eur J Haematol 2018;100(4):325–34.

54. Byrd JC, Furman RR, Coutre SE, et al. Three-year follow-up of treatment-naïve and previously treated patients with CLL and SLL receiving single-agent ibrutinib. Blood 2015;125(16):2497–506.

55. Chanan-Khan A, Cramer P, Demirkan F, et al. Ibrutinib combined with bendamustine and rituximab compared with placebo, bendamustine, and rituximab for previously treated chronic lymphocytic leukaemia or small lymphocytic lymphoma (HELIOS): a randomised, double-blind, phase 3 study. Lancet Oncol 2016;17(2):200–11.

56. Byrd JC, Harrington B, O'Brien S, et al. Acalabrutinib (ACP-196) in relapsed chronic lymphocytic leukemia. N Engl J Med 2016;374(4):323–32.

57. Davids MS, Hallek M, Wierda W, et al. Comprehensive safety analysis of venetoclax monotherapy for patients with relapsed/refractory chronic lymphocytic leukemia. Clin Cancer Res 2018;24(18):4371–9.

58. DiNardo CD, Pratz KW, Letai A, et al. Safety and preliminary efficacy of venetoclax with decitabine or azacitidine in elderly patients with previously untreated acute myeloid leukaemia: a non-randomised, open-label, phase 1b study. Lancet Oncol 2018;19(2):216–28.

59. Hilal T, Gea-Banacloche JC, Leis JF. Chronic lymphocytic leukemia and infection risk in the era of targeted therapies: linking mechanisms with infections. Blood Rev 2018;32(5):387–99.

60. Sehn LH, Hallek M, Jurczak W, et al. A retrospective analysis of pneumocystis jirovecii pneumonia infection in patients receiving idelalisib in clinical trials. Blood 2016;128(22):3705.

61. Cooper N, Arnold DM. The effect of rituximab on humoral and cell mediated immunity and infection in the treatment of autoimmune diseases. Br J Haematol 2010;149(1):3–13.

62. Mikulska M, Lanini S, Gudiol C, et al. ESCMID Study Group for Infections in Compromised Hosts (ESGICH) Consensus Document on the safety of targeted and biological therapies: an infectious diseases perspective (Agents targeting lymphoid cells surface antigens [I]: CD19, CD20 and CD52). Clin Microbiol Infect 2018;24:S71–82.

63. Schuh E, Berer K, Mulazzani M, et al. Features of human CD3+CD20+ T cells. J Immunol 2016;197(4):1111–7.

64. Pfreundschuh M, Trümper L, Österborg A, et al. CHOP-like chemotherapy plus rituximab versus CHOP-like chemotherapy alone in young patients with good-prognosis diff use large-B-cell lymphoma: a randomised controlled trial by the MabThera International Trial. MInT) Group. Lancet Oncol 2006;7(5):379–91.

65. Ertrand Oiffier BC, Ric Epage EL, Osette Rière JB, et al. CHOP chemotherapy plus rituximab compared with CHOP alone in elderly patients with diffuse large-B-cell lymphoma. N Engl J Med 2002;346(4):235–42.

66. Hua Q, Zhu Y, Liu H. Severe and fatal adverse events risk associated with rituximab addition to B-cell non-Hodgkin's lymphoma (B-NHL) chemotherapy: a meta-analysis Anticancer Original Research Paper severe and fatal adverse events risk associated with rituximab addition to B-. J Chemother 2015;27(6):365–70.

67. Lanini S, Molloy AC, Fine PE, et al. Risk of infection in patients with lymphoma receiving rituximab: systematic review and meta-analysis. BMC Med 2011; 9(1):36.

68. Bauer K, Rancea M, Roloff V, et al. Rituximab, ofatumumab and other mono-clonal anti-CD20 antibodies for chronic lymphocytic leukaemia. Cochrane Database Syst Rev 2012;(11). https://doi.org/10.1002/14651858.CD008079.pub2.

69. Aksoy S, Dizdar Ö, Hayran M, et al. Infectious complications of rituximab in patients with lymphoma during maintenance therapy: a systematic review and meta-analysis. Leuk Lymphoma 2009;50(3):357–65.

70. Vidal L, Gafter-Gvili A, Leibovici L, et al. Rituximab maintenance for the treatment of patients with follicular lymphoma: systematic review and meta-analysis of randomized trials. J Natl Cancer Inst 2009;101(4):248–55.

71. Gentile G, Andreoni M, Antonelli G, et al. Systematic review Screening, monitoring, prevention, prophylaxis and therapy for hepatitis B virus reactivation in patients with haematologic malignancies and patients who underwent haematologic stem cell transplantation: a systematic review. Clin Microbiol Infect 2017; 23(12):916–23.

72. Barreto JN, Ice LL, Thompson CA, et al. Low incidence of pneumocystis pneumonia utilizing PCR-based diagnosis in patients with B-cell lymphoma receiving rituximab-containing combination chemotherapy. Am J Hematol 2016;91(11): 1113–7.

73. Jiang X, Mei X, Feng D, et al. Prophylaxis and treatment of pneumocystis jiroveci pneumonia in lymphoma patients subjected to rituximab-contained therapy: a systemic review and meta-analysis. PLoS One 2015;10(4):e0122171.

74. Hillmen P, Robak T, Janssens A, et al. Chlorambucil plus ofatumumab versus chlorambucil alone in previously untreated patients with chronic lymphocytic leukaemia (COMPLEMENT 1): a randomised, multicentre, open-label phase 3 trial. Lancet 2015;385:1873–83.

75. Sehn LH, Goy A, Offner FC, et al. Randomized phase II trial comparing obinutuzumab (GA101) with rituximab in patients with relapsed CD20+ indolent B-cell non-hodgkin lymphoma: final analysis of the GAUSS study. J Clin Oncol 2015; 33(30):3467–74.

76. Connors JM, Jurczak W, Straus DJ, et al. Brentuximab vedotin with chemotherapy for stage III or IV hodgkin's lymphoma. N Engl J Med 2017. https://doi.org/10.1056/NEJMoa1708984.

77. Moskowitz CH, Nademanee A, Masszi T, et al. Brentuximab vedotin as consolidation therapy after autologous stem-cell transplantation in patients with Hodgkin's lymphoma at risk of relapse or progression (AETHERA): a randomised, double-blind, placebo-controlled, phase 3 trial. Lancet 2015;385(9980): 1853–62.

78. Tudesq JJ, Vincent L, Lebrun J, et al. Cytomegalovirus infection with retinitis after brentuximab vedotin treatment for CD30+lymphoma. Open Forum Infect Dis 2017;4(2):12–4.

79. Drgona L, Gudiol C, Lanini S, et al. ESCMID study group for infections in compromised hosts (ESGICH) consensus document on the safety of targeted and biological therapies: an infectious diseases perspective (Agents targeting lymphoid or myeloid cells surface antigens [II]: CD22, CD30, CD33. Clin Microbiol Infect 2018;24:S83–94.

80. Palumbo A, Chanan-Khan A, Weisel K, et al. Daratumumab, bortezomib, and dexamethasone for multiple myeloma. N Engl J Med 2016;375(8):754–66.

81. Dimopoulos MA, Oriol A, Nahi H, et al. Daratumumab, lenalidomide, and dexamethasone for multiple myeloma. N Engl J Med 2016;375(14):1319–31.

82. Lundin J, Porwit-MacDonald A, Rossmann ED, et al. Cellular immune reconstitution after subcutaneous alemtuzumab (anti-CD52 monoclonal antibody, CAMPATH-1H) treatment as first-line therapy for B-cell chronic lymphocytic leukaemia. Leukemia 2004;18(3):484–90.

83. Skoetz N, Bauer K, Elter T, et al. Alemtuzumab for patients with chronic lymphocytic leukaemia. Cochrane Database Syst Rev 2012;(2). https://doi.org/10.1002/14651858.CD008078.pub2.

84. Treon SP, Soumerai JD, Hunter ZR, et al. Long-term follow-up of symptomatic patients with lymphoplasmacytic lymphoma/Waldenström macroglobulinemia treated with the anti-CD52 monoclonal antibody alemtuzumab. Blood 2011;118(2):276–81.

85. Sloand EM, Olnes MJ, Shenoy A, et al. Alemtuzumab treatment of intermediate-1 myelodysplasia patients is associated with sustained improvement in blood counts and cytogenetic remissions. J Clin Oncol 2010;28(35):5166–73.

86. Fink EC, Ebert BL. The novel mechanism of lenalidomide activity. Blood 2015;126(21):2366–9.

87. Durie BGM, Hoering A, Abidi H, et al. Bortezomib with lenalidomide and dexamethasone versus lenalidomide and dexamethasone alone in patients with newly diagnosed myeloma without intent for immediate autologous stem-cell transplant (SWOG S0777): a randomised, open-label, phase 3 trial. Lancet 2017;389. https://doi.org/10.1016/S0140-6736(16)31594-X.

88. Teh BW, Harrison SJ, Worth LJ, et al. Infection risk with immunomodulatory and proteasome inhibitorebased therapies across treatment phases for multiple myeloma: a systematic review and meta-analysis. Eur J Cancer 2016;67:21–37.

89. Chen M, Zhao Y, Xu C, et al. Immunomodulatory drugs and the risk of serious infection in multiple myeloma: systematic review and meta-analysis of randomized and observational studies. Ann Hematol 2018;97(6):925–44.

90. McCarthy PL, Owzar K, Hofmeister CC, et al. Lenalidomide after stem-cell transplantation for multiple myeloma. N Engl J Med 2012;366(19):1770–81.

91. Wang Y, Yang F, Shen Y, et al. Maintenance therapy with immunomodulatory drugs in multiple myeloma: a meta-analysis and systematic review. J Natl Cancer Inst 2016;108(3). https://doi.org/10.1093/jnci/djv342.

92. Miguel JS, Weisel K, Moreau P, et al. Pomalidomide plus low-dose dexamethasone versus high-dose dexamethasone alone for patients with relapsed and refractory multiple myeloma (MM-003): a randomised, open-label, phase 3 trial. Lancet Oncol 2013;14(11):1055–66.

93. Redelman-Sidi G, Michielin O, Cervera C, et al. ESCMID Study Group for Infections in Compromised Hosts (ESGICH) Consensus Document on the safety of targeted and biological therapies: an infectious diseases perspective (Immune checkpoint inhibitors, cell adhesion inhibitors, sphingosine-1-phosphate rece. Clin Microbiol Infect 2018;24:S95–107.

94. Dimopoulos MA, Goldschmidt H, Niesvizky R, et al. Carfilzomib or bortezomib in relapsed or refractory multiple myeloma (ENDEAVOR): an interim overall survival analysis of an open-label, randomised, phase 3 trial. Lancet Oncol 2017;18:1327–37.

95. Moreau P, Masszi T, Grzasko N, et al. Oral ixazomib, lenalidomide, and dexamethasone for multiple myeloma. N Engl J Med 2016;374(17):1621–34.

96. Kantarjian H, Stein A, Gökbuget N, et al. Blinatumomab versus chemotherapy for advanced acute lymphoblastic leukemia. N Engl J Med 2017;376(9):836–47.

97. So W, Pandya S, Quilitz R, et al. Infectious risks and complications in adult leukemic patients receiving blinatumomab. Mediterr J Hematol Infect Dis 2018;10(1):e2018029.

98. Picchi H, Mateus C, Chouaid C, et al. Infectious complications associated with the use of immune checkpoint inhibitors in oncology: reactivation of tuberculosis after anti PD-1 treatment. Clin Microbiol Infect 2018;24(3):216–8.

99. Brudno JN, Kochenderfer JN. Toxicities of chimeric antigen receptor T cells: recognition and management. Blood 2016;127(26):3321–30.

100. Hill JA, Li D, Hay KA, et al. Infectious complications of CD19-targeted chimeric antigen receptor-modified T-cell immunotherapy. Blood 2018;131(1):121–30.

101. Zhu Y, Tan Y, Ou R, et al. Anti-CD19 chimeric antigen receptor-modified T cells for B-cell malignancies: a systematic review of efficacy and safety in clinical trials. Eur J Haematol 2016;96(4):389–96.

102. Maude SL, Laetsch TW, Buechner J, et al. Tisagenlecleucel in children and young adults with B-Cell lymphoblastic leukemia. N Engl J Med 2018;378(5): 439–48.

103. Schuster SJ, Svoboda J, Chong EA, et al. Chimeric antigen receptor T cells in refractory B-cell lymphomas. N Engl J Med 2017;377(26):2545–54.

Host and Graft Factors Impacting Infection Risk in Hematopoietic Cell Transplantation

Roy L. Kao, MD*, Shernan G. Holtan, MD

KEYWORDS

- Hematopoietic cell transplantation • Transplant-related mortality
- Nonrelapse mortality • Transplant infectious disease • Immune reconstitution
- Infection risk factors

KEY POINTS

- A complex interplay of host, graft, and technical factors contributes to infectious risk in the hematopoietic cell transplantation recipient.
- Many of these factors contribute to delays in immune reconstitution, graft-versus-host disease, mucosal injury, and/or organ dysfunction, which in turn predispose the hematopoietic cell transplantation recipient to infection.
- Prior exposures and posttransplant environmental factors must also be taken into consideration when assessing infectious risk.
- Risk for infection must often be balanced against treatment of underlying disease and risk for graft-versus-host disease for each individual being evaluated for hematopoietic cell transplantation.
- Future directions may include risk stratification based on genetic and microbiota profiling.

CASE STUDIES

A 4-month-old boy with eczema, hematochezia, and thrombocytopenia is diagnosed with Wiskott-Aldrich syndrome and referred for transplant. Infectious prophylaxis against pneumocystis and immunoglobulin replacement are started. He has no siblings but a 5/6 cord and 19-year-old male 10/10 unrelated donor are identified. He undergoes busulfan and cyclophosphamide myeloablative conditioning, followed by

Disclosures: R L. Kao has no commercial or financial conflicts of interest. S.G. Holtan has served as consultant for Incyte and served on an advisory board for Bristol Myers Squibb.
Division of Hematology, Oncology, and Transplantation, Department of Medicine, University of Minnesota, 420 Delaware Street Southeast, MMC 480, Minneapolis, MN 55455, USA
* Corresponding author.
E-mail address: rkao@umn.edu

bone marrow infusion from the 10/10 unrelated donor. He develops pseudomonal bacteremia on day +10 while awaiting engraftment.

A 49-year-old man is now in his second complete remission after multiple lines of chemotherapy and targeted therapy for diffuse large B-cell lymphoma. He has no cord or matched unrelated donors, but does have a haploidentical brother. He receives cyclophosphamide, melphalan, fludarabine, and total body irradiation followed by peripheral blood stem cells collected from his brother. He engrafts by day +14 but develops graft-versus-host disease of the gut, treated with steroids. Later he develops confusion and hematuria and is found to have BK viremia and human herpes virus-6 (HHV-6) in the cerebrospinal fluid.

INTRODUCTION

Hematopoietic cell transplantation (HCT) is defined as the infusion of hematopoietic progenitor cells from any of various sources to reconstitute the bone marrow (BM) and immune system. HCT has been an important, and often curative, component of therapy for patients with a variety of acquired and inherited malignant and nonmalignant disorders. Although transplant outcomes continue to improve, serious infectious complications remain one of the major sources of morbidity and mortality in HCT recipients.[1,2]

A complex interplay of pre-HCT variables contribute to infection risk after HCT (**Fig. 1**). These variables can be divided into host (ie, the HCT recipient), graft (ie, the HCT cell product), and preparative regimen factors. These factors are, in turn, associated with variations in various aspects of immune reconstitution, the major factor in susceptibility to infection. Pre-HCT and post-HCT exposure to infectious organisms and host mucosal barrier integrity also play a major role in determining risk of infection after transplantation. After HCT, both acute graft-versus-host disease (GHVD) and chronic GVHD are complications that are known for end-organ damage, but can also severely affect immune reconstitution.[3] Various pre-HCT factors affect risk for acute GVHD and chronic GVHD, thus indirectly affecting a patient's post-HCT infection risk. Infection after HCT, in turn, can lead to transplant-related morbidity and mortality as well as itself contributing to mucosal injury (herpes simplex virus [HSV]-1 and mucositis, for example), triggering GVHD[4,5] or delaying engraftment.[6]

HEMATOPOIETIC CELL TRANSPLANTATION BASICS AND IMMUNE RECONSTITUTION AFTER HEMATOPOIETIC CELL TRANSPLANTATION

An HCT recipient's susceptibility to infection at various stages in their pre-HCT and post-HCT course correlates directly with levels of immune compromise and immune reconstitution or recovery.

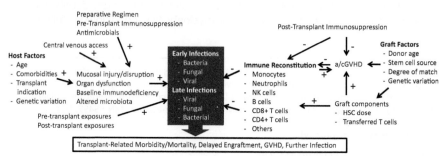

Fig. 1. Complex interplay of host, graft, and technical factors for infection in HCT. a/cGVHD, acute/chronic GVHD; HSC, hematopoietic stem cell; NK, natural killer.

Table 1 summarizes the prototypical relationship between phases of a myeloablative allogeneic HCT, recipient immune status, and risk of infection. Classically, the goals of treatment before transplantation have been to (1) eradicate malignant disease, or alternatively, (2) eradicate a defective hematopoietic system in nonmalignant disease, and (3) decrease risk of nonengraftment (ie, graft rejection) by sufficient host immunosuppression and cytoreduction of the BM space.

Treatment before Hematopoietic Cell Transplantation and Preparative Regimens

For patients with nonmalignant disease, preparative (conditioning) regimens may involve high doses of immunosuppressive therapies, chemotherapy, and/or total body irradiation. For patients with malignant disease, preparative conditioning is usually preceded by multiple cycles of disease-directed chemotherapy and/or immunotherapy to achieve—ideally—a minimal residual disease–negative state. The preparative regimen would also ideally have activity against the disease. Autologous HCT is similar in that recipients have usually received multiple cycles of disease-directed therapies before HCT. Autologous HCT, however, is primarily used to rescue the recipient's hematopoietic system, allowing for higher doses of myelotoxic chemotherapy as a way to improve antitumor activity. In this case, immunosuppression is not needed.

Nonmyeloablative (NMA) and reduced intensity conditioning preparative regimens have become an important strategy for patients with advanced age or comorbidities, with a goal of using more of the immune-mediated effects of the HCT to eradicate disease and replace host hematopoiesis, while decreasing the toxicity associated with myeloablative regimens, including infectious complications.

Hematopoietic Cell Transplantation Cell Product

The HCT cell product itself can be derived from various donors and sources, depending on what is available to each individual patient through family members or donor registries. Allogeneic donors may be siblings, other family members, or unrelated donors. Autologous HCT involves prior collection of hematopoietic cells from the patient/recipient, usually some months before the actual HCT. Donors can be fully matched (conventionally, at least 8/8 or 10/10 human leukocyte antigen [HLA] alleles), mismatched (matched on 7/8 or 9/10 HLA alleles or fewer), or haploidentical (parent, child, or sibling matching at least 5/10 HLA alleles). A matched sibling donor is also known as an HLA-identical donor.

Regardless of the donor, hematopoietic cells can be obtained (hematopoietic cell source) through either (1) apheresis of donor peripheral blood (PB), usually after mobilization with granulocyte colony-stimulating factor; (2) repeated bilateral aspiration of donor posterior iliac crest BM, usually under anesthesia; or (3) collection of a infant donor's umbilical cord blood (UCB) from the placenta after cord clamping. As detailed elsewhere in this article, the characteristics of each of these donor sources contribute to variations in infectious risk.

Preengraftment Phase

As a result of the preparative regimen, the recipient is likely near the nadir of her or his immunologic function at the time of HCT. Although the HCT itself can contain some mature donor immune cells, a persistent hematopoietic and immune system will need to be reconstituted from donor progenitor and stem cells to control infections.

Occurring during the first part of immune reconstitution, the preengraftment phase is usually characterized by severe to profound neutropenia and lymphodepletion, with resulting susceptibility to bacterial and fungal infections, as well as HSV infection. This

Table 1
Summary of the prototypical relationship between phases of a myeloablative allogeneic HCT, recipient immune status, and risk of infection

	Before HCT	Preengraftment	Postengraftment	Late Phase
Approx. Timing	Before HCT, including receipt of preparative regimen	The first 15–45 d after HCT	From engraftment to approximately day +100 after HCT	After day +100	After 1–2 y after HCT
Immune status	Depends on prior treatment and immune status	Lymphodepletion, myelosuppression, mucosal injury	Recovery of neutrophils, monocytes	Recovery of natural killer cells, CD8 T cells, but restricted T-cell repertoire	Recovery of B cells and CD4 T cells, diversifying T-cell repertoire
Most prevalent infections	Variable	Bacterial and fungal infections, HSV	Pneumocystis, fungal, viral infections/reactivations	Viral infections, encapsulated bacteria	
GVHD risk	-	-	Acute GVHD	Chronic GVHD	

phase is also associated with mucosal injury resulting from the preparative regimen; thus, many infections present as febrile neutropenia and are the result of bacterial translocation through the gut and oral mucosa. Maintenance immunosuppression (eg, a calcineurin inhibitor, mycophenolate, and/or corticosteroids), with or without posttransplant immunosuppression (eg, doses of methotrexate or cyclophosphamide), is given during this time.

The preengraftment phase lasts between the transplant and neutrophil recovery (absolute neutrophil count of $\geq 0.5 \times 10^9$/L). The exact length of this phase, and thus relative susceptibility to infection, depends greatly on the total nucleated cell dose (including mature immune cells) and T-cell dose. These factors depend on the cell product donor and source, lasting about 2 weeks with PB, 2 to 3 weeks after BM, and 3 to 4 weeks after UCB. Granulocyte colony-stimulating factor or granulocyte monocyte-colony stimulating factor are sometimes used to try to decrease the duration of severe neutropenia. Rarely, donor granulocytes can be transfused as a temporary adjunct to treat life-threatening infections during this phase.[7]

Postengraftment Phase and Late Phase

Engraftment occurs as donor-derived elements of the innate immune system, such as neutrophils, other granulocytes, and monocytes, are detected in the PB and gradually regain their full function. Mucosal injury from the preparative regimen begins to improve. Because of this, the likelihood of many bacterial and fungal infections decreases. Natural killer cells, a subset of lymphocytes that influence both innate and adaptive immune responses, appear in the first few months after HCT, and play a protective role against several viral, bacterial, and possibly fungal infections.

During the late phase (roughly after day +100), adaptive immunity may take months to years to fully recover both counts and immune competence. Some B and T lymphocytes are passively transferred along with the HCT; however, other B and T lymphocytes must follow normal ontogeny in developing from stem and progenitor cells. Total B-cell counts may take 6 to 12 months to recover, with total immunoglobulin levels not reaching normal numbers for 12 to 18 months or more. Prolonged deficiency of IgG2, in particular, may explain the susceptibility of HCT recipients to late bacterial infections.[8] IgA seems to be the last to recover, likely contributing to the risk of recurrent sinopulmonary and gastrointestinal tract infections. Because of the functional immaturity of donor-derived lymphocytes, revaccination against vaccine-preventable diseases (eg, tetanus, polio, *Haemophilus influenzae* type b infection, pneumococcal infection) is recommended for both autologous and allogeneic HCT recipients.[9]

Initially, T cells infused with the graft expand after HCT with a limited repertoire, usually generating some CD8[+] T cells and memory T cells. These cells can achieve normal counts by 1 year. Donor stem cell-derived T cells, however, must undergo thymopoiesis in the recipient thymus, a process that may take several years before producing fully functional T-cell immunity with a full T-cell repertoire. Several reviews summarize further knowledge about post-HCT immune reconstitution.[10,11]

Of the measurable components of immune reconstitution, the recovery of neutrophils and the recovery of lymphocytes, specifically CD4[+] T cells, have been most closely linked with transplant-related mortality and infectious outcomes in HCT recipients. A longer duration and depth of neutropenia has long been associated with a risk for infection.[12] For this reason, NMA conditioning, which is associated with much less neutropenia, has become an attractive option for older individuals who would not have tolerated more intense conditioning and prolonged neutropenia. More recently, lymphocyte and lymphocyte subset recovery have also been related to better HCT outcomes, including fewer infections.[13–16]

VARIABLES CONTRIBUTING TO INFECTIOUS RISK BEFORE HEMATOPOIETIC CELL TRANSPLANTATION
Host Factors

Disease indication for transplantation

HCT has a wide range of indications, including various hematologic malignancies, nonmalignant hematologic disorders, some solid tumors, and even certain autoimmune diseases.[17] Because of this, HCT recipients will have undergone a diverse range of disease-directed therapies before HCT, have a varying level of immune competence, and have the potential for previous infection with opportunistic pathogens.

For example, some HCT recipients may have one of several congenital primary immunodeficiencies involving T-cell dysfunction, such as Wiskott-Aldrich syndrome, ataxia-telangiectasia, and severe combined immunodeficiency. Early HCT is advocated if possible in many of these patients because the development of autoimmunity, such as in Wiskott-Aldrich syndrome, and certain infections can be associated with poor prognosis after HCT.[18,19] In contrast, certain groups of HCT recipients, including those with sickle cell disease and thalassemia, will have had a relatively low risk of severe or opportunistic infections before HCT.

Even patients with hematologic malignancy will present for HCT with a wide range of diagnoses and disease statuses, a wide range of previous therapies (including chemotherapy, immunotherapy and other targeted therapies, radiation, prolonged courses of steroids, and even prior HCT), and a variable time between diagnosis and HCT. These factors can all affect each patient's individual risk for infection both before and after HCT. For example, higher rates of early bacteremia and cytomegalovirus (CMV) disease have been found in groups of patients with "high-risk" disease, including active acute myeloid leukemia, myelodysplastic syndrome (refractory anemia with excess blasts or excess of blasts in transformation), acute lymphocytic leukemia, chronic lymphocytic leukemia, Hodgkin disease, multiple myeloma, renal cell carcinoma, and chronic myeloid leukemia in accelerated phase or blast crisis.[20,21]

Comorbidities

Comorbidity indexes for HCT have been developed, such as the hematopoietic stem cell transplantation-specific comorbidity index,[22] and comorbidities that are more significant can be associated with a higher incidence of aspergillosis.[23] Pulmonary dysfunction (as defined by abnormalities on pulmonary function testing) is a major contributor to the HCT comorbidity index. Along the same lines, smoking (tobacco or marijuana) has been identified as a risk factor for invasive mold infections in patients undergoing allogeneic HCT.[24]

Age

Because donor T-cell progenitors must undergo thymopoiesis in the recipient thymus, age-related thymic involution is a significant barrier to generating a full T-cell repertoire after allogeneic transplantation in elderly adults.[25,26] Lower CD4 T-cell counts, in turn, are associated with higher rates of infection during the late phase of engraftment.[13,27] This factor may contribute to the association of invasive aspergillosis and other infections with advanced age.[23,28] In contrast, pediatric patients may be more likely to develop adenovirus infection and viremia than adults, partly from a lack of previous immunity.[29]

Previous exposures

Many younger pediatric patients are especially at risk for complications of primary viral infection, which can be either transmitted through close contacts or directly through blood transfusion or the HCT itself.[30] To prevent primary viral infections in all recipients, donors are screened for several blood borne viral infections such as hepatitis B virus, hepatitis C virus, and human immunodeficiency virus. Although donation from human immunodeficiency virus-infected individuals is avoided, even detectable levels of hepatitis B virus and hepatitis C virus in a donor can be acceptable with careful monitoring and appropriate preemptive antiviral therapy.[9,31]

However, many HCT recipients are more likely to have complications from reactivation of latent infections from pathogens they have previously been exposed to. This is especially the case for viral infections, such as with CMV, Epstein-Barr virus (EBV), HSV-1 and HSV-2, HHV-6, varicella zoster virus, BK polyomavirus, and others. Latent tuberculosis can also reactivate after HCT. HCT candidates living with hepatitis B virus, hepatitis C virus, and human immunodeficiency virus infections warrant special consideration, but may still derive benefit from HCT as long as their infection is kept under control.[9]

CMV provides an example of using information about previous exposures for the prevention of disease-related complications. HCT recipients and donors are tested for CMV IgG antibodies before transplantation. Seronegative recipients, who are at risk for primary infection, are given blood products from CMV-negative donors or CMV-safe leukocyte-reduced blood products. If possible, the HCT donor for a seronegative recipient would ideally also be seronegative (D$^-$/R$^-$). Seropositive recipients (D$^+$/R$^+$ or D$^-$/R$^+$), as well as seronegative recipients with a CMV seropositive donor (D$^+$/R$^-$) are monitored closely for both CMV asymptomatic viremia and disease. Because CMV prophylaxis is poorly tolerated, preemptive therapy is given for CMV viremia with acceptable results.[32]

Finally, HCT candidates have often undergone chemotherapy and received other immunosuppressive medications and may have developed opportunistic or other treatment-related infections that can affect HCT outcome. For example, HCT recipients with pre-HCT invasive fungal infections such as those with *Candida* spp. and *Aspergillus* spp. were found to have higher nonrelapse mortality rates and worse overall survival compared with controls.[33]

Environmental factors

Seasonal variation plays a role in HCT recipient infectious risk, with influenza, respiratory syncytial virus, and other respiratory viruses usually peaking in the winter. The incidence of invasive aspergillosis in HCT recipients can also vary by season in some geographies, corresponding with weather changes (such as high temperature and low precipitation).[34]

HCT recipients with lower socioeconomic status have also been found to have worse overall survival at 1 year or more after HCT, driven by nonrelapse mortality. Infection plays a major role in this outcome.[35,36] The mechanisms for this finding are unclear, but differences in the home environment and the ability to adhere to advice about infection prevention, as well as the ability to return to the transplant center in case of serious infection, may contribute.

Central venous access

Central venous access devices (CVAD) are indispensable in the care of the HCT recipient. Not only are they required for infusion of the HCT product, but they also provide access for frequent laboratory testing, as well as the infusion of blood products, fluids, and medications. In addition, an autologous HCT recipient may have needed a specialized CVAD for apheresis during PB hematopoietic cell collection.

By the time of HCT, some CVADs will have been in place for months to facilitate the delivery of pretransplant chemotherapy. However, they compromise the integrity of the skin as a physical barrier to potential pathogens on the skin. They also can become colonized by bacteria or fungi disseminated through the bloodstream from another site. CVAD infections can cause significant morbidity and mortality. Thus, it is important to consider methods of decreasing the risk of CVAD infection, including rigorous infection prevention practices during CVAD insertion and maintenance, limiting the period of time that a CVAD is in place, and considering the benefits and risks of different types of CVADs.

Peripherally inserted central venous catheter lines have been shown in hematology-oncology populations to have a lower risk for CVAD-associated bloodstream infections compared with tunneled lines.[37] They also have the benefit of being able to be placed and removed by trained nursing staff. Externally tunneled catheters, however, are historically preferred for hematopoietic stem cell infusions and are necessary for apheresis in the setting of autologous donation.

Graft Factors

Donor characteristics

Several donor characteristics affect infectious risk, most importantly the degree of histocompatibility. Sibling donor HCT has comparatively lower rates of bacterial and fungal infection compared with HCT from matched unrelated, mismatched unrelated, or haploidentical donors.[38,39] In contrast, donor mismatch has been associated with an increased likelihood of life-threatening opportunistic infection, as well as transplant-related mortality, including infectious mortality.[27,40,41] Compared with mismatched or matched unrelated donor HCT recipients, haploidentical HCT recipients receiving recent posttransplant cyclophosphamide regimens have been found in different series to have a high incidence of viral infections, including CMV, BK and JC polyomaviruses, and HHV-6.[42–47] Rates of EBV reactivation and EBV-related lymphoproliferative disorders seemed to be decreased.[43,44,47] Preengraftment bacterial bloodstream infections have been reported to be more frequent in haploidentical HCT.[48]

As in allogeneic HCT, infection related to prolonged neutropenia remains a concern in autologous HCT. In contrast with allogeneic HCT, however, autologous HCT does not require an immunosuppressive regimen for either the prevention of graft rejection or for GVHD prophylaxis or treatment. Because of this, T-cell and B-cell compartments reconstitute at a faster rate in autologous HCT.[49] The age of the donor can be a risk factor for transplant-related mortality, including infection.[40] This finding is likely from decreases in repopulating ability, especially in T cells, and impaired homing ability in cells from older donors.[50]

Stem cell source

Compared with BM HCT, PB HCT has the advantage of easier collection (apheresis rather than a surgical procedure), a higher potential cell yield, and a faster neutrophil and T-cell recovery because of a significant number of transferred mature and progenitor lymphoid and myeloid cells. The drawback to the higher number of transferred donor lymphocytes (approximately 1 log more) has been a higher rate of chronic GVHD.[51] PB is the stem cell source of choice for autologous transplant, because GVHD is not a concern in the autologous setting, and PB is frequently used in the adult allogeneic setting. Pediatric PB HCT, however, has been associated with higher mortality, transplant-related mortality, treatment failure, and chronic GVHD compared with BM HCT, and is thus used less frequently.[52] In terms of infection, PB and BM HCT have similar overall fungal and viral infection rates. BM HCT, however, has been associated with higher rates of bacterial and preengraftment viral infections, likely related to a longer period of neutropenia before neutrophil engraftment.[53]

With lower HLA matching requirements (6 alleles rather than 8–10), a decreased risk of chronic GVHD, and the ready availability of cryopreserved UCB units, UCB HCT has become an attractive alternative for patients without an HLA-matched donor. Compared with PB and BM, however, UCB contains fewer hematopoietic stem cells and immune cells, and these immune cells are more immature.[54] Thus, it is expected that immune reconstitution in UCB HCT, as measured in either neutrophil engraftment and T-cell recovery, is more prolonged than in BM and PB HCT.[55–57] Consequently, viral infections, including HHV-6, BK virus, EBV, and adenovirus,[6,58,59] have especially been more frequent in adult UCB HCT, because immunity depends on antigen-specific T cells. In contrast, a similar increase in infections after pediatric UCB HCT has not been seen compared with BM HCT.[60,61]

Newer studies have shown, however, that some of the delay in immune reconstitution with UCB may be from use of antithymocyte globulin (ATG) in the preparative regimen. UCB HCT without ATG in 1 study was shown to have prompt T-cell recovery ($CD3^+CD4^+$ T-cell count of >200 cells/μL by day 120 after HCT), with a decreased infectious mortality.[62]

Cell dose

Cell dose, defined as number of either total nucleated cells or $CD34^+$ (hematopoietic stem and progenitor) cells in an HCT product per kilogram of patient weight, is associated with decreased transplant-related mortality in HCT from BM sources. This outcome is partly from a decreased rate of fungal and viral infections in the first month.[63–65] Experimental models suggest that this effect is from more rapid regeneration of donor-derived immune cells and enhanced thymopoiesis, as well as a greater ability of hematopoietic stem cell clones to produce multiple lineages of lymphoid cells.[66,67]

Stem cell product manipulation

Because of the finding that a greater T-cell dose in PB HCT is associated with greater risk of GVHD, T-cell depletion and $CD34^+$ cell selection have been explored as methods to decrease the risk for GVHD. The initial experience with T-cell depletion showed increased incidence of invasive aspergillosis and CMV.[28,68,69] This method has also been seen in the autologous setting, where $CD34^+$ selection is used to reduce incidence of relapse owing to contaminant tumor cells in the product.[70,71] More recent protocols have not shown a difference compared with T-cell–replete protocols.[72–74]

Donor vaccination

The vaccination of donors before HCT has been studied as a strategy for improving immune reconstitution in HCT recipients. Although there have been individual reports of efficacy in improving serologic titers against vaccine-preventable diseases in HCT recipients, a systematic review showed inconsistent results and a lack of long-term benefit.[75]

Preparative Regimen Factors

Myeloablative versus nonmyeloablative conditioning

Whereas myeloablative HCT uses high-dose chemotherapy and radiation to eradicate disease and immunoablate the host in preparation for donor cell infusion, NMA and reduced intensity conditioning regimens aim to (1) control disease through graft-versus-tumor effects and (2) prevent GVHD and graft failure (host-versus-graft) through immunosuppression, while (3) minimizing myelosuppression. This approach decreases the duration and depth of neutropenia with a corresponding decrease in rates of many infections, including bacteremia and invasive aspergillosis.[20,76–78] Recipients of NMA conditioning had similar rates of CMV disease compared with recipients of myeloablative conditioning; however, the onset of CMV disease was delayed in recipients of NMA conditioning.[21]

Chemotherapy and radiation

Besides the immunosuppressive and myelosuppressive effects mentioned elsewhere in this article, chemotherapy and radiation can each specifically cause mucosal injury and organ dysfunction, which can lead to a higher risk for infection. Total body irradiation is often included as a part of the preparative regimen because of its excellent immunosuppressive properties, activity against a wide variety of malignancies even if resistant to chemotherapy, as well as the ability to penetrate sanctuary sites, such as the central nervous system and testes. Large doses of radiation, however, are associated with pulmonary, liver, and gut toxicity. Pulmonary injury in turn can affect pulmonary clearance of pathogenic organisms, and gut epithelial injury can lead to the translocation of gut flora into the bloodstream. Thymic epithelial cell injury from radiation can also delay full immune reconstitution of the T-cell compartment.[79]

Chemotherapy can also contribute to both mucosal injury as well as organ dysfunction. For example, cyclophosphamide, a common component of many preparative regimens, is associated with oral and gut mucositis, as well as with bladder toxicity. Oral mucositis is especially associated with bacterial and fungal bloodstream infections, especially alpha-hemolytic streptococcal bacteria and Candida spp., as well as with oral HSV reactivation.[80–82] Gut mucositis can both predispose to bacteremia from bacterial translocation as well as be associated with neutropenic enterocolitis.[83] Conditioning with cyclophosphamide, known to cause bladder injury, may also contribute to the reactivation of BK polyomavirus and adenovirus in the setting of hemorrhagic cystitis after HCT.[84] Besides radiation and cyclophosphamide, methotrexate, busulfan, etoposide, melphalan, and cytarabine have also been known to cause mucositis.

Immunosuppression as a part of the preparative regimen

Preparative regimens may also contain primarily immunosuppressive agents, such as ATG and anti-CD52 antibody alemtuzumab. These agents are useful for preventing graft rejection, and have been found to have beneficial effects on acute GVHD and chronic GVHD. They can also have significant effects on immune reconstitution. ATG given before HCT can be detected in recipient plasma several weeks after HCT.[85] This finding is especially relevant to T-cell recovery after UCB HCT because of the lower number and relatively naïve T cells in the UCB, and in this setting ATG has been associated with greater risk for EBV, CMV, and adenovirus infections and death from viral infection.[86] Earlier timing of ATG or alemtuzumab use and using equine instead of rabbit ATG may also improve T-cell recovery, and, with good supportive care and antimicrobial prophylaxis, infection-related mortality in UCB HCT is approaching that of matched sibling donor PB HCT.[54,87]

Posttransplant Immunosuppression and Maintenance Therapy

Posttransplant immunosuppression

After HCT, GVHD prophylaxis is usually achieved with one or more of the following agents: calcineurin inhibitors (such as tacrolimus and cyclosporine), sirolimus, mycophenolate mofetil, methotrexate, and prednisone/methylprednisolone. Although each agent causes immunosuppression or delayed immune reconstitution to varying degrees, a systematic review did not show a difference in infection rates between regimens.[88] Other studies have specifically noted increases in invasive fungal infections with the addition of steroids to GVHD prophylaxis regimens.[89,90]

Posttransplant cyclophosphamide has also gained interest as another measure to prevent GVHD. It has mostly been used as part of GVHD prophylaxis for haploidentical transplant, as mentioned elsewhere in this article; however, more recently, posttransplant cyclophosphamide has been reported in use for HLA-matched donors either as a single post-HCT GVHD agent or in combination with standard calcineurin inhibitors. With single-agent posttransplantation cyclophosphamide, immune reconstitution was relatively rapid. Infection rates have been low or similar to other GVHD preventative measures.[91,92]

Posttransplant maintenance therapy

Finally, because disease relapse remains as one of the major contributors to post-HCT mortality, various pharmacologic interventions may be used to maintain remission. Examples include tyrosine kinase inhibitors for Philadelphia chromosome–positive acute lymphocytic leukemia, rituximab for non-Hodgkin lymphoma, azacitidine for acute myeloid leukemia, sorafenib for FLT3-mutated acute myeloid leukemia, and various regimens for multiple myeloma.[93–96] The effect of each regimen on immunosuppression and infection is varied and few data are available specific to the posttransplant setting.

FUTURE DIRECTIONS

Despite controlling for factors such as stem cell source, donor, and preparative and immunosuppressive regimens, certain HCT recipients seem to develop more severe infections compared with others. Recent work in 2 major areas of inquiry—immunogenetics and the host microbiome—may significantly affect clinical evaluation and management of infectious risk in HCT recipients in the near future.

Candidate gene studies in this area have focused on innate immune system-related genetic polymorphisms. So far, genes—both recipient and donor—encoding pattern recognition receptors such as Toll-like receptor-4, nucleotide-binding oligomerization domain containing 2, and Dectin-1, among others, have shown the strongest associations with susceptibility to severe bacterial, fungal, or viral infections in HCT recipients.[97,98] Other variations may help to explain race variations in HCT infectious outcomes.[99,100] These findings may be supplemented by genome-wide association studies, which suggest that variations in noncoding RNAs and in epigenetics may also play significant roles.[101]

Characteristics of the host microbiome, and the changes incurred on host microbiota by chemotherapy and antibiotic exposure, have also been associated with HCT outcomes, including infection. The gut microbiota in particular contributes to colonization resistance, reconstitution of the gut barrier, and development of the mucosal immune system in a symbiotic relationship with the host.[102,103] Suppression of gut microbiota diversity both by HCT-related therapies—especially antibiotics before time of HCT—and by inflammation can result in a higher risk for bloodstream infection[104,105] and progression of respiratory viral infections.[106] Here, too, genetic variation can play a role, because nucleotide-binding oligomerization domain containing 2 variants, which are already associated with severe infections in HCT recipients, are also associated with shifts in bacterial colonization in other populations.[98]

Significant confirmatory work still needs to be done in these 2 areas. Future directions for translation to clinical practice may include using or developing prophylactic and therapeutic antimicrobials with less deleterious effects on bacterial diversity, using differential antimicrobial prophylaxis regimens informed by genetic risk assessment and molecular microbiota profiling, and considering fecal microbiota transplantation to reestablish bacterial diversity and protective commensal microbiota after HCT.[97,103,107,108]

SUMMARY

A wide range of host, graft, and technical factors contributes to infectious risk in the HCT recipient. As one of the major contributors to transplant-related, nonrelapse mortality, each HCT candidate's risk for infection must be balanced against treatment of the underlying disease, GVHD, and other HCT toxicities when evaluating for a patient's best options for donor selection, stem cell source, preparative regimen, and posttransplant immunosuppression. Substantial progress has been made in prophylaxis and preemptive monitoring of infections in HCT recipients, although several innovations, including next-generation pathogen sequencing to identify pathogens in blood and stool before clinical symptoms manifest, and other techniques may further refine posttransplant care in the years ahead.

REFERENCES

1. Gooley TA, Chien JW, Pergam SA, et al. Reduced mortality after allogeneic hematopoietic-cell transplantation. N Engl J Med 2010;363:2091–101.
2. Patel SS, Rybicki LA, Corrigan D, et al. Prognostic factors for mortality among day +100 survivors after allogeneic hematopoietic cell transplantation. Biol Blood Marrow Transplant 2018;24(5):1029–34.
3. Clave E, Busson M, Douay C, et al. Acute graft-versus-host disease transiently impairs thymic output in young patients after allogeneic hematopoietic stem cell transplantation. Blood 2009;113:6477–84.
4. Cantoni N, Hirsch HH, Khanna N, et al. Evidence for a bidirectional relationship between cytomegalovirus replication and acute graft-versus-host disease. Biol Blood Marrow Transplant 2010;16:1309–14.
5. Dulery R, Salleron J, Dewilde A, et al. Early human herpesvirus type 6 reactivation after allogeneic stem cell transplantation: a large-scale clinical study. Biol Blood Marrow Transplant 2012;18:1080–9.
6. Chevallier P, Hebia-Fellah I, Planche L, et al. Human herpes virus 6 infection is a hallmark of cord blood transplant in adults and may participate to delayed engraftment: a comparison with matched unrelated donors as stem cell source. Bone Marrow Transplant 2009;45:1204–11.
7. Morton S, Mijovic A, Marks DI, et al. Use of granulocyte transfusions among haematology units in England and North Wales. Transfus Med 2018;28(3):243–8.
8. Kelsey SM, Lowdell MW, Newland AC. IgG subclass levels and immune reconstitution after T cell-depleted allogeneic bone marrow transplantation. Clin Exp Immunol 1990;80(3):409–12.

9. Tomblyn M, Chiller T, Einsele H, et al. Guidelines for preventing infectious complications among hematopoietic cell transplantation recipients: a global perspective. Biol Blood Marrow Transplant 2009;15(10):1143–238.
10. Mehta RS, Rezvani K. Immune reconstitution post allogeneic transplant and the impact of immune recovery on the risk of infection. Virulence 2016;7(8):901–16.
11. Ogonek J, Kralj Juric M, Ghimire S. Immune reconstitution after allogeneic hematopoietic stem cell transplantation. Front Immunol 2016;7:507.
12. Bodey GP, Buckley M, Sathe YS, et al. Quantitative relationships between circulating leukocytes and infection in patients with acute leukemia. Ann Intern Med 1966;64:328–40.
13. Storek J, Gooley T, Witherspoon RP, et al. Infectious morbidity in long-term survivors of allogeneic marrow transplantation is associated with low CD4 T cell counts. Am J Hematol 1997;54:131–8.
14. Kim HT, Armand P, Frederick D, et al. Absolute lymphocyte count recovery after allogeneic hematopoietic stem cell transplantation predicts clinical outcome. Biol Blood Marrow Transplant 2015;2(5):873–80.
15. Buhlmann L, Buser AS, Cantoni N, et al. Lymphocyte subset recovery and outcome after T-cell replete allogeneic hematopoietic SCT. Bone Marrow Transplant 2011;46:1357–62.
16. Berger M, Figari O, Bruno B, et al. Lymphocyte subsets recovery following allogeneic bone marrow transplantation (BMT): CD4+ cell count and transplant-related mortality. Bone Marrow Transplant 2008;41:52–62.
17. Sureda A, Bader P, Cesaro S, et al. Indications for allo- and auto-SCT for haematological diseases, solid tumors, and immune disorders: current practice in Europe, 2015. Bone Marrow Transplant 2015;50(8):1037–56.
18. Pai S, Notarangelo LD. Hematopoietic cell transplantation for Wiskott-Aldrich syndrome: advances in biology and future directions for treatment. Immunol Allergy Clin North Am 2010;30(2):179–94.
19. Pai S, Logan BR, Griffith LM, et al. Transplantation outcomes for severe combined immunodeficiency, 2000-2009. N Engl J Med 2014;371:434–46.
20. Junghanss C, Marr KA, Carter RA, et al. Incidence and outcome of bacterial and fungal infections following nonmyeloablative compared with myeloablative allogeneic hematopoietic stem cell transplantation: a matched control study. Biol Blood Marrow Transplant 2002;8:512–20.
21. Junghanss C, Boeckh M, Carter RA, et al. Incidence and outcome of cytomegalovirus infections following nonmyeloablative compared with myeloablative allogeneic stem cell transplantation, a matched control study. Blood 2002;99(6):1978–85.
22. Sorror ML, Maris MB, Storb R, et al. Hematopoietic cell transplantation (HCT)-specific comorbidity index: a new tool for risk assessment before allogeneic HCT. Blood 2005;106(8):2912–9.
23. Blennow O, Remberger M, Torlen J, et al. Risk factors for invasive mold infections and implications for choice of prophylaxis after allogeneic stem cell transplantation. Biol Blood Marrow Transplant 2016;22(9):1684–9.
24. Chien SH, Liu YC, Liu CJ, et al. Invasive mold infections in acute leukemia patients undergoing allogeneic hematopoietic stem cell transplantation. J Microbiol Immunol Infect 2018. https://doi.org/10.1016/j.jmii.2018.09.006 [pii:S1684-1182(18)30404-3].
25. Weinberg K, Annett G, Kashyap A, et al. The effect of thymic function on immunocompetence following bone marrow transplantation. Biol Blood Marrow Transplant 1995;1:18–23.

26. Storek J, Witherspoon RP, Storb R. T cell reconstitution after bone marrow transplantation into adult patients does not resemble T cell development in early life. Bone Marrow Transplant 1995;16:413–25.

27. Small TN, Papadopoulos EB, Boulad F, et al. Comparison of immune reconstitution after unrelated and related T-cell-depleted bone marrow transplantation: effect of patient age and donor leukocyte infusions. Blood 1999;93(2):467–80.

28. Wald A, Leisenring W, van Burik JA, et al. Epidemiology of Aspergillus infections in a large cohort of patients undergoing bone marrow transplantation. J Infect Dis 1997;175(6):1459–66.

29. Sedlacek P, Petterson T, Robin M, et al. Incidence of adenovirus infection in hematopoietic stem cell transplantation recipients: findings from the AdVance study. Biol Blood Marrow Transplant 2018. https://doi.org/10.1016/j.bbmt.2018.12.753 [pii:S1083-8791(18)31575-1].

30. Lau YL, Peiris M, Chan GC, et al. Primary human herpes virus 6 infection transmitted from donor to recipient through bone marrow infusion. Bone Marrow Transplant 1998;21:1063–6.

31. Tomblyn M, Chen M, Kukreja M, et al. No increased mortality from donor or recipient hepatitis B- and/or hepatitis C-positive serostatus after related-donor allogeneic hematopoietic cell transplantation. Transpl Infect Dis 2012;14(5):468–78.

32. Boeckh M, Gooley TA, Myerson D, et al. Cytomegalovirus pp65 antigenemia guided early treatment with ganciclovir versus ganciclovir at engraftment after allogeneic marrow transplantation: a randomized double-blind study. Blood 1996;88:4063–71.

33. Maziarz RT, Brazauskas R, Chen M, et al. Pre-existing invasive fungal infection is not a contraindication for allogeneic HCST for patients with hematologic malignancies: a CIBMTR study. Bone Marrow Transplant 2017;52(2):270–8.

34. Panackal AA, Li H, Kontoyiannis DP, et al. Geoclimactic influences on invasive aspergillosis after hematopoietic stem cell transplantation. Clin Infect Dis 2010;50:1588–97.

35. Baker KS, Davies SM, Majhail NS, et al. Race and socioeconomic status influence outcomes of unrelated donor hematopoietic cell transplantation. Biol Blood Marrow Transplant 2009;15(12):1543–54.

36. Fu S, Rybicki L, Abounader D, et al. Association of socioeconomic status with long-term outcomes in 1-year survivors of allogeneic hematopoietic cell transplantation. Bone Marrow Transplant 2015;50:1326–30.

37. Mollee P, Jones M, Stackelroth J, et al. Catheter-associated bloodstream infection incidence and risk factors in adults with cancer: a prospective cohort study. J Hosp Infect 2011;78:26–30.

38. Raiola AM, Dominetto A, di Grazia C, et al. Unmanipulated haploidentical transplants compared with other alternative donors and matched sibling grafts. Biol Blood Marrow Transplant 2014;20(10):1573–9.

39. Saber W, Opie S, Rizzo JD, et al. Outcomes after matched unrelated donor versus identical sibling hematopoietic cell transplantation in adults with acute myelogenous leukemia. Blood 2012;119:3908–16.

40. Castro-Malaspina H, Harris RE, Gajewski J, et al. Unrelated donor marrow transplantation for myelodysplastic syndromes: outcome analysis in 510 transplants facilitated by the national marrow donor program. Blood 2002;99:1943–51.

41. Servais S, Lengline E, Porcher R, et al. Long-term immune reconstitution and infection burden after mismatched hematopoietic stem cell transplantation. Biol Blood Marrow Transplant 2014;20(4):507–17.

42. Baker M, Wang H, Rowley SD, et al. Comparative outcomes after haploidentical or unrelated donor bone marrow or blood stem cell transplantation in adult patients with hematological malignancies. Biol Blood Marrow Transplant 2016; 22(11):2047–55.

43. Crocchiolo R, Bramanti S, Vai A. Infections after T-replete haploidentical transplantation and high-dose cyclophosphamide as graft-versus-host disease prophylaxis. Transpl Infect Dis 2015;17(2):242–9.

44. Kanakry JA, Kasamon YL, Bolanos-Meade J, et al. Absence of post-transplant lymphoproliferative disorder after allogeneic blood or marrow transplantation using post-transplantation cyclophosphamide as graft-versus-host disease prophylaxis. Biol Blood Marrow Transplant 2013;19:1514–7.

45. Luznik L, O'Donnell PV, Symons HJ, et al. HLA-haploidentical bone marrow transplantation for hematologic malignancies using nonmyeloablative conditioning and high-dose, post transplantation cyclophosphamide. Biol Blood Marrow Transplant 2008;14(6):641–50.

46. Ruggeri A, Roth-Guepin G, Battipaglia G. Incidence and risk factors for hemorrhagic cystitis in unmanipulated haploidentical transplant recipients. Transpl Infect Dis 2015;17(6):822–30.

47. Slade M, Goldsmith S, Romee R, et al. Epidemiology of infections following haploidentical peripheral blood hematopoietic cell transplantation. Transpl Infect Dis 2017;19(1). https://doi.org/10.1111/tid.12629.

48. Mikulska M, Raiola AM, Galaverna F, et al. Pre-engraftment bloodstream infections after allogeneic hematopoietic cell transplantation: impact of T-cell-replete transplantation from a haploidentical donor. Biol Blood Marrow Transplant 2018; 24(1):109–18.

49. Wiegering V, Eyrich M, Winkler B, et al. Comparison of immune reconstitution after allogeneic vs. autologous stem cell transplantation in 182 pediatric recipients. J Pediatr Hematol Oncol 2017;2(1):2–6.

50. Liang Y, Van Zant G, Szilvassy SJ. Effects of aging on the homing and engraftment of murine hematopoietic stem and progenitor cells. Blood 2005;106: 1479–87.

51. Mehta RS, Peffault de Latour R, DeFor TE, et al. Improved graft-versus-host disease-free, relapse-free survival associated with bone marrow as the stem cell source in adults. Haematologica 2016;101(6):764–72.

52. Eapen M, Horowitz MM, Klein JP, et al. Higher mortality after allogeneic peripheral-blood transplantation compared with bone marrow in children and adolescents: the Histocompatibility and Alternate Stem Cell Source Working Committee of the International Bone Marrow Transplant Registry. J Clin Oncol 2004;22(24):4872–80.

53. Young JH, Logan BR, Wu J, et al. Infections after transplantation of bone marrow or peripheral blood stem cells from unrelated donors. Biol Blood Marrow Transplant 2016;22(2):359–70.

54. Szabolcs P, Niedzwiecki D. Immune reconstitution after unrelated cord blood transplantation. Cytotherapy 2007;9(2):111–22.

55. Bejanyan N, Brunstein CG, Cao Q, et al. Delayed immune reconstitution after allogeneic transplantation increases the risks of mortality and chronic GVHD. Blood Adv 2018;2(8):909–22.

56. Inoue H, Yasuda Y, Hattori K, et al. The kinetics of immune reconstitution after cord blood transplantation and selected CD34+ stem cell transplantation in children: comparison with bone marrow transplantation. Int J Hematol 2003; 77:399–407.

57. Klein AK, Patel DD, Gooding ME, et al. T-cell recovery in adults and children following umbilical cord blood transplantation. Biol Blood Marrow Transplant 2001;7:454–66.

58. Cahu X, Rialland F, Touzeau C, et al. Infectious complications after unrelated umbilical cord blood transplantation in adult patients with hematologic malignancies. Biol Blood Marrow Transplant 2009;15(12):1531–7.

59. Ballen K, Ahn KW, Chen M, et al. Infection rates among acute leukemia patients receiving alternative donor hematopoietic cell transplantation. Biol Blood Marrow Transplant 2016;22(9):1636–45.

60. Barker JN, Hough RE, van Burik JA, et al. Serious infections after unrelated donor transplantation in 136 children: impact of stem cell source. Biol Blood Marrow Transplant 2005;11(5):362–70.

61. van Burik JA, Brunstein CG. Infectious complications following unrelated cord blood transplantation. Vox Sang 2007;92(4):289–96.

62. Sauter C, Abboud M, Jia X. Serious infection risk and immune recovery after double-unit cord blood transplantation without antithymocyte globulin. Biol Blood Marrow Transplant 2011;17(10):1460–71.

63. Bittencourt H, Rocha V, Chevret S, et al. Association of CD34 cell dose with hematopoietic recovery, infections, and other outcomes after HLA-identical sibling bone marrow transplantation. Blood 2002;99:2726–33.

64. Dominietto A, Lamperlli T, Raiola AM, et al. Transplant-related mortality and long-term graft function are significantly influenced by cell dose in patients undergoing allogeneic marrow transplantation. Blood 2002;100:3930–4.

65. Miyakoshi S, Kusumi E, Matsumura T, et al. Invasive fungal infection following reduced-intensity cord blood transplantation for adult patients with hematologic diseases. Biol Blood Marrow Transplant 2007;13(7):771–7.

66. Chen BJ, Cui X, Sempowski GD, et al. Hematopoietic stem cell dose correlates with the speed of immune reconstitution after stem cell transplantation. Blood 2004;103:4344–52.

67. Brewer C, Chu E, Chin M. Transplantation dose alters the differentiation program of hematopoietic stem cells. Cell Rep 2016;15(8):1848–57.

68. Pirsch JD, Maki DG. Infectious complications in adults with bone marrow transplantation and T-cell depletion of donor marrow. Increased susceptibility to fungal infections. Ann Intern Med 1986;104:619–31.

69. van Burik JA, Carter SL, Freifeld AG, et al. Higher risk of cytomegalovirus and aspergillus infections in recipients of T cell-depleted unrelated bone marrow: analysis of infectious complications in patients treated with T cell depletion versus immunosuppressive therapy to prevent graft-versus-host disease. Biol Blood Marrow Transplant 2007;13:1487–98.

70. Crippa F, Holmberg L, Carter RA, et al. Infectious complications after autologous CD34-selected peripheral blood stem cell transplantation. Biol Blood Marrow Transplant 2002;8(5):281–9.

71. Holmberg LA, Boeckh M, Hooper H, et al. Increased incidence of cytomegalovirus disease after autologous CD34-selected peripheral stem cell transplantation. Blood 1999;94:4029–35.

72. Devine SM, Carter S, Soiffer RJ, et al. Low risk of chronic graft-versus-host disease and relapse associated with T cell-depleted peripheral blood stem cell transplantation for acute myelogenous leukemia in first remission: results of the blood and marrow transplant clinical trials network protocol 0303. Biol Blood Marrow Transplant 2011;17(9):1343–51.

73. Jakubowski AA, Small TN, Kernan NA, et al. T cell-depleted unrelated donor stem cell transplantation provides favorable disease-free survival for adults with hematologic malignancies. Biol Blood Marrow Transplant 2011; 17(9):1335–42.

74. Pasquini MC, Devine S, Mendizabal A, et al. Comparative outcomes of donor graft CD34+ selection and immune suppressive therapy as graft-versus-host disease prophylaxis for patients with acute myeloid leukemia in complete remission undergoing HLA-matched sibling allogeneic hematopoietic cell transplantation. J Clin Oncol 2012;30(26):3194–201.

75. Muhsen IN, Aljurf M, Wingard JR, et al. Vaccinating donors for hematopoietic cell transplantation: a systematic review and future perspectives. Vaccine 2018;36(41):6043–52.

76. Pulsipher MA, Chitphakdithai P, Logan BR, et al. Donor, recipient, and transplant characteristics as risk factors after unrelated donor PBSC transplantation: beneficial effects of higher CD34+ dose. Blood 2009;114:2606–16.

77. Bachanova V, Brunstein CG, Burns LJ, et al. Fewer infections and lower infection-related mortality following non-myeloablative versus myeloablative conditioning for allotransplantation of patients with lymphoma. Bone Marrow Transplant 2009;43:237–44.

78. Wingard JR, Carter SL, Walsh TJ, et al. Randomized, double-blind trial of fluconazole versus voriconazole for prevention of invasive fungal infection after allogeneic hematopoietic cell transplantation. Blood 2010;116:111–8.

79. Kelly RM, Highfill SL, Panoskaltsis-Mortari A, et al. Keratinocyte growth factor and androgen blockade work in concert to protect against conditioning regimen-induced thymic epithelial damage and enhance T-cell reconstitution after murine bone marrow transplantation. Blood 2008;111(12):5734–44.

80. Stiff P. Mucositis associated with stem cell transplantation: current status and innovative approaches to management. Bone Marrow Transplant 2001; 27(Suppl 2):S3–11.

81. Wingard JR. Fungal infections after bone marrow transplant. Biol Blood Marrow Transplant 1999;5:55–68.

82. Eisen D, Essell J, Broun ER. Oral cavity complications of bone marrow transplantation. Semin Cutan Med Surg 1997;16:265–72.

83. Avigan D, Richardson P, Elias A, et al. Neutropenic enterocolitis as a complication of high dose chemotherapy with stem cell rescue in patients with solid tumors: a case series with a review of the literature. Cancer 1998;83:409–14.

84. Lunde LE, Dasaraju S, Cao Q, et al. Hemorrhagic cystitis after allogeneic hematopoietic cell transplantation: risk factors, graft source and survival. Bone Marrow Transplant 2015;50(11):1432–7.

85. Remberger MM, Persson MM, Mattsson JJ, et al. Effects of different serumlevels of ATG after unrelated donor umbilical cord blood transplantation. Transpl Immunol 2012;27(1):59–62.

86. Lindemans CA, Chiesa R, Amrolla PJ, et al. Impact of thymoglobulin prior to pediatric unrelated umbilical cord blood transplantation on immune reconstitution and clinical outcome. Blood 2014;123:126–32.

87. Bhatt ST, Bednarski JJ, Berg J, et al. Immune reconstitution and infection patterns after early alemtuzumab and reduced intensity transplantation for nonmalignant disorders in pediatric patients. Biol Blood Marrow Transplant 2018. https://doi.org/10.1016/j.bbmt.2018.10.008 [pii:S1083-8791(18)30641-30644].

88. Ram R, Gafter-Gvili A, Yeshurun M, et al. Prophylaxis regimens for GVHD: systemic review and meta-analysis. Bone Marrow Transplant 2009;43:643–53.

89. O'Donnell MR, Schmidt GM, Tegtmeier BR, et al. Prediction of systemic fungal infection in allogeneic marrow recipients: impact of amphotericin prophylaxis in high-risk patients. J Clin Oncol 1994;12(4):827–34.

90. Martino R, Subira M, Rovira M, et al. Invasive fungal infections after allogeneic peripheral blood stem cell transplantation: incidence and risk factors in 395 patients. Br J Haematol 2002;116(2):475–82.

91. Kanakry CG, O'Donnell PV, Furlong T, et al. Multi-institutional study of post-transplantation cyclophosphamide as single-agent graft-versus-host disease prophylaxis after allogeneic bone marrow transplantation using myeloablative busulfan and fludarabine conditioning. J Clin Oncol 2014;32(31):3497–505.

92. Ruggeri A, Labopin M, Bacigalupo A, et al. Post-transplant cyclophosphamide for graft-versus-host disease prophylaxis in HLA matched sibling or matched unrelated donor transplant for patients with acute leukemia, on behalf of ALWP-EBMT. J Hematol Oncol 2018;11:40.

93. Hourigan CS, McCarthy P, de Lima M. Back to the Future! The evolving role of maintenance therapy after hematopoietic stem cell transplantation. Biol Blood Marrow Transplant 2014;20:154–63.

94. Craddock C, Jilani N, Siddique S, et al. Tolerability and clinical activity of post-transplantation azacitidine in patients allografted for acute myeloid leukemia treated on the RICAZA trial. Biol Blood Marrow Transplant 2016;22(2):385–90.

95. Antar A, Otrock ZK, El-Cheikh J, et al. Inhibition of FLT3 in AML: a focus on sorafenib. Bone Marrow Transplant 2017;52(3):344–51.

96. Sengsayadeth S, Malard F, Savani BN, et al. Posttransplant maintenance therapy in multiple myeloma: the changing landscape. Blood Cancer J 2017;7(3):e545.

97. Wojtowicz A, Bochud PY. Risk stratification and immunogenetic risk for infections following stem cell transplantation. Virulence 2016;7(8):917–29.

98. Espinoza JL, Wadasaki Y, Takami A. Infection complications in hematopoietic stem cells transplant recipients: do genetics really matter? Front Microbiol 2018;9:2317.

99. Sano H, Hilinski JA, Applegate K, et al. African American race is a newly identified risk factor for postengraftment blood stream infections in pediatric allogeneic blood and marrow transplantation. Biol Blood Marrow Transplant 2017;23(2):357–60.

100. Saleh M, Vaillancourt JP, Graham RK, et al. Differential modulation of endotoxin responsiveness by human caspase-12 polymorphisms. Nature 2004;429:75–9.

101. Ramsuran V, Ewy R, Nguyen H, et al. Variation in the untranslated genome and susceptibility to infections. Front Immunol 2018;9:2046.

102. Shi N, Li N, Duan X, et al. Interaction between the gut microbiome and mucosal immune system. Mil Med Res 2017;4:14.

103. Khoruts A, Hippen KL, Lemire AM, et al. Toward revision of antimicrobial therapies in hematopoietic stem cell transplantation: target the pathogens, but protect the indigenous microbiota. Transl Res 2017;179:116–25.

104. Taur Y, Jenq RR, Perales M, et al. The effects of intestinal tract bacterial diversity on mortality following allogeneic hematopoietic stem cell transplantation. Blood 2014;124:1174–82.

105. Montassier E, Al-Ghalith GA, Ward T, et al. Pretreatment gut microbiome predicts chemotherapy-related bloodstream infection. Genome Med 2016;8(1):49.

106. Haak BW, Littman ER, Chaubard JL, et al. Impact of gut colonization with butyrate-producing microbiota on respiratory viral infections following allo-HCT. Blood 2018;131(26):2978–86.

107. Weber D, Hiergeist A, Weber M, et al. Detrimental effect of broad-spectrum antibiotics on intestinal microbiome diversity in patients after allogeneic stem cell transplantation: lack of commensal sparing antibiotics. Clin Infect Dis 2018. https://doi.org/10.1093/cid/ciy711.

108. Taur Y, Coyte K, Schluter J, et al. Reconstitution of the gut microbiota of antibiotic-treated patients by autologous fecal microbiota transplant. Sci Transl Med 2018;10(460) [pii:eaap9489].

Complications of Stem Cell Transplantation that Affect Infections in Stem Cell Transplant Recipients, with Analogies to Patients with Hematologic Malignancies

Sunita Nathan, MD, Celalettin Ustun, MD*

KEYWORDS

- Stem cell transplantation • Hematopoietic stem cell transplantation
- Complications of stem cell transplantation
- Infections affecting stem cell transplantation complications

KEY POINTS

- HSCT is associated with different complications either directly or indirectly due to the conditioning regimen used, ensuing immunosuppressed state or immune- mediated injury post-HSCT.
- These impact the integrity of the affected organ and predispose to different infectious complications.
- Type of infections is impacted by the timing from the HSCT and type of immune component (humoral or cellular) affected.
- Early detection and appropriate intervention is required to reverse and prevent deleterious outcomes such as severe morbidity and mortality.

MUCOSITIS

Key Points

1. Mucositis is common after either autologous or allogeneic hematopoietic stem cell transplant.
2. The frequency of mucositis is affected by both transplant-specific and patient-related factors.

Section of Bone Marrow Transplant and Cellular Therapy, Division of Hematology, Oncology and Cell Therapy, Rush University Medical Center, 1725 West Harrison Street, Suite 809, Chicago, IL 60612, USA
* Corresponding author.
E-mail address: celalettin_ustun@rush.edu

Infect Dis Clin N Am 33 (2019) 331–359
https://doi.org/10.1016/j.idc.2019.01.002
0891-5520/19/© 2019 Elsevier Inc. All rights reserved.

3. Although there is no good treatment therapy, recombinant human keratinocyte growth factor-1 can be used to prevent oral mucositis.
4. Oral mucositis increases the risk for infections, especially gram-positive bacterial, anaerobic bacterial, and fungal infections.

Mucositis refers to the inflammatory and/or ulcerative lesions of the oral and/or gastrointestinal tract (mouth, larynx, pharynx, stomach, duodenum, small and large bowel, to the anus). Mucosal injury may be caused by high-dose chemotherapy with or without radiotherapy, medications, infectious diseases, and immune deficiency that ensues in either an autologous or allogeneic hematopoietic stem cell transplant (HSCT) setting.[1]

The incidence of World Health Organization (WHO) grade 2 to 4 is about 75% to 80% in patients undergoing HSCT.[1,2] Risk factors are shown in **Box 1.**

Inflammatory processes ensuing during stem cell transplant are responsible for the development of oral mucositis and include a 5-phase process of initiation, upregulation/activation, signal amplification, ulceration, and healing involving the epithelial and connective tissue of the mucosa.[3–5]

Oral mucositis manifests with pain, erythema, and ulceration with various degrees of inability to tolerate oral intake (fluids, solids, and pills), and gastrointestinal mucositis manifests with pain, nausea and emesis, and diarrhea. The WHO oral toxicity scale and the National Cancer Institute Common Terminology Criteria for Adverse Events grading scale have been used to grade symptoms that develop based on clinical changes and ability to tolerate oral intake of solids and liquids.[5,6]

Development of mucositis with disruption of mucosal barrier in the setting of immunosuppressive therapy (IST) facilitates access of oral and gastrointestinal flora to the blood stream and cause infections ranging from bacteremia, fungal blood stream infections, to sepsis. Bacteremia is more common after myeloablative than reduced-intensity conditioning regimens of HSCT.[7] The most common organisms include gram-positive bacteria (coagulase-negative *Staphylococcus*, *Staphylococcus aureus*, and *Enterococcus* [all species]); gram-negative bacteria (*Escherichia coli*, *Klebsiella* species, *Pseudomonas* species, *Enterobacter*, *Stenotrophomonas*); *Clostridium difficile*, *Nocardia*, and nontuberculous mycobacterial infections.[8] Anaerobic bacterial organisms, *Enterococcus*, and *Candida* species have also been reported.[9]

Several preventive and treatment measures have been identified. The current guidelines recommend (ie, strong evidence supports effectiveness in the treatment setting)[1,2]:

- Use of recombinant human keratinocyte growth factor-1 (palifermin) to prevent oral mucositis (at a dose of 60 μg/kg/d for 3 days before conditioning treatment and for 3 days after transplant).

Box 1
Risk factors for mucositis

Transplant related
   Conditioning intensity (myeloablative)
   Total body irradiation (TBI)
   Graft-versus-host disease (GVHD) prophylaxis (use of methotrexate)

Patient related
   Malnutrition
   Salivary hypofunction/xerostomia caused by antiemetics, prior radiation
   Genetic polymorphisms

- Low-level laser therapy (wavelength 650 nm, power 40 mW, and each square centimeter treated with the required time to a tissue energy dose of 2 J/cm^2) in patients receiving high-dose chemotherapy with or without TBI, followed by auto-HSCT.
- Patient-controlled analgesia with morphine be used to treat pain caused by oral mucositis in patients undergoing HSCT in addition to mouth care.
- Oral cryotherapy has been used to prevent oral mucositis in patients receiving high-dose melphalan.
- Prevention of infections is facilitated by use of appropriate prophylactic antimicrobials with onset of neutropenia.
- Treatment of associated infections involves specific antimicrobial therapy based on identification/speciation and sensitivities.

TYPHLITIS
Key Points

1. A life-threatening complication in HSCT affecting the small and large bowel.
2. Typhlitis is usually caused by disruptions of the mucosal barrier by a conditioning regimen.
3. Bloodstream infections with gram-negative bacteria, anaerobic bacteria, and *Candida* are common.
4. Treatment usually includes antibiotics covering anaerobes and gram-negative bacteria and conservative measures.

Neutropenic enterocolitis (NE), also known as typhlitis, is a life-threatening complication of chemotherapy in patients undergoing high-dose chemotherapy and HSCT.[10] Risk factors are shown in **Box 2**.

Symptoms of NE involve fevers, abdominal pain, and diarrhea in the setting of neutropenia. NE usually develops with onset of neutropenia at a median days 3 to 7 following transplant.[11,12] The ascending colon is often involved, but other portions of the large and small intestine may also be involved.[13–15] Abdominal ultrasonography or computed tomography (CT) scan with greater than 4 mm bowel thickening in this scenario is diagnostic.[13,16–18] In severe cases, ileus and pneumatosis intestinalis with bowel perforation and life-threatening sepsis may occur.

Bacteremia with translocation of gut flora may be seen.[11,12] The microbiologic cause of typhlitis is rarely determined, but typhlitis is presumed to be caused mostly by gram-negative and anaerobic bacteria. Invasion of the compromised bowel wall by *Candida* species has been noted.[19,20]

Rapid identification and timely, aggressive medical and/or surgical intervention are the cornerstones of survival for these patients, who are usually managed conservatively with good supportive care, which includes bowel rest and total parenteral

---

Box 2
Risk factors for typhlitis

Transplant related
    Conditioning regimen (etoposide, thiotepa, and melphalan)[11,12]
    TBI

Patient related
    Hematologic malignancy (lymphoma, multiple myeloma, and leukemia)[10]
    Neutropenia
    Underlying inflammatory bowel disorders (eg, ulcerative colitis, Crohn's disease)

nutrition (TPN), pain management, antibiotics against gram-negative bacteria and anaerobes, and avoidance of antidiarrheals.[11,12,16–22]

ENGRAFTMENT SYNDROME
Key Points

1. Noninfectious complication seen primarily in autologous HSCT and on occasion in allo-HSCT during engraftment.
2. Engraftment syndrome (ES) is a clinical syndrome characterized by noninfectious fever, rash, and diarrhea.
3. The most important clinical point is to recognize ES and eliminate the presence of infection.
4. ES may be associated with an increased risk of infection caused by low levels of CD4+ T cells.
5. ES is treated with high-dose steroids, which are generally tapered rapidly.

ES has been recognized as an inflammatory condition during neutrophil recovery after HSCT characterized by noninfectious fever and skin rash.[23–26] In addition, ES may manifest with diarrhea; hepatic dysfunction; renal dysfunction; transient encephalopathy; and capillary leak features, such as noncardiogenic pulmonary infiltrates, hypoxia, and weight gain with no alternative causal basis other than engraftment.[24] The criteria by Spitzer[27] and Maiolino and colleagues[28] are used to identify ES.[24,27,28] Median onset is 7 days post-HSCT; however, it highly varies per donor source.

Risk factors reported include stem cell source (peripheral blood), use of granulocyte colony-stimulating factor (G-CSF),[29–31] number of infused CD34+ cells,[32] female gender, underlying disease (higher incidence in solid tumors or autoimmune disorders), number of therapies before HSCT, early phases of disease, limited or no prior treatment, and use of melphalan as in amyloidosis and polyneuropathy, organomegaly, endocrinopathy, monoclonal gammopathy, and skin changes (POEMS) syndrome.[33] Use of fewer therapies pre-HSCT is associated with less damaged stem cells, endothelial cells, and tissues that release excessive proinflammatory cytokines at the time of engraftment resulting in the development of ES.

Diagnosis of ES is usually clinical. Infections can cause the same symptoms and signs, therefore eliminating infection is critical. Cultures and necessary images (eg, CT of the chest) should be obtained as part of the investigation to assess for a possible infectious focus. C-reactive protein level is usually increased.[34,35]

Treatment of ES includes the use of methylprednisolone at the dose of 1 mg/kg every 12 hours to be started as soon as possible but always after stopping G-CSF, administering 24 to 48 hours of broad-spectrum antibiotics (based on neutropenic fever guidelines or definitive diagnosis of infection), and after confirming the negativity of the microbiological tests. This dose is maintained for 3 days and then tapered over 7 to 8 days.[33]

Most patients have a low CD4(+)/CD8(+) ratio during at least the first year posttransplant, caused by a persistent increase of CD8(+) and a reduction of CD4(+) lymphocytes, making the patients susceptible to infections for a prolonged period of time posttransplant.[36,37]

GRAFT-VERSUS-HOST DISEASE
Key Points

1. Acute and chronic graft-versus-host disease (GVHD) result from alloreactive donor T cell–mediated tissue damage.

2. Diagnosis of GVHD is usually clinical and the mainstay of its treatment is composed of optimizing immunosuppressive drugs and high-dose steroids.
3. GVHD is associated with impaired cell-mediated immunity in recipients and hypogammaglobulinemia.
4. Most common infections include endogenous organism reactivation, such as cytomegalovirus and Epstein-Barr virus; and exogenous infections, including pneumocystis, aspergillosis, other molds, encapsulated organisms, and respiratory viruses.
5. Prophylaxis, surveillance, and preemptive treatment are the main approach to managing these infections.

Acute graft-versus-host disease (GVHD) is an immune-triggered (alloreactive donor T cells) process, leading to profound immune dysregulation and organ dysfunction.[38] It is a clinical syndrome that affects the skin, gut, or liver, manifesting with skin rash of variable degree, intractable nausea/emesis, large-volume diarrhea, and hyperbilirubinemia. Chronic GVHD has commonly seen diagnostic features, as outlined by the National Institutes of Health (NIH) consensus criteria,[14] include skin disorder varying from lichen planus–like lesions to full sclerosis, bronchiolitis obliterans syndrome (BOS), and oral lichen planus–like lesions (ie, skin, lung, and mouth involvement). Esophageal webs and strictures and muscle or joint fasciitis are also diagnostic.[39]

Pathogenesis of acute GVHD involves 3 phases in the development of acute GVHD: an afferent phase, an efferent phase, and an effector phase.[40] The afferent phase begins with activation of host antigen-presenting cells (APCs) by danger signals expressed on damaged tissues (damage-associated molecular patterns) and/or pathogens (pathogen-associated molecular patterns, eg, lipopolysaccharide).[41] Activated host APCs then present host antigens to donor T cells, leading to alloactivation and inflammatory cytokine release in the efferent phase. These inflammatory cytokines then recruit and induce proliferation of additional immune effector cells, perpetuating the cycle of alloreactive tissue injury and inflammation constituting the effector phase.[38–43]

Risk factors include extent of human leukocyte antigen (HLA) disparity, increased age of both the recipient and the donor, gender disparity, multiparous female donors, ineffective GVHD prophylaxis, and the intensity of the transplant conditioning regimen and the source of graft.[44–47] Less commonly reported are higher intensity of the conditioning regimen (irradiation),[44,48] prior cytomegalovirus (CMV) infection in the recipient,[48,49] donor age,[50] and grafting with growth factor–mobilized blood cells.[50,51] For chronic GVHD, risk factors include prior acute GVHD,[52–54] grafting with growth factor–mobilized blood cells,[51,55,56] the use of a female donor for male recipients,[53,54] older patient age,[52–54,57] and mismatched and unrelated donors.[54,58]

Diagnosis of GVHD is usually clinically suspected and confirmed by a biopsy of skin or gastrointestinal tract. The severity of acute and chronic GVHD is graded clinically. Chronic GVHD is graded as mild, moderate, or severe based on number and extent of organ involvement.[59–62] Prevention involves use of GVHD prophylaxis using a combination of various agents, such as calcineurin inhibitor (CNI), methotrexate, sirolimus, mycophenolate mofetil, T-cell depletion techniques with antithymocyte globulin (ATG), and alemtuzumab.[63]

Corticosteroids are the backbone of the management of acute and chronic GVHD.[64–69] In resistant cases, more immunosuppressive, lympholytic modalities/drugs (ATG, mycophenolate mofetil, anti–interleukin (IL)-2 receptor, anti–CD5-specific immunotoxin, pan T-cell ricin A-chain immunotoxin, ABX-CBL, etanercept, infliximab, daclizumab, visilizumab and pentostatin, extracorporeal photopheresis, Bruton tyrosine kinase inhibitors) have been used.[64–70] GVHD treatment further increases the risk of infections.

Infectious risk associated with GVHD, both acute and chronic, is secondary to immune dysfunction and enhanced immunosuppression. Immunosuppression is also caused by GVHD therapy (eg, steroids). Patients with chronic GVHD are functionally asplenic. Immune defects observed in patients with GVHD include both impaired cell-mediated immunity and hypogammaglobulinemia. Infections seen include reactivation of endogenous herpes virus infections such as CMV, varicella zoster virus, and Epstein-Barr virus (EBV). There is also increased potential for exogenously acquired infections, such as *Pneumocystis*; *Aspergillus*; other inhaled molds; encapsulated bacterial organisms, the most common being *Streptococcus pneumoniae*; and respiratory viruses (eg, influenza, parainfluenza, and respiratory syncytial virus [RSV]). Candida infections, especially oral thrush, and catheter-related infections are also noted.[71]

During immunosuppressive therapy, patients at risk should be on a surveillance plan to identify early herpes virus reactivation, receive appropriate prophylaxis for commonly expected infections, and receive preemptive therapy for CMV before the development of end-organ infection. CMV-seropositive patients should be monitored weekly with quantitative CMV (and sometimes EBV testing) through at least day +180 following transplant.[72] Prophylaxis against *Pneumocystis jiroveci* pneumonia (PJP) (eg, trimethoprim/sulfamethoxazole, dapsone, atovaquone, or inhaled pentamidine), encapsulated bacteria (penicillin or levofloxacin), and molds (voriconazole or posaconazole) is continued during IST or even until 3 months after the cessation of IST. Prophylactic antibacterial agents should be used indefinitely for patients who are anatomically or functionally asplenic (chronic GVHD). In responding patients with limited chronic GVHD symptoms, on prednisone equivalents of 0.5 mg/kg every other day, ongoing monitoring for reactivation of CMV and prophylactic fungal medication is less critical. Prophylaxis for PJP and encapsulated bacteria should continue until 3 to 6 months after discontinuation of immunosuppressive therapy.[71–83]

Standard therapy applies for CMV and EBV infections. Important to note is that intravenous (IV) immune globulin can be used as an adjunct to antiviral therapy up to every other day for 3 weeks along with induction treatment therapy with life-threatening infections. These patients usually have severe hypogammaglobulinemia (ie, immunoglobulin G levels of <400 mg/dL), which can be very common in patients with GVHD.[73]

Reactivation of varicella zoster virus and hepatitis B and C virus may also be seen during GVHD and treated per guidelines mentioned earlier.

Candida infections may develop during GVHD treatment. *Candida albicans* usually is replaced by *Candida krusei* or *Candida Glabrata*, which are most likely be resistant to fluconazole and hence therapy should be guided by testing sensitivities.[71]

PJP prophylaxis should be maintained until the CD4 is count greater than 200 cells/mm^3. First-line treatment is with trimethoprim/sulfamethoxazole, which could also provide protection against nocardiosis, toxoplasmosis, salmonellosis, infection with *Haemophilus* species, and *S aureus* infection.[71] Dosage is usually a double-strength tablet twice daily on 2 days of the week. Alternative prophylaxis and treatment regimens include dapsone, pentamidine aerosolized or IV, trimethoprim-dapsone, clindamycin-primaquine, and oral atovaquone. Duration is usually at least 1 year (or until 3 months after the cessation of IST).[71]

Aspergillus fumigatus and *Aspergillus flavus* are more commonly inhaled mold infections in the GVHD setting. High-risk patients for aspergillosis are those who have been exposed to construction/renovations close to hospitals or clinics and potted plants, especially exposure to marijuana. Incidence is about 15%.[73] Surveillance involves checking *Aspergillus* galactomannan antigen levels in bronchoalveolar lavage (BAL) or serum (least sensitive) and useful if serial tests are done (but expensive) and in the absence of antimold therapy. Prophylaxis is the best practice and involves the use of posaconazole[76,77] or voriconazole[78] during GVHD treatment. Invasive aspergillosis infections manifest as lung nodules, although tracheobronchitis and skin nodules have been seen. Upfront diagnosis and aggressive initiation of antifungal monotherapy are vitally important, especially with voriconazole dosed twice daily as oral (preferred for creatinine clearance <50 mL/min) or IV (loading with 6 mg/kg/dose for 2 doses, followed by a decrease to 3–4 mg/kg/dose). Voriconazole also has good central nervous system (CNS) penetration, which can be important for patients with CNS disease.

Other mold infections during GVHD presenting most often as pulmonary or disseminated disease are *Rhizopus*, *Rhizomucor*, and *Mucor*.[69] Posaconazole and isavuconazole are oral drugs that have activity in the treatment of Mucorales infections.[82,83] IV amphotericin products are also active against the Mucorales. *Fusarium* spp, most commonly *Fusarium moniliforme* and *Fusarium oxysporum*, resemble *Aspergillus* in pathologic tissue sections and are recoverable from the blood stream in blood culture. Frequent sites of infection include skin, nails, the airways, and eyes. Blood cultures become positive for 40% to 60% of patients with disseminating infection. The most important host defense risk factor for invasive fusariosis is neutropenia.[82–84] Systemic corticosteroids used in GVHD therapy are also linked to infection.[85] Invasive disease is usually prevented and/or treated with voriconazole.[86] Secondary prophylaxis should be continued during GVHD if there is prior history and presence of neutropenia.

Routine use of quinolones or macrolides decreases risk of infections with encapsulated organisms, especially penicillin-resistant pneumococci, during GVHD. In initial series of immunizations, conjugate pneumococcal and *Haemophilus influenzae* type b vaccines are given after IST therapy is discontinued.[71,87]

Respiratory viral infections (RSV), such as influenza, parainfluenza, adenovirus, human metapneumovirus, enteroviruses, herpes viruses (including human herpesvirus 6 [HHV-6]), and rhinovirus are common during GVHD and can involve both the upper and lower respiratory tract. There is no diagnostic monitoring schedule for respiratory viruses among asymptomatic patients undergoing GVHD treatment. Local rapid diagnostic nucleic acid–based methods include seasonal use of rapid antigen studies and/or shell vial assays. The historical gold standard for diagnosis is a 21-day incubation respiratory virus culture, which is performed year-round on request. However, nucleic acid–based testing is used for adenovirus, HHV-6, and human metapneumovirus. Preferred diagnostic specimens include nasopharyngeal specimens and BAL fluid instead of throat swabs. Both suspected and documented infection require initiation of contact and droplet isolation precautions. Prevention of exposure to respiratory viruses is critical given that no effective therapy is available for most respiratory viruses. Antiviral treatment choices vary depending on which virus is involved: influenza is most often treated with oseltamivir, RSV and parainfluenza viruses are most often treated with aerosolized ribavirin, and adenovirus is at times treated with cidofovir (although evidence of efficacy is lacking).[71,87]

HEMORRHAGIC CYSTITIS
Key Points

1. Hemorrhagic cystitis (HC) is frequently observed after each autologous and allogeneic HSCT.
2. HC results from direct chemotherapy-associated injury or infections.
3. Viral infections (BK virus, adenovirus, and CMV) are the most commonly implicated infectious causes of HC.

4. Treatment incudes supportive care and antiviral therapy against specific viruses (although its efficacy is not clear in all patients).

Hemorrhagic cystitis (HC) is a serious and frequent complication of HSCT affecting both allogeneic HSCT and autologous HSCT recipients.[88–92] Early-onset hematuria after transplant is usually attributed to toxic effects of the preparative regimens or GVHD prophylaxis, especially those using high-dose cyclophosphamide (HD-Cy). Late-onset hematuria, occurring 2 weeks after HSCT, is often caused by viral infections.[88] Polyoma BK virus, CMV, and adenovirus are associated with HC in both adults and children.[89,93–100]

The incidence of HC in the HSCT setting varies from 16% to 41% in the literature.[101–103] Risk factors are shown in **Box 3**.[88,89,95,96,99,102,104–114]

Prevention of HC includes hyperhydration and mesna with regimens involving HD-Cy and has proved to be beneficial.[88,115,116] Treatment of HC comprises intravascular hydration and constant bladder irrigation, and cystoscopy can be considered for evacuation of blood clots in severe cases.

Virus-specific antiviral therapy has been used with ganciclovir for CMV infection or cidofovir as intravesicular or IV (with or without probenecid to prevent renal toxicity) in BK and adenovirus infection.[117–120] Cidofovir can improve viral-induced HC in 50% to 70% of patients.[120]

Hyperbaric oxygen therapy has also been found to be a safe and effective therapeutic option for treatment-resistant radiogenic and chemotherapy-induced HC.[121] The effect of HC on survival remains controversial, but its morbidity can be substantial, even in survivors.

SINUSOIDAL OBSTRUCTIVE SYNDROME
Key Points

1. Sinusoidal obstructive syndrome (SOS) is a life-threatening complication affecting the liver.
2. Prior therapies and exposure, underlying chronic hepatitis (hepatitis B and C viruses) infections, and iron overload increase the risk of developing SOS.
3. An association with fungal infections in patients with SOS has been reported.
4. Early identification, supportive care, and use of defibrotide are the mainstay of treatment.

Hepatic sinusoidal obstruction syndrome (SOS), previously called hepatic venoocclusive disease (VOD), is characterized by hepatomegaly, right upper quadrant pain, jaundice, and ascites. It is most commonly seen in patients undergoing HSCT, and

---

Box 3
Risk factors for hemorrhagic cystitis

Transplant related
  Donor source (unrelated and cord blood)
  Conditioning regimens
    High-dose cyclophosphamide
    TBI containing
    Intensity (myeloablative conditioning [MAC] > reduced-intensity conditioning [RIC])

Patient related
  Older age in pediatric and younger age in adult patients
  Presence of GVHD

less commonly following the use of certain chemotherapeutic agents in nontransplant settings, ingestion of alkaloid toxins, high-dose radiation therapy, or liver transplant.[122]

Overactivation of the hepatic sinusoidal epithelium after injury is suggested to lead to formation of microemboli (sloughed epithelium) causing occlusion of the terminal hepatic venules and hepatic sinusoids. As a result, hepatic venous outflow obstruction occurs. Preexisting liver disease, such chronic hepatitis, may impair metabolism of drugs and render these patients more susceptible to the cytoreductive regimen–induced endothelial cell injury. Moreover, endothelial cells in patients with hepatitis may abnormally express adhesion molecules and procoagulant factors.[123–125]

The incidence of SOS is about 11.6% and severe SOS with multiorgan dysfunction may be associated with greater than 80% mortality. Risk factors are as shown in **Box 4**.

VOD/SOS has been diagnosed using modified Seattle criteria ($\geq$2 of bilirubin level >2 mg/dL, hepatomegaly, or >2% weight gain [sometimes >5%]) or Baltimore criteria (bilirubin level $\geq$2 mg/dL and $\geq$2 of hepatomegaly, ascites, $\geq$5% weight gain)[136]; the European Society for Blood and Marrow Transplantation proposed new adult criteria in 2016. Early predictors of impending VOD/SOS identified include increased tacrolimus levels, renal dysfunction, and platelet transfusion refractoriness in the week before VOD/SOS diagnosis. It develops at a median of 12 to 14 days post-HSCT but can occur though day 21.[135–139] Late cases are seen beyond days 21 to 40 to 50 days.

Association of VOD/SOS with increased risk for invasive fungal infections has been reported, which is presumed to be caused by iron overload and risk for SOS and the association of increased risk for fungal pulmonary infections in the setting of iron overload (IO).[140,141]

Diagnosis includes specific criteria of new onset of ultrasonography-confirmed ascites and/or hepatomegaly and attenuated or reversed hepatic venous flow and nonspecific criteria of gall bladder wall thickening.[142] Measurement of the hepatic venous gradient pressure through the jugular vein and liver biopsy helps make the definitive diagnosis of SOS/VOD but is invasive and difficult to perform in routine practice.[143]

Reversal of SOS/VOD risk factors and pharmacologic prevention may decrease risk of VOD/SOS.[135] Although the reversal of patient-related and hepatic disease-related risk factors are difficult to change, therapy-related risk factors can be altered (eg, dosage of conditioning regimen or replacing the order of administration of medications

---

Box 4
Risk factors for sinusoidal obstruction syndrome

Prior therapies or exposures
  Monoclonal antibodies conjugated with calicheamicin (gemtuzumab, inotuzumab)[126–128]
  High-dose radiation to liver (usually >30 Gy) without cytoreductive chemotherapy[129,130]
  Radioembolization of liver tumors[131]
  Ingestion of pyrrolizidine alkaloids (from herbal sources; eg, bush tea)[132]
  After liver transplant[133,134]

Patient related[135]
  Underlying liver disease, especially chronic hepatitis (eg, viral, alcohol, iron overload)

Transplant related[135]
  MAC>RIC
  High-dose cyclophosphamide
  TBI

[eg, cyclophosphamide-busulfan instead of busulfan-cyclophosphamide]; hyperfractionated doses of TBI).[135] Pharmacologic preventive interventions include use of heparin (although most studies had a negative impact) and use of ursodeoxycholic acid has been shown to be protective against development of SOS/VOD.[136,143–145] In a pediatric population, defibrotide effectively decreased SOS rates in high-risk patients.

Treatment involves early detection and symptom management in a timely fashion.[146] Fluid and sodium balance, careful use of diuretics (spironolactone or furosemide) alleviate ascites, pleural effusion, and supplemental oxygen where needed. Paracentesis, respiratory/ventilatory support, and hemodialysis/hemofiltration should be used as required.[146] Severe SOS/VOD treatment requires transfer to an intensive care unit. A transjugular intrahepatic portosystemic shunt can be considered in patients with less advanced SOS/VOD,[147] and hepatic transplant is needed in the most severe cases.[148] The only proven curative treatment is the use of defibrotide. Defibrotide is a polydisperse oligonucleotide with local antithrombotic, anti-ischemic, and antiinflammatory activity[149] that has protective effects on the small vessel endothelium. It potentially facilitates protection of endothelial cells and restoration of the thrombotic-fibrinolytic balance. Several studies done in the past 15 years led to approval of this drug at 25 mg/kg/d because of safety, improved complete response rates, and 100-day survival.[149–152]

HEPATITIS, NOT OTHERWISE SPECIFIED
Key Points

1. IO and drug-induced liver injury are other noninfectious complications of the liver in the HSCT patients.
2. IO and hyperferritinemia have been associated with increased risk for bacterial and invasive fungal infections.

The most frequent noninfectious complications of liver following allogeneic HSCT include SOS, GVHD, IO, and drug-induced liver injury (DILI).[153] SOS and GVHD are described elsewhere.

IO is common in patients with hematologic malignancies who require chemotherapy and transfusion support. IO can cause liver dysfunction and induce fibrosis, and thereby potentiate other transplant-associated complications, such as SOS,[154–158] infections, cardiac toxicity, and mortality. In addition, there is an association between IO and acute GVHD.[159–161]

Risk factors of IO include frequent red blood cell transfusions and hemochromatosis (acquired or hereditary). IO is usually asymptomatic and manifests with abnormal blood tests. Pretransplant IO may adversely affect overall survival and nonrelapse mortality.[162–164]

DILI is a diagnosis of exclusion. Many drugs used during hematopoietic cell transplant (HCT) can cause abnormal liver function tests. CNIs; (predominantly increase direct bilirubin levels because of inhibition of bilirubin transport), total parenteral nutrition (TPN), antimicrobials such as trimethoprim/sulfamethoxazole (mainly cholestasis), and antifungal azoles (itraconazole, voriconazole, posaconazole) are well known for hepatotoxicity. Most patients with IO do not have any symptoms on presentation.

Transaminitis is more prominent than cholestasis (bilirubin and alkaline phosphatase) in viral hepatitis and DILI. Cholestasis is more prominent than transaminitis in acute and chronic GVHD, sepsis, extrahepatic biliary duct obstruction, and cyclosporine A and TPN use.

Blood cultures and virus-specific tests should be ordered to rule out viral or other infections (eg, bacterial stream infections, systemic candidiasis). IO (ferritin levels greater than 1000 ng/mL). Ferritin levels can be increased as an acute phase reactant, and transferrin saturation should also be ordered if it is. MRI of the liver is used for quantitative iron measures. Liver biopsy can be considered in patients if IO or DILI is suspected. Iron levels are tested on the biopsy (normal levels are 530–900 µg/g dry weight).

IO is associated with increased risk for fungal infections and bloodstream infections in the first 100 days post-HSCT.[140,165,166] The most common organisms identified in patients with IO were gram-positive bacteria, gram-negative bacteria, and fungi.

Treatment of IO is evolving. Treatment options depend on hemoglobin and erythropoiesis. If normal, use phlebotomy, and, if anemic, use iron chelation therapy (oral deferasirox or parenteral deferoxamine, both of which are US Food and Drug Administration approved), which may help with iron depletion but the impact on survival is unknown. Treatment guidelines are not standardized. Current recommendations are based on liver iron content (LIC). If LIC is more than 7000 to 15,000 mg/g dry weight, phlebotomy preferred; if LIC is less than 7000 mg/g dry weight, treatment is indicated only if there is evidence of liver disease. If there are ongoing transfusion needs after HCT, concurrent chelation therapy is indicated.[167-175]

Treatment of DILI involves holding or replacing the culprit drugs. Transaminases may improve promptly (within 7–10 days) but drug-induced cholestasis resolves longer periods.

DIFFUSE ALVEOLAR HEMORRHAGE
Key Points

1. Life-threatening pulmonary complication in allo-HSCT patients.
2. Transplant-related factors and respiratory infections are considered contributing factors.
3. Various bacterial, fungal, and viral organisms have been identified as associated with diffuse alveolar hemorrhage.

Diffuse alveolar hemorrhage (DAH) is a life-threatening pulmonary complication of HSCT with unclear pathogenesis.[176,177] It usually presents with acute-onset hypoxemia and pulmonary infiltrates on chest radiograph or CT chest, and definitive diagnosis involves progressively bloodier BAL in the absence of an infectious source on bronchoscopy. A similar clinical syndrome with an identifiable infectious source is referred to as infection-associated alveolar hemorrhage (IAH).[176-179] Therefore, whether DAH and IAH are different complications can be questioned.

Incidence of DAH after HSCT ranges from 1% to 5% in autologous HSCT and from 3% to 7% in allogeneic HSCT.[180-182] Most patients develop severe respiratory failure, and mortalities are 70% or higher.[180-184] The exact cause of DAH is unknown; however, DAH originates from the pulmonary microvasculature in response to alveolar injury. Vascular damage and inflammation from chemoradiotherapy used in the conditioning regimen (especially myeloablative TBI) and immune-mediated events, including GVHD, have been considered as predisposing factors.[177-186]

Risk factors after HSCT include older age, allogeneic donor source, umbilical cord blood, use of myeloablative conditioning including TBI, delayed engraftment, and presence of severe acute GVHD caused by direct injury or increasing the susceptibility to other insults. Infections (particularly respiratory infections) may be an important contributing factor.[176,177] Microorganisms isolated in patients with DAH/IAH include coagulase-negative *Staphylococcus* spp, *Enterococcus* spp, CMV, *C albicans* and *C glabrata*, *Pseudomonas aeruginosa*, *S aureus*, RSV, *Enterobacter cloacae*,

Streptococcus viridans, adenovirus, *H influenzae, Saccharomyces cerevisiae*, and *P jirovecii*.[176] HHV-6 infection is an emerging viral pathogen.

Treatment involves early detection and early intervention. Intervention includes supportive care involving oxygen supplementation, preventing cough, correcting coagulopathy and maintaining adequate platelet goal, use of factor VIIa, DDAVP, and aminocaproic acid where indicated. High-dose steroids are the cornerstone of treatment, presumably because of their antiinflammatory effect.[187,188] Appropriate antimicrobial and antiviral therapy are also indicated. Early-onset DAH has lower mortality and hence better survival outcomes than late-onset cases. Despite all efforts, the mortality at 60 days remains high, at approximately 80%.

POSTERIOR REVERSIBLE ENCEPHALOPATHY SYNDROME
Key Points

1. Posterior reversible encephalopathy syndrome (PRES) is a neurologic syndrome most commonly associated with the use of CNIs as GVHD prophylaxis.
2. Certain bacterial and viral infections are suggested to have indirect or direct association with PRES.
3. Treatment of PRES comprises stopping or eradicating the inciting agent or infection.

Posterior reversible encephalopathy syndrome (PRES) is a serious adverse event associated with CNIs used for GVHD prophylaxis in patients undergoing allogeneic HSCT.[189–193] It is a clinical syndrome that is characterized by neurologic symptoms and distinct neuroradiologic changes. Symptoms are usually mild, such as headache, tremors, paresthesia, insomnia, photophobia, and mood disturbances, and in severe cases altered mental status, cognitive deficits, seizures, visual disturbances, and coma. Radiologic findings are distinct for edema involving the white matter in the posterior portions of the cerebral hemispheres.[189–193]

The pathophysiology with immunosuppressive agents is possibly caused by an acute episode of vasogenic edema in the vertebral white matter with a predilection for the posterior temporal, parietal, and occipital regions. The extracellular edema is attributed to autoregulatory dysfunction in the posterior circulation and a transient breakdown of the blood-brain barrier with a leakage of protein/fluids causing the neuronal injury.[190] Polymorphisms in drug metabolizing genes, such as Multidrug Resistance Gene 1, can enhance tacrolimus-associated neurotoxocity.[194,195]

Incidence is about 1.6%.[196] Risk factors include use of CNIs such as tacrolimus and cyclosporine. Of note, increased levels do not correlate to development of PRES. GVHD has been associated with PRES, most commonly seen in matched unrelated donor and cord blood HSCT.[197,198] Increase of blood pressure on average 25% more than baseline associated with tacrolimus may predispose to PRES.[199] Renal dysfunction possibly from tacrolimus-induced renal vasoconstriction, fluid weight gain ~10%, hypomagnesemia, and fludarabine have also been associated with PRES.[199–202]

PRES can also be seen in patients with other diseases or clinical conditions, including after chemotherapy, infections/sepsis/shock, eclampsia, and autoimmune disorders. Regarding infections, in 23 patients, significant infection and/or bacteremia occurred in close association with the development of PRES. In 11 of the 23 patients with infection, clinical sepsis was noted or suspected during their illness before development of PRES. In 21 of these 23 patients with infection, PRES developed immediately after or coincident with the severe infection or bacteremia. In 18 of these 21 patients, PRES occurred within 2 weeks of the infection and, in 3 patients, neurotoxicity developed between 20 and 30 days of infection identification (overall average, 6.7 days; range, 0–30 days).[203,204]

Treatment includes early recognition of symptom profile, and timely confirmation with imaging studies and intervention is prudent to avoid long-term effects. Supportive therapy includes optimizing blood pressure control, fluid status, electrolyte replacement, and especially magnesium and antiseizure medications. Discontinuation of CNIs and switching to an alternative immunosuppressant regimen including mycophenolate mofetil, steroids, and sirolimus is indicated.[190–203,205,206] Concomitant antimicrobial therapy and antiviral therapy is indicated to treat the underlying associated infection as identified.

BRONCHIOLITIS OBLITERANS SYNDROME AND BRONCHIOLITIS OBLITERANS WITH ORGANIZING PNEUMONIA
Key Points

1. These complications result from attack from donor immune cells to recipient lung tissue.
2. Infections, especially resistant infections, cause increased lung injury.
3. Infections may be the cause of death in many patients with severe BOS.
4. Some studies suggest that infections may increase risk for BOS.

Pulmonary complications occur in 25% to 50% of allogeneic HSCT recipients, and can account for approximately 50% of transplant-related deaths.[207–213] These complications can be acute, as in idiopathic pulmonary syndrome, a noninfectious lung injury, or subacute or late onset, as in BOS and bronchiolitis obliterans with organizing pneumonia (BOOP).

BOS is also referred to as constrictive bronchiolitis. It manifests clinically by the presence of airflow obstruction presenting as progressive dyspnea, nonproductive cough, and wheezing. Median time to development is 1 year.[214] Pulmonary function studies show an irreversible decline in forced expiratory volume in 1 second (FEV_1) of at least 20% from baseline, and it is graded using the International Society for Heart and Lung Transplantation (ISHLT) criteria.[215] Chest radiographs are often normal; however, hyperinflation has been described.[216] High-resolution CT or thin-section CT in the diagnosis of BOS may show air trapping, mosaic perfusion, bronchial dilatation (bronchiectasis), and bronchial wall thickening.[217–220] BAL is usually done to eliminate an infectious cause.[221] Lung biopsy, if possible, is characterized by submucosal bronchiolar fibrosis along with luminal narrowing and obliteration.[222–224]

The incidence varies from 1.7% to 26%. Risk factors are shown in **Box 5**.[217,225–231]

The pathogenesis has not been well defined. It is presumed to be a multifactorial process involving both alloimmunologic reactions, as in chronic GVHD, and nonalloimmunologic inflammatory conditions, such as viral infections (parainfluenza and RSV), recurrent aspiration, and conditioning chemoradiotherapy.[229,232,233] Strong association between respiratory viral infection early after HSCT and the development of life-threatening acute and chronic alloimmune lung syndromes, including BOS, has been shown. It is possible that early viral respiratory infections render the lungs a target for alloimmune reactions/tissue destruction.[230]

Infections are common in patients with BOS. In a study, in addition to baseline infections (24 out of 25 patients), 45 infections occurred during the study period. These infections were bacterial (36%, most commonly gram-negative bacteria), viral (47%, most commonly influenza), fungal (16%, mostly *Aspergillus*), and mycobacterial infections (2%). Adenovirus infection was found to be a risk factor.[234] Nontuberculosis

---

Box 5
Risk factors for bronchiolitis obliterans syndrome and bronchiolitis obliterans with organizing pneumonia

Transplant related
  Donor
    Source (peripheral blood stem cells > bone marrow)
    Female donor to male recipient
    Older age
  Conditioning regimens
    Busulfan-containing conditioning regimens
    Intensity (MAC>RIC)
  GVHD prophylaxis (use of methotrexate)

Patient related
  Decreased immunoglobulin levels
  Lower pretransplant FEV_1/forced vital capacity ratio
  Prior episode of interstitial pneumonitis

Infections
  Respiratory viral infections within the first 100 days

---

mycobacterium (NTM) infections are more common in patients with BOS. However, it is not clear whether NTMs are the cause or result of BOS. Moreover, NTMs can be contaminant micrganisms.[235]

The mainstay of treatment involves increased immunosuppression, which involves high-dose corticosteroids.[232] Inhaled cyclosporine may be effective both in the prevention and treatment of BOS after lung transplant,[230,232–236] and is now in HSCT trials. Azithromycin[237,238] has been reported to have efficacy because of antiinflammatory effects (IL-8 and airway neutrophilia).[239,240] A study cautions that long-term use of macrolide antibiotics for BOS may induce resistant NTMs.[241]

Tumor necrosis factor alpha (TNFα) neutralizing agents such as etanercept represent a novel therapy.[242] Infliximab, monoclonal antibody for human TNFα,[243] has been used successfully. Anti-TNF drugs are risk factors for infections, especially mycobacterial infections. Extracorporeal photochemotherapy, which has been shown to be a promising treatment of chronic GVHD,[244,245] has been used with some success for BOS after HSCT. Lung transplant has been increasingly reported as a possible therapeutic option for end-stage BOS after HSCT.[246]

BOOP is a disorder involving bronchioles, alveolar ducts, and alveoli, the lumens of which become filled with buds of granulation tissue consisting of fibroblasts and an associated matrix of loose connective tissue. The bronchiolitis in BOOP is of the proliferative type, and generally includes mild inflammation of the bronchiolar walls.[247]

Incidence is about 1%[248] in the setting of acute or chronic GVHD, 1.6% in matched related donor HSCT,[249] and 10.3% in matched unrelated donor AHCT.[250] Median time to occurrence is 108 days.[248] BOOP presents with fever, nonproductive cough, and dyspnea. Radiology findings include CT with diffuse, fluffy consolidations, ground-glass opacity, and nodules.[207] Bronchoscopy and BAL are useful in ruling out pulmonary infection and establishing the diagnosis of BOOP. Transbronchial lung biopsy shows organizing pneumonia.

Treatment is not standardized and corticosteroid is the mainstay of therapy. The role of macrolides has also been explored in the treatment in BOOP.[251]

REFERENCES

1. Peterson DE, Bensadoun RJ, Roila F, ESMO Guidelines Working Group. Management of oral and gastrointestinal mucositis: ESMO Clinical Practice Guidelines. Ann Oncol 2011;22(Suppl 6):vi78–84.
2. Lalla RV, Bowen J, Barasch A, et al. MASCC/ISOO clinical practice guidelines for the management of mucositis secondary to cancer therapy. Cancer 2014; 120(10):1453–61.
3. Oral complications in hematopoietic stem cell transplantation recipients: the role of inflammation. Mediators Inflamm 2014;2014:18. Article ID 378281.
4. Sonis ST. The pathobiology of mucositis. Nat Rev Cancer 2004;4:277–84.
5. Sonis ST, Elting LS, Keefe D, et al, Mucositis Study Section of the Multinational Association for Supportive Care in Cancer, International Society for Oral Oncology. Perspectives on cancer therapy-induced mucosal injury: pathogenesis, measurement, epidemiology, and consequences for patients. Cancer 2004;100(9 Suppl):1995–2025.
6. National Cancer Institute. Common terminology criteria for adverse events v4.0. NCI, NIH, DHHS; 2009. NIH publication # 09-7473.
7. Kim SH. Transpl Infect Dis 2013.
8. Young JH, Logan BR, Wu J, et al, Blood and Marrow Transplant Clinical Trials Network Trial 0201. Infections after transplantation of bone marrow or peripheral-blood stem cells from unrelated donors. Biol Blood Marrow Transplant 2016;22(2):359–70.
9. Osakabe L, Utsumi A, Saito B, et al. Influence of oral anaerobic bacteria on hematopoietic stem cell transplantation patients: oral mucositis and general condition. Transplant Proc 2017;49:2176–82.
10. Davila ML. Neutropenic enterocolitis. Curr Opin Gastroenterol 2006;22(1):44.
11. Rodrigues FG, Dasilva G, Wexner SD. Neutropenic enterocolitis. World J Gastroenterol 2017;23(1):42–7.
12. Gil L, Poplawski D, Mol A, et al. Neutropenic enterocolitis after high-dose chemotherapy and autologous stem cell transplantation: incidence, risk factors, and outcome. Transpl Infect Dis 2013;15(1):1–7.
13. Gorschlüter M, Mey U, Strehl J, et al. Neutropenic enterocolitis in adults: systematic analysis of evidence quality. Eur J Haematol 2005;75(1):1–13.
14. Cardona AF, Ramos PL, Casasbuenas A. From case reports to systematic reviews in neutropenic enterocolitis. Eur J Haematol 2005;75(5):445–6.
15. Aksoy DY, Tanriover MD, Uzun O, et al. Diarrhea in neutropenic patients: a prospective cohort study with emphasis on neutropenic enterocolitis. Ann Oncol 2007;18(1):183–9.
16. Kirkpatrick ID, Greenberg HM. Gastrointestinal complications in the neutropenic patient: characterization and differentiation with abdominal CT. Radiology 2003; 226(3):668–74.
17. Cronin CG, O'Connor M, Lohan DG, et al. Imaging of the gastrointestinal complications of systemic chemotherapy. Clin Radiol 2009;64(7):724–33.
18. Coy DL, Ormazabal A, Godwin JD, et al. Imaging evaluation of pulmonary and abdominal complications following hematopoietic stem cell transplantation. Radiographics 2005;25(2):305–17 [discussion: 318].
19. Cardona Zorrilla AF, Reveiz Herault L, Casasbuenas A, et al. Systematic review of case reports concerning adults suffering from neutropenic enterocolitis. Clin Transl Oncol 2006;8(1):31–8.

20. Gorschluter M, Mey U, Strehl J, et al. Invasive fungal infections in neutropenic enterocolitis: a systematic analysis of pathogens, incidence, treatment and mortality in adult patients. BMC Infect Dis 2006;6:35.

21. Cloutier RL. Neutropenic enterocolitis. Hematol Oncol Clin North Am 2010;24(3): 577–84.

22. Jimenez AM, et al. Favorable outcomes of neutropenic enterocolitis following hematopoietic stem cell transplantation (HSCT) using a conservative medical therapy approach. Blood 2010;116:1283.

23. Spitzer TR. Engraftment syndrome: double-edged sword of hematopoietic cell transplants. Bone Marrow Transplant 2015;50(4):469–75.

24. Cornell RF, Hari P, Drobyski WR. Engraftment syndrome after autologous stem cell transplantation: an update unifying the definition and management approach. Biol Blood Marrow Transplant 2015;21(12):2061–8.

25. Omer AK, Kim HT, Yalamarti B, et al. Engraftment syndrome after allogeneic hematopoietic cell transplantation in adults. Am J Hematol 2014;89(7):698–705.

26. Schmid I, Stachel D, Pagel P, et al. Incidence, predisposing factors, and outcome of engraftment syndrome in pediatric allogeneic stem cell transplant recipients. Biol Blood Marrow Transplant 2008;14:438–44.

27. Spitzer TR. Engraftment syndrome following hematopoietic stem cell transplantation. Bone Marrow Transplant 2001;27(9):893–8.

28. Maiolino A, Biasoli I, Lima J, et al. Engraftment syndrome following autologous hematopoietic stem cell transplantation: definition of diagnostic criteria. Bone Marrow Transplant 2003;31(5):393–7.

29. Edenfield WJ, Moores LK, Goodwin G, et al. An engraftment syndrome in autologous stem cell transplantation related to mononuclear cell dose. Bone Marrow Transplant 2000;25(4):405–9.

30. Akasheh M, Eastwood D, Vesole DH. Engraftment syndrome after autologous hematopoietic stem cell transplant supported by granulocyte-colony-stimulating factor (G-CSF) versus granulocyte-macrophage colony-stimulating factor (GM-CSF). Bone Marrow Transplant 2003;31(2):113–6.

31. Tuazon S, Daskalakis C, Mandala A, et al. Comparison of Engraftment Syndrome with G-CSF Versus GM-CSF after Autologous Hematopoietic Progenitor Cell Transplantation for Multiple Myeloma. Poster presented at: American Society for Blood and Marrow Transplantation BMT Tandem Meetings; San Diego, CA, 2015.

32. Carreras E, Saiz A, Marin P, et al. CD34+ selected autologous peripheral blood stem cell transplantation for multiple sclerosis: report of toxicity and treatment results at one year of follow-up in 15 patients. Haematologica 2003;88(3): 306–14.

33. Carreras E, Fernández-Avilés F, Silva L, et al. Engraftment syndrome after auto-SCT: analysis of diagnostic criteria and risk factors in a large series from a single center. Bone Marrow Transplant 2010;45(9):1417–22.

34. Fassas AB, Miceli MH, Grazzlutti M, et al. Serial measurement of serum C-reactive protein levels can identify patients at risk for severe complications following autologous stem cell transplantation. Leuk Lymphoma 2005;46(8):1159–61.

35. Ortega M, Rovira M, Almela M, et al. Measurement of C-reactive protein in adults with febrile neutropenia after hematopoietic cell transplantation. Bone Marrow Transplant 2004;33(7):741–4.

36. Steingrimsdottir H, Gruber A, Björkholm M, et al. Immune reconstitution after autologous hematopoietic stem cell transplantation in relation to underlying

disease, type of high-dose therapy and infectious complications. Haematologica 2000;85(8):832–8.

37. Gale RP, Lazarus HM. Engraftment syndrome, the Emperor's new clothes and the artist formerly known as prince. Bone Marrow Transplant 2015;50(4):483–4.

38. Nassereddine S, Rafei H, Elbahesh E, et al. Acute graft *Versus* host disease: a comprehensive review. Anticancer Res 2017;37(4):1547–55.

39. Flowers ME, Inamoto Y, Carpenter PA, et al. Comparative analysis of risk factors for acute graft-*versus*-host disease and for chronic graft-*versus*-host disease according to National institutes of Health consensus criteria. Blood 2011; 117(11):3214–9.

40. Ball LM, Egeler R. Acute GvHD: pathogenesis and classification. Bone Marrow Transplant 2008;41:S58–64.

41. Holtan SG, Pasquini M, Weisdorf DJ. Acute graft-versus-host disease: a bench-to-bedside update. Blood 2014;124:363–73.

42. Blazar BR, Murphy WJ, Abedi M. Advances in graft-versus-host disease biology and therapy. Nat Rev Immunol 2012;12(6):443–58.

43. Paczesny S, Hanauer D, Reddy P, et al. New perspectives on the biology of acute GVHD. Bone Marrow Transplant 2009;45(1):1–11.

44. Nash RA, Deeg HJ, Doney K, et al. Acute graft-*versus*-host disease: analysis of risk factors after allogeneic marrow transplantation and prophylaxis with cyclosporine and methotrexate. Blood 1992;80(7):1838–45.

45. Gale RP, Kersey JH, Marmont A, et al. Risk factors for acute graft-*versus*-host disease. Br J Haematol 1987;67(4):397–406.

46. Anasetti C, Couban S, Ehninger G, et al. Peripheral-blood stem cells *versus* bone marrow from unrelated donors for the blood and marrow transplant clinical trials network. N Engl J Med 2012;367(16):1487–96.

47. Lee SE, Lee S, Min CK, et al. Risk and prognostic factors for acute GVHD based on NIH consensus criteria. Bone Marrow Transplant 2012;48(4):587–92.

48. Hahn T, McCarthy PL Jr, Zhang MJ, et al. Risk factors for acute graft-versus-host disease after human leukocyte antigen-identical sibling transplants for adults with leukemia. J Clin Oncol 2008;26(35):5728–34.

49. Jacobsen N, Badsberg JH, Lonnqvist B, et al. Graft-versus-leukaemia activity associated with CMV-seropositive donor, post-transplant CMV infection, young donor age and chronic graft-versus-host disease in bone marrow allograft recipients. The Nordic Bone Marrow Transplantation Group. Bone Marrow Transplant 1990;5(6):413–8.

50. Kollman C, Howe CW, Anasetti C, et al. Donor characteristics as risk factors in recipients after transplantation of bone marrow from unrelated donors: the effect of donor age. Blood 2001;98(7):2043–51.

51. Cutler C, Giri S, Jeyapalan S, et al. Acute and chronic graft-versus-host disease after allogeneic peripheral-blood stem-cell and bone marrow transplantation: a meta-analysis. J Clin Oncol 2001;19(16):3685–91.

52. Storb R, Prentice RL, Sullivan KM, et al. Predictive factors in chronic graft-versus-host disease in patients with aplastic anemia treated by marrow transplantation from HLA-identical siblings. Ann Intern Med 1983;98(4):461–6.

53. Carlens S, Ringden O, Remberger M, et al. Risk factors for chronic graft-versus-host disease after bone marrow transplantation: a retrospective single centre analysis. Bone Marrow Transplant 1998;22(8):755–61.

54. Lee SJ, Vogelsang G, Flowers ME. Chronic graft-versus-host disease. Biol Blood Marrow Transplant 2003;9(4):215–33.

55. Körbling M, Anderlini P. Peripheral blood stem cell versus bone marrow allo-transplantation: does the source of hematopoietic stem cells matter? Blood 2001;98(10):2900–8.
56. Eapen M, Logan BR, Confer DL, et al. Peripheral blood grafts from unrelated donors are associated with increased acute and chronic graft-versus-host disease without improved survival. Biol Blood Marrow Transplant 2007;13(12):1461–8.
57. Atkinson K, Horowitz MM, Gale RP, et al. Risk factors for chronic graft-versus-host disease after HLA-identical sibling bone marrow transplantation. Blood 1990;75(12):2459–64.
58. Lee SJ, Klein JP, Barrett AJ, et al. Severity of chronic graft-versus-host disease: association with treatment-related mortality and relapse. Blood 2002;100(2): 406–14.
59. Baird K, Steinberg SM, Grkovic L, et al. National Institutes of Health chronic graft-versus-host disease staging in severely affected patients: organ and global scoring correlate with established indicators of disease severity and prognosis. Biol Blood Marrow Transplant 2013;19(4):632–9.
60. Curtis LM, Grkovic L, Mitchell SA, et al. NIH response criteria measures are associated with important parameters of disease severity in patients with chronic GVHD. Bone Marrow Transplant 2014;49(12):1513–20.
61. Pidala J, Kim J, Anasetti C, et al. The global severity of chronic graft-versus-host disease, determined by National Institutes of Health consensus criteria, is associated with overall survival and non-relapse mortality. Haematologica 2011; 96(11):1678–84.
62. Inamoto Y, Martin PJ, Storer BE, et al, Chronic GVHD Consortium. Association of severity of organ involvement with mortality and recurrent malignancy in patients with chronic graft-versus-host disease. Haematologica 2014;99(10):1618–23.
63. Ruutu T, Van Biezen A, Hertenstein B, et al. Prophylaxis and treatment of GVHD after allogeneic haematopoietic SCT: a survey of centre strategies by the European Group for Blood and Marrow Transplantation. Bone Marrow Transplant 2012;47(11):1459–64.
64. Mielcarek M, Boeckh M, Martin PJ. Effectiveness and safety of lower dose prednisone for initial treatment of acute graft-*versus*-host disease: a randomized controlled trial. Haematologica 2015;100(6):842–8.
65. Chen X, Wang C, Zhang Y, et al. Efficacy of mesenchymal stem cell therapy for steroid-refractory acute graft-*versus*-host disease following allogeneic hematopoietic stem cell transplantation: a systematic review and meta-analysis. PloS One 2015;10(8):e0136991.
66. Kitko CL, Levine JE. Extracorporeal photopheresis in prevention and treatment of acute GVHD. Transfus Apher Sci 2015;52(2):151–6.
67. Flowers ME, Martin PJ. How we treat chronic graft-versus-host disease. Blood 2015;125:606–15.
68. Martin PJ, Inamoto Y, Carpenter PA, et al. Treatment of chronic graft-versus-host disease: past, present and future. Korean J Hematol 2011;46(3):153–63.
69. Wolff D, Schleuning M, von Harsdorf S, et al. Consensus conference on clinical practice in chronic GVHD: second-line treatment of chronic graft-versus-host disease. Biol Blood Marrow Transplant 2011;17(1):1–17.
70. Flowers MED, Deeg HJ. Chronic graft-versus-host disease. In: Treleaven J, Barrett AJ, editors. Hematopoietic stem cell transplantation in clinical practice. Edinburgh (United Kingdom): Elsevier Ltd; 2009. p. 401–7.
71. Young JH. Infectious complications of acute and chronic GVHD. Best Pract Res Clin Haematol 2008;21(2):343–56.

72. Boeckh M, Nichols WG. The impact of cytomegalovirus serostatus of donor and recipient before hematopoietic stem cell transplantation in the era of antiviral prophylaxis and preemptive therapy. Blood 2004;103:2003–8.

73. Emanuel D, Cunningham I, Jules-Elysee K. Cytomegalovirus pneumonia after bone marrow transplantation successfully treated with the combination of ganciclovir and high-dose intravenous immunoglobulin. Ann Intern Med 1988;109: 777–82.

74. Bogunia-Kubik K, Mlynarczewska A, Jaskula E, et al. The presence of IFNG 3/3 genotype in the recipient associates with increased risk for Epstein-Barr virus reactivation after allogeneic haematopoietic stem cell transplantation. Br J Haematol 2006;132:326–32.

75. Wald A, Leisenring W, van Burik JA, et al. Epidemiology of Aspergillus infections in a large cohort of patients undergoing bone marrow transplantation. J Infect Dis 1997;175:1459–66.

76. Cornely OA, Maertens J, Winston DJ, et al. Posaconazole vs. fluconazole or itraconazole prophylaxis in patients with neutropenia. N Engl J Med 2007;356: 348–59.

77. Ullmann AJ, Lipton JH, Vesole DH, et al. Posaconazole or fluconazole for prophylaxis in severe graft-versus-host disease. N Engl J Med 2007;356:335–47.

78. Wingard J, Carter S, Walsh T, et al. Results of a randomized, double-blind trial of fluconazole vs. voriconazole for the prevention of invasive fungal infections in 600 allogeneic blood and marrow transplant patients. Blood 2007;11 [abstract: 163].

79. Herbrecht R, Denning DW, Patterson TF, et al. Voriconazole versus amphotericin B for primary therapy of invasive aspergillosis. N Engl J Med 2002;347:408–15.

80. van Burik JA, Hare RS, Solomon HF, et al. Posaconazole is effective as salvage therapy in zygomycosis: a retrospective summary of 91 cases. Clin Infect Dis 2006;42:e61–5.

81. Greenberg RN, Mullane K, van Burik JA, et al. Posaconazole as salvage therapy for zygomycosis. Antimicrob Agents Chemother 2006;50:126–33.

82. Gamis AS, Gudnason T, Giebink GS, et al. Disseminated infection with Fusarium in recipients of bone marrow transplants. Rev Infect Dis 1991;13:1077–88.

83. Boutati EI, Anaissie EJ. Fusarium, a significant emerging pathogen in patients with hematologic malignancy: ten years' experience at a cancer center and implications for management. Blood 1997;90:999–1008.

84. Prins C, Chavaz P, Tamm K, et al. Ecthyma gangrenosum-like lesions: a sign of disseminated Fusarium infection in the neutropenic patient. Clin Exp Dermatol 1995;20:428–30.

85. Sampathkumar P, Paya CV. Fusarium infection after solid-organ transplantation. Clin Infect Dis 2001;32:1237–40.

86. Baden LR, Katz JT, Fishman JA, et al. Salvage therapy with voriconazole for invasive fungal infections in patients failing or intolerant to standard antifungal therapy. Transplantation 2003;76:1632–7.

87. Tomblyn M, Young JA, Boeckh MJ, et al, Center for International Blood and Marrow Research; National Marrow Donor program; European Blood and Marrow Transplant Group; American Society of Blood and Marrow Transplantation; Canadian Blood and Marrow Transplant Group; Infectious Diseases Society of America; Society for Healthcare Epidemiology of America; Association of Medical Microbiology and Infectious Disease Canada; Centers for Disease Control and Prevention. Guidelines for preventing infectious complications

among hematopoietic cell transplantation recipients: a global perspective. Biol Blood Marrow Transplant 2009;15(10):1143–238.

88. Lunde LE, Dasaraju S, Cao Q, et al. Hemorrhagic cystitis after allogeneic hematopoietic cell transplantation: risk factors, graft source and survival. Bone Marrow Transplant 2015;50(11):1432–7.

89. Silva Lde P, Patah PA, Saliba RM, et al. Hemorrhagic cystitis after allogeneic hematopoietic stem cell transplants is the complex result of BK virus infection, preparative regimen intensity and donor type. Haematologica 2010;95(7):1183–90.

90. Ilhan O, Koç H, Akan H, et al. Hemorrhagic cystitis as a complication of bone marrow transplantation. J Chemother 1997;9(1):56–61.

91. Cesaro S, Brugiolo A, Faraci M, et al. Incidence and treatment of hemorrhagic cystitis in children given hematopoietic stem cell transplantation: a survey from the Italian association of pediatric hematology oncology-bone marrow transplantation group. Bone Marrow Transplant 2003;32(9):925–31.

92. Mori Y, Miyamoto T, Kamezaki K, et al. Low incidence of adenovirus hemorrhagic cystitis following autologous hematopoietic stem cell transplantation in the rituximab era. Am J Hematol 2012;87(8):828–30.

93. Fioriti D, Degener AM, Mischitelli M, et al. BKV infection and hemorrhagic cystitis after allogeneic bone marrow transplant. Int J Immunopathol Pharmacol 2005; 18(2):309–16.

94. Mori T, Aisa Y, Shimizu T, et al. Hemorrhagic cystitis caused by adenovirus type 34 after allogeneic bone marrow transplantation. Transplantation 2005;79(5): 624.

95. van Aalderen MC, Heutinck KM, Huisman C, et al. BK virus infection in transplant recipients: clinical manifestations, treatment options and the immune response. Neth J Med 2012;70(4):172–83.

96. Bogdanovic G, Priftakis P, Giraud G, et al. Association between a high BK virus load in urine samples of patients with graft-versus-host disease and development of hemorrhagic cystitis after hematopoietic stem cell transplantation. J Clin Microbiol 2004;42(11):5394–6.

97. Dropulic LK, Jones RJ. Polyomavirus BK infection in blood and marrow transplant recipients. Bone Marrow Transplant 2008;41(1):11–8.

98. Megged O, Stein J, Ben-Meir D, et al. BK-virus-associated hemorrhagic cystitis in children after hematopoietic stem cell transplantation. J Pediatr Hematol Oncol 2011;33(3):190–3.

99. Haines HL, Laskin BL, Goebel J, et al. Blood, and not urine, BK viral load predicts renal outcome in children with hemorrhagic cystitis following hematopoietic stem cell transplantation. Biol Blood Marrow Transplant 2011;17(10):1512–9.

100. Mori Y, Miyamoto T, Kato K, et al. Different risk factors related to adenovirus- or BK virus-associated hemorrhagic cystitis following allogeneic stem cell transplantation. Biol Blood Marrow Transplant 2012;18(3):458–65.

101. El-Zimaity M, Saliba R, Chan K, et al. Hemorrhagic cystitis after allogeneic hematopoietic stem cell transplantation: donor type matters. Blood 2004; 103(12):4674–80.

102. Giraud G, Bogdanovic G, Priftakis P, et al. The incidence of hemorrhagic cystitis and BK-viruria in allogeneic hematopoietic stem cell recipients according to intensity of the conditioning regimen. Haematologica 2006;91(3):401–4.

103. Uhm J, Hamad N, Michelis FV, et al. The risk of polyomavirus BK-associated hemorrhagic cystitis after allogeneic hematopoietic SCT is associated with myeloablative conditioning, CMV viremia and severe acute GVHD. Bone Marrow Transplant 2014;49(12):1528–34.

104. Gorczynska E, Turkiewicz D, Rybka K, et al. Incidence, clinical outcome, and management of virus-induced hemorrhagic cystitis in children and adolescents after allogeneic hematopoietic cell transplantation. Biol Blood Marrow Transplant 2005;11(10):797–804.

105. Seber A, Shu XO, Defor T, et al. Risk factors for severe hemorrhagic cystitis following BMT. Bone Marrow Transplant 1999;23(1):35–40.

106. Sencer SF, Haake RJ, Weisdorf DJ. Hemorrhagic cystitis after bone-marrow transplantation. Risk-factors and complications. Transplantation 1993;56(4): 875–9.

107. Arai Y, Maeda T, Sugiura H, et al. Risk factors for and prognosis of hemorrhagic cystitis after allogeneic stem cell transplantation: retrospective analysis in a single institution. Hematology 2012;17(4):207–14.

108. Kopterides P, Theodorakopoulou M, Mentzelopoulos S, et al. Cyclophosphamide-induced hemorrhagic cystitis successfully treated with conjugated estrogens. Am J Hematol 2005;80(2):166–7.

109. Walker RD. Cyclophosphamide induced hemorrhagic cystitis. J Urol 1999; 161(6):1747.

110. Russell SJ, Vowels MR, Vale T. Haemorrhagic cystitis in paediatric bone marrow transplant patients: an association with infective agents, GVHD and prior cyclophosphamide. Bone Marrow Transplant 1994;13(5):533–9.

111. Ayas M, Siddiqui K, Al-Jefri A, et al. Factors affecting the outcome of related allogeneic hematopoietic cell transplantation in patients with Fanconi anemia. Biol Blood Marrow Transplant 2014;20(10):1599–603.

112. Alesawi AM, El-Hakim A, Zorn KC, et al. Radiation-induced hemorrhagic cystitis. Curr Opin Support Palliat Care 2014;8(3):235–40.

113. Hale GA, Rochester RJ, Heslop HE, et al. Hemorrhagic cystitis after allogeneic bone marrow transplantation in children: clinical characteristics and outcome. Biol Blood Marrow Transplant 2003;9(11):698–705.

114. Gilis L, Morisset S, Billaud G, et al. High burden of BK virus-associated hemorrhagic cystitis in patients undergoing allogeneic hematopoietic stem cell transplantation. Bone Marrow Transplant 2014;49(5):664–70.

115. Meisenberg B, Lassiter M, Hussein A, et al. Prevention of hemorrhagic cystitis after high-dose alkylating agent chemotherapy and autologous bone marrow support. Bone Marrow Transplant 1994;14(2):287–91.

116. Droller MJ, Saral R, Santos G. Prevention of cyclophosphamide-induced hemorrhagic cystitis. Urology 1982;20(3):256–8.

117. Gurman G, Atilla E, Ozen M, et al. Management of hemorrhagic cystitis after allogeneic hematopoietic stem cell transplantation. Biol Blood Marrow Transplant 2014;20(2):S194–5.

118. Foster J, Cheng WS, Leung K, et al. Intravesicular cidofovir for BK hemorrhagic cystitis in pediatric patients after hematopoietic stem cell transplant. Biol Blood Marrow Transplant 2016;22(3):S163–4.

119. Coomes EA, Wolfe Jacques A, Michelis FV, et al. Efficacy of cidofovir in treatment of BK virus–induced hemorrhagic cystitis in allogeneic hematopoietic cell transplant recipients. Biol Blood Marrow Transplant 2018;24(9):1901–5.

120. Yoshimura T, Nishimoto M, Nakamae H, et al. Cidofovir treatment for adenovirus-associated hemorrhagic cystitis in adult recipients of allogeneic hematopoietic stem cell transplantation: a retrospective comparative study. Biol Blood Marrow Transplant 2017;23(3):S202.

121. Degener S, Pohle A, Strelow H, et al. Long-term experience of hyperbaric oxygen therapy for refractory radio- or chemotherapy-induced haemorrhagic cystitis. BMC Urol 2015;15:38.

122. Coppell JA, Richardson PG, Soiffer R, et al. Hepatic veno-occlusive disease following stem cell transplantation: incidence, clinical course, and outcome. Biol Blood Marrow Transplant 2010;16(2):157–68.

123. Zeniya M, Fukata H, Toda G. Thrombomodulin expression of sinusoidal endothelial cells in chronic viral hepatitis. J Gastroenterol Hepatol 1995;10(S1):S77–80.

124. Scoazec JY, Feldmann G. In situ immunophenotyping study of endothelial cells of the human hepatic sinusoid: results and functional implications. Hepatology 1991;14(5):789–97.

125. Volpes R, Van Den Oord JJ, Desmet VJ. Distribution of the VLA family of integrins in normal and pathological human liver tissue. Gastroenterology 1991; 101(1):200–6.

126. McKoy JM, Angelotta C, Bennett CL, et al. Gemtuzumab ozogamicin-associated sinusoidal obstructive syndrome (SOS): an overview from the research on adverse drug events and reports (RADAR) project. Leuk Res 2007;31(5):599–604.

127. Wadleigh M, Richardson PG, Zahrieh D, et al. Prior gemtuzumab ozogamicin exposure significantly increases the risk of veno-occlusive disease in patients who undergo myeloablative allogeneic stem cell transplantation. Blood 2003; 102(5):1578–82.

128. Kebriaei P, Wilhelm K, Ravandi F, et al. Feasibility of allografting in patients with advanced acute lymphoblastic leukemia after salvage therapy with inotuzumab ozogamicin. Clin Lymphoma Myeloma Leuk 2013;13(3):296–301.

129. Willemart S, Nicaise N, Struyven J, et al. Acute radiation-induced hepatic injury: evaluation by triphasic contrast enhanced helical CT. Br J Radiol 2000;73(869): 544–6.

130. Sempoux C, Horsmans Y, Geubel A, et al. Severe radiation-induced liver disease following localized radiation therapy for biliopancreatic carcinoma: activation of hepatic stellate cells as an early event. Hepatology 1997;26(1):128–34.

131. Sangro B, Gil-Alzugaray B, Rodriguez J, et al. Liver disease induced by radioembolization of liver tumors: description and possible risk factors. Cancer 2008; 112:1538–46.

132. Brown AC. Liver toxicity related to herbs and dietary supplements: online table of case reports. Part 2 of 5 series. Food Chem Toxicol 2017;107(Pt A):472–501.

133. Sebagh M, Debette M, Samuel D, et al. "Silent" presentation of veno-occlusive disease after liver transplantation as part of the process of cellular rejection with endothelial predilection. Hepatology 1999;30(5):1144–50.

134. Nakazawa Y, Chisuwa H, Mita A, et al. Life-threatening veno-occlusive disease after living-related liver transplantation. Transplantation 2003;75(5):727–30.

135. Mohty M, Malard F, Abecassis M, et al. Sinusoidal obstruction syndrome/veno-occlusive disease: current situation and perspectives—a position statement from the European Society for Blood and Marrow Transplantation (EBMT). Bone Marrow Transplant 2015;50(6):781–9.

136. Roeker LE, Kim HT, Glotzbecker B, et al. Early clinical predictors of hepatic veno-occlusive disease/sinusoidal obstruction syndrome after myeloablative stem cell transplantation. Biol Blood Marrow Transplant 2019. https://doi.org/10.1016/j.bbmt.2018.07.039.

137. McDonald GB, Sharma P, Matthews DE, et al. Venocclusive disease of the liver after bone marrow transplantation: diagnosis, incidence, and predisposing factors. Hepatology 1984;4(1):116–22.

138. McDonald GB, Hinds MS, Fisher LD, et al. Veno-occlusive disease of the liver and multiorgan failure after bone marrow transplantation: a cohort study of 355 patients. Ann Intern Med 1993;118(4):255–67.

139. Jones RJ, Lee KS, Beschorner WE, et al. Venoocclusive disease of the liver following bone marrow transplantation. Transplantation 1987;44(6):778–83.

140. Ozyilmaz E, Aydogdu M, Sucak G, et al. Risk factors for fungal pulmonary infections in hematopoietic stem cell transplantation recipients: the role of iron overload. Bone Marrow Transplant 2010;45(10):1528–33.

141. Rosetti F, Schoch HG, Fisher L, et al. Fungal liver infection in marrow transplant recipients: prevalence at autopsy, predisposing factors, and clinical features. Clin Infect Dis 1995;20:801–11.

142. Dignan FL, Wynn RF, Hadzic N, et al, Haemato-oncology Task Force of British Committee for Standards in Haematology, British Society for Blood and Marrow Transplantation. BCSH/BSBMT guideline: diagnosis and management of veno-occlusive disease (sinusoidal obstruction syndrome) following haematopoietic stem cell transplantation. Br J Haematol 2013;163(4):444–57.

143. Carreras E, Grañena A, Navasa M, et al. On the reliability of clinical criteria for the diagnosis of hepatic veno-occlusive disease. Ann Hematol 1993;66(2): 77–80.

144. Imran H, Tleyjeh IM, Zirakzadeh A, et al. Use of prophylactic anticoagulation and the risk of hepatic veno-occlusive disease in patients undergoing hematopoietic stem cell transplantation: a systematic review and meta-analysis. Bone Marrow Transplant 2006;37(7):677–86.

145. Ruutu T, Eriksson B, Remes K, et al, Nordic Bone Marrow Transplantation Group. Ursodeoxycholic acid for the prevention of hepatic complications in allogeneic stem cell transplantation. Blood 2002;100(6):1977–83.

146. Carreras E. Review How I manage sinusoidal obstruction syndrome after haematopoietic cell transplantation. Br J Haematol 2015;168(4):481–91.

147. Azoulay D, Castaing D, Lemoine A, et al. Transjugular intrahepatic portosystemic shunt (TIPS) for severe veno-occlusive disease of the liver following bone marrow transplantation. Bone Marrow Transplant 2000;25(9):987–92.

148. Kim ID, Egawa H, Marui Y, et al. A successful liver transplantation for refractory hepatic veno-occlusive disease originating from cord blood transplantation. Am J Transplant 2002;2(8):796–800.

149. Richardson PG, Corbacioglu S, Ho VT, et al. Drug safety evaluation of defibrotide. Expert Opin Drug Saf 2013;12(1):123–36.

150. Richardson PG, Soiffer RJ, Antin JH, et al. Defibrotide for the treatment of severe hepatic veno-occlusive disease and multiorgan failure after stem cell transplantation: a multicenter, randomized, dose-finding trial. Biol Blood Marrow Transplant 2010;16(7):1005–17.

151. Richardson P, et al. Results of a Phase 3 study utilizing a historical control. Defibrotide (DF) in the treatment of severe hepatic veno-occlusive disease (VOD) with multi-organ failure (MOF) following stem cell transplantation (SCT) ASH Annual Meeting Abstracts. 2009;114:654.

152. Richardson PG, et al. Results of the large prospective study on the use of defibrotide (DF) in the treatment of hepatic veno-occlusive disease (VOD) in hematopoietic stem cell transplant (HSCT). Early intervention improves

outcome – updated results of a treatment IND (T-IND) expanded access protocol. ASH Annual Meeting Abstracts. 2013;122:700.

153. Ustun C, Weisdorf D. Non-infectious complications after bone marrow transplant: liver complications. Cancer Therapy Advisor.

154. Armand P, Kim HT, Cutler CS, et al. Prognostic impact of elevated pretransplantation serum ferritin in patients undergoing myeloablative stem cell transplantation. Blood 2007;109(10):4586–8.

155. Sucak GT, Yegin ZA, Ozkurt ZN, et al. Iron overload: predictor of adverse outcome in hematopoietic stem cell transplantation. Transplant Proc 2010;42: 1841–8.

156. Morado M, Ojeda E, Garcia-Bustos J, et al. BMT: Serum Ferritin as Risk Factor for Veno-occlusive Disease of the Liver. Prospective Cohort Study. Hematology 2000;4:505–12.

157. Maradei SC, Maiolino A, de Azevedo AM, et al. Serum ferritin as risk factor for sinusoidal obstruction syndrome of the liver in patients undergoing hematopoietic stem cell transplantation. Blood 2009;114:1270–5.

158. Lee SH, Yoo KH, Sung KW, et al. Hepatic veno-occlusive disease in children after hematopoietic stem cell transplantation: incidence, risk factors, and outcome. Bone Marrow Transplant 2010;45(8):1287–93.

159. Alessandrino EP, Della Porta MG, Bacigalupo A, et al. Prognostic impact of pretransplantation transfusion history and secondary iron overload in patients with myelodysplastic syndrome undergoing allogeneic stem cell transplantation: a GITMO study. Haematologica 2010;95:476–84.

160. Platzbecker U, Bornhauser M, Germing U, et al. Red blood cell transfusion dependence and outcome after allogeneic peripheral blood stem cell transplantation in patients with de novo myelodysplastic syndrome (MDS). Biol Blood Marrow Transplant 2008;14:1217–25.

161. Pullarkat V, Blanchard S, Tegtmeier B, et al. Iron overload adversely affects outcome of allogeneic hematopoietic cell transplantation. Bone Marrow Transplant 2008;42:799–805.

162. Barba P, López Corral L, Sierra J, et al. Impact of hyperferritinemia on the outcome of reduced-intensity conditioning allogeneic hematopoietic cell transplantation for lymphoid malignancies. Biol Blood Marrow Transplant 2013; 19(4):597–601.

163. Mahindra A, Bolwell B, Sobecks R, et al. Elevated ferritin is associated with relapse after autologous hematopoietic stem cell transplantation for lymphoma. Biol Blood Marrow Transplant 2008;14(11):1239–44.

164. Nakamae M, Nakamae H, Koh S, et al. Prognostic value and clinical implication of serum ferritin levels following allogeneic hematopoietic cell transplantation. Acta Haematol 2015;133(3):310–6.

165. Kontoyiannis DP, Chamilos G, Lewis RE, et al. Increased bone marrow iron stores is an independent risk factor for invasive aspergillosis in patients with high-risk hematologic malignancies and recipients of allogeneic hematopoietic stem cell transplantation. Cancer 2007;110:1303–6.

166. Tachibana T, Tanaka M, Takasaki H, et al. Pretransplant serum ferritin is associated with bloodstream infections within 100 days of allogeneic stem cell transplantation for myeloid malignancies. Int J Hematol 2011;93:368–74.

167. Altes A, Remacha AF, Sureda A, et al. Iron overload might increase transplant-related mortality in haematopoietic stem cell transplantation. Bone Marrow Transplant 2002;29:987–9.

168. Kataoka K, Nannya Y, Hangaishi A, et al. Influence of pretransplantation serum ferritin on nonrelapse mortality after myeloablative and nonmyeloablative allogeneic hematopoietic stem cell transplantation. Biol Blood Marrow Transplant 2009;15:195–204.
169. Lee JW, Kang HJ, Kim EK, et al. Effect of iron overload and iron-chelating therapy on allogeneic hematopoietic SCT in children. Bone Marrow Transplant 2009; 44:793–7.
170. Mahindra A, Bolwell B, Sobecks R, et al. Elevated pretransplant ferritin is associated with a lower incidence of chronic graft-versus-host disease and inferior survival after myeloablative allogeneic haematopoietic stem cell transplantation. Br J Haematol 2009;146:310–6.
171. Storey JA, Connor RF, Lewis ZT, et al. The transplant iron score as a predictor of stem cell transplant survival. J Hematol Oncol 2009;2:44.
172. Kim YR, Kim JS, Cheong JW, et al. Transfusion-associated iron overload as an adverse risk factor for transplantation outcome in patients undergoing reduced-intensity stem cell transplantation for myeloid malignancies. Acta Haematol 2008;120:182–9.
173. Lim ZY, Fiaccadori V, Gandhi S, et al. Impact of pre-transplant serum ferritin on outcomes of patients with myelodysplastic syndromes or secondary acute myeloid leukaemia receiving reduced intensity conditioning allogeneic haematopoietic stem cell transplantation. Leuk Res 2009;34:723–7.
174. Chow JK, Werner BG, Ruthazer R, et al. Increased serum iron levels and infectious complications after liver transplantation. Clin Infect Dis 2010;51:e16–23.
175. Bazuave GN, Buser A, Gerull S, et al. Prognostic impact of iron parameters in patients undergoing allo-SCT. Bone Marrow Transplant 2012;47(1):60–4.
176. Majhail NS, Parks K, Defor TE, et al. Diffuse alveolar hemorrhage (DAH) is a noninfectious pulmonary complication of hematopoietic stem cell transplantation (HSCT) with unclear pathogenesis and treatment. Biol Blood Marrow Transplant 2006;12(10):1038–46.
177. Keklik F, Alrawi EB, Cao Q, et al. Diffuse alveolar hemorrhage is most often fatal and is affected by graft source, conditioning regiment toxicity, and engraftment kinetics. Haematologica 2018;103(12):2109–15.
178. Specks U. Diffuse alveolar hemorrhage syndromes. Curr Opin Rheumatol 2001; 13:12–7.
179. Yen KT, Lee AS, Krowka MJ, et al. Pulmonary complications in bone marrow transplantation: a practical approach to diagnosis and treatment. Clin Chest Med 2004;25(1):189–201.
180. Afessa B, Tefferi A, Litzow MR, et al. Diffuse alveolar hemorrhage in hematopoietic stem cell transplant recipients. Am J Respir Crit Care Med 2002;166(5): 641–5.
181. Lewis I, DeFor T, Weisdorf D. Increasing incidence of diffuse alveolar hemorrhage following allogeneic bone marrow transplantation: cryptic etiology and uncertain therapy. Bone Marrow Transplant 2000;26(5):539–43.
182. Weisdorf DJ. Diffuse alveolar hemorrhage: an evolving problem? Leukemia 2003;17:1049–50.
183. Metcalf JP, Rennard SI, Reed EC, et al. Corticosteroids as adjunctive therapy for diffuse alveolar hemorrhage associated with bone marrow transplantation. University of Nebraska Medical Center Bone Marrow Transplant Group. Am J Med 1994;96(4):327–34.
184. Robbins RA, Linder J, Stahl MG, et al. Diffuse alveolar hemorrhage in autologous bone marrow transplant recipients. Am J Med 1989;87:511–8.

185. Ho VT, Weller E, Lee SJ, et al. Prognostic factors for early severe pulmonary complications after hematopoietic stem cell transplantation. Biol Blood Marrow Transplant 2001;7(4):223–9.

186. Wojno KJ, Vogelsang GB, Bescnorner WE, et al. Pulmonary hemorrhage as a cause of death in allogeneic bone marrow recipients with severe acute graft-versus-host disease. Transplantation 1994;57(1):88–92.

187. Chao NJ, Duncan SR, Long GD, et al. Corticosteroid therapy for diffuse alveolar hemorrhage in autologous bone marrow transplant recipients. Ann Intern Med 1991;114(2):145–6.

188. Raptis A, Mavroudis D, Suffredini A, et al. High-dose corticosteroid therapy for diffuse alveolar hemorrhage in allogeneic bone marrow stem cell transplant recipients. Bone Marrow Transplant 1999;24(8):879–83.

189. Gaziev J, Marziali S, Paciaroni K, et al. Posterior reversible encephalopathy syndrome after hematopoietic cell transplantation in children with hemoglobinopathies. Biol Blood Marrow Transplant 2017;23(9):1531–40.

190. Mishaw K, de Lima M, Giralt S, et al. Be impressed with PRES. Biol Blood Marrow Transplant 2004;(suppl 1):94.

191. Hinchey J, Caplan LR. A reversible posterior leukoencephalopathy syndrome Reply. N Eng J Med 1996;334:1746.

192. Stott VL, Hurrell MA, Anderson TJ. Reversible posterior leukoencephalopathy syndrome: a misnomer reviewed. Intern Med J 2005;35(2):83–90.

193. Wu Q, Marescaux C, Wolff V, et al. Tacrolimus-associated posterior reversible encephalopathy syndrome after solid organ transplantation. Eur Neurol 2010;64(3):169–77.

194. Yamauchi A, Ieiri I, Kataoka Y, et al. Neurotoxicity induced by tacrolimus after liver transplantation: Relation to genetic polymorphisms of the ABCB1 (MDR1) gene. Transplantation 2002;74(4):571–2.

195. Yanagimachi M, Naruto T, Tanoshima R, et al. Influence of CYP3A5 and ABCB1 gene polymorphisms on calcineurin inhibitor-related neurotoxicity after hematopoietic stem cell transplantation. Clin Transplant 2010;24(6):855–61.

196. Wong R, Beguelin GZ, de Lima M, et al. Tacrolimus-associated posterior reversible encephalopathy syndrome after allogeneic haematopoietic stem cell transplantation. Br J Haematol 2003;122(1):128–34.

197. Misawa A, Takeuchi Y, Hibi S, et al. FK506-induced intractable leukoencephalopathy following allogeneic bone marrow transplantation. Bone Marrow Transplant 2000;25(3):331–4.

198. Kanekiyo T, Hara J, Matsuda-Hashii Y, et al. Tacrolimus-related encephalopathy following allogeneic stem cell transplantation in children. Int J Hematol 2005;81(3):264–8.

199. Tam CS, Galanos J, Seymour JF, et al. Reversible posterior leukoencephalopathy syndrome complicating cytotoxic chemotherapy for hematologic malignancies. Am J Hematol 2004;77(1):72–6.

200. Oliverio PJ, Restrepo L, Mitchell SA, et al. Reversible tacrolimus-induced neurotoxicity isolated to the brain stem. AJNR Am J Neuroradiol 2000;21:1251–4.

201. Beitinjaneh A, McKinney AM, Cao Q, et al. Toxic leukoencephalopathy following fludarabine-associated hematopoietic cell transplantation. Biol Blood Marrow Transplant 2011;17(3):300–8.

202. Naesens M, Kuypers DR, Sarwal M. Calcineurin inhibitor nephrotoxicity. Clin J Am Soc Nephrol 2009;4:481–508.

203. Bartynski WS. Cerebral adenovirus endotelitis as PRES was reported in patient. AJNR Am J Neuroradiol 2006;27(10):2179–90.

204. Steg RE, Kessinger A, Wszolek ZK. Cortical blindness and seizures in a patient receiving FK506 after bone marrow transplantation. Bone Marrow Transplant 1999;23(9):959–62.

205. Moskowitz A, Nolan C, Lis E, et al. Posterior reversible encephalo syndrome due to sirolimus. Bone Marrow Transplant 2007;39:653–4.

206. Cutler C, Antin JH. Sirolimus immunosuppression f or graft-versus-host disease prophylaxis and therapy: an update. Curr Opin Hematol 2010;17:500–4.

207. Yoshihara S, Yanik G, Cooke KR, et al. Bronchiolitis obliterans syndrome (BOS), bronchiolitis obliterans organizing pneumonia (BOOP), and other late-onset noninfectious pulmonary complications following allogeneic hematopoietic stem cell transplantation. Biol Blood Marrow Transplant 2007;13(7):749–59.

208. Clark JG, Madtes DK, Martin TR, et al. Idiopathic pneumonia after bone marrow transplantation: cytokine activation and lipopolysaccharide amplification in the bronchoalveolar compartment. Crit Care Med 1999;27:1800–6.

209. Crawford SW, Hackman RC. Clinical course of idiopathic pneumonia after bone marrow transplantation. Am Rev Respir Dis 1993;147:1393–400.

210. Weiner RS, Bortin MM, Gale RP, et al. Interstitial pneumonitis after bone marrow transplantation (assessment of risk factors). Ann Intern Med 1986;104:168–75.

211. Quabeck K. The lung as a critical organ in marrow transplantation. Bone Marrow Transplant 1994;14:S19–28.

212. Crawford SW, Longton G, Storb R. Acute graft-versus-host disease and the risks for idiopathic pneumonia after marrow transplantation for severe aplastic anemia. Bone Marrow Transplant 1993;12:225–31.

213. Kantrow SP, Hackman RC, Boeckh M, et al. Idiopathic pneumonia syndrome: changing spectrum of lung injury after marrow transplantation. Transplantation 1997;63:1079–86.

214. Curtis DJ, Smale A, Thien F, et al. Chronic airflow obstruction in long-term survivors of allogeneic bone marrow transplantation. Bone Marrow Transplant 1995; 16:169–73.

215. Chan CK, Hyland RH, Hutcheon MA, et al. Small-airways disease in recipients of allogeneic bone marrow transplants (An analysis of 11 cases and a review of the literature). Medicine (Baltimore) 1987;66:327–40.

216. Clark JG, Crawford SW, Madtes DK, et al. Obstructive lung disease after allogeneic marrow transplantation (clinical presentation and course). Ann Intern Med 1989;111:368–76.

217. Worthy SA, Park CS, Kim JS, et al. Bronchiolitis obliterans after lung transplantation: high-resolution CT findings in 15 patients. AJR Am J Roentgenol 1997; 169:673–7.

218. Leung AN, Fisher K, Valentine V, et al. Bronchiolitis obliterans after lung transplantation: detection using expiratory HRCT. Chest 1998;113:365–70.

219. Bankier AA, Van Muylem A, Knoop C, et al. Bronchiolitis obliterans syndrome in heart-lung transplant recipients: diagnosis with expiratory CT. Radiology 2001; 218:533–9.

220. Siegel MJ, Bhalla S, Gutierrez FR, et al. Post-lung transplantation bronchiolitis obliterans syndrome: usefulness of expiratory thin-section CT for diagnosis. Radiology 2001;220:455–62.

221. St John RC, Gadek JE, Tutschka PJ, et al. Analysis of airflow obstruction by bronchoalveolar lavage following bone marrow transplantation (implications for pathogenesis and treatment). Chest 1990;98:600–7.

222. Ralph DD, Springmeyer SC, Sullivan KM, et al. Rapidly progressive air-flow obstruction in marrow transplant recipients (possible association between

obliterative bronchiolitis and chronic graft-versus-host disease). Am Rev Respir Dis 1984;129:641–4.

223. Clark JG, Schwartz DA, Flournoy N, et al. Risk factors for airflow obstruction in recipients of bone marrow transplants. Ann Intern Med 1987;107:648–56.

224. Crawford SW, Clark JG. Bronchiolitis associated with bone marrow transplantation. Clin Chest Med 1993;14:741–9.

225. Holland HK, Wingard JR, Beschorner WE, et al. Bronchiolitis obliterans in bone marrow transplantation and its relationship to chronic graft-v-host disease and low serum IgG. Blood 1988;72:621–7.

226. Schwarer AP, Hughes JM, Trotman-Dickenson B, et al. A chronic pulmonary syndrome associated with graft-versus-host disease after allogeneic marrow transplantation. Transplantation 1992;54:1002–8.

227. Chien JW, Martin PJ, Gooley TA, et al. Airflow obstruction after myeloablative allogeneic hematopoietic stem cell transplantation. Am J Respir Crit Care Med 2003;168:208–14.

228. Santo Tomas LH, Loberiza FR, Klein JP, et al. Risk factors for bronchiolitis obliterans in allogeneic hematopoietic stem-cell transplantation for leukemia. Chest 2005;128:153–61.

229. Yoshihara S, Tateishi U, Ando T, et al. Lower incidence of Bronchiolitis obliterans in allogeneic hematopoietic stem cell transplantation with reduced-intensity conditioning compared with myeloablative conditioning. Bone Marrow Transplant 2005;35:1195–200.

230. Versluys AB, Rossen JW, van Ewijk B, et al. Strong association between respiratory viral infection early after hematopoietic stem cell transplantation and the development of life-threatening acute and chronic alloimmune lung syndromes. Biol Blood Marrow Transplant 2010;16(6):782–91.

231. Au BK, Au MA, Chien JW. Bronchiolitis obliterans syndrome epidemiology after allogeneic hematopoietic cell transplantation. Biol Blood Marrow Transplant 2011;17(7):1072–8.

232. Ratjen F, Rjabko O, Kremens B. High-dose corticosteroid therapy for bronchiolitis obliterans after bone marrow transplantation in children. Bone Marrow Transplant 2005;36:135–8.

233. Iacono AT, Corcoran TE, Griffith BP, et al. Aerosol cyclosporin therapy in lung transplant recipients with bronchiolitis obliterans. Eur Respir J 2004;23:384–90.

234. Colom AJ, Teper AM, Vollmer WM, et al. Risk factors for the development of bronchiolitis obliterans in children with bronchiolitis. Thorax 2006;61:503–6.

235. Shah SK, McAnally KJ, Seoane L, et al. Analysis of pulmonary non-tuberculous mycobacterial infections after lung transplantation. Transpl Infect Dis 2016; 18(4):585–91.

236. Iacono AT, Johnson BA, Grgurich WF, et al. A randomized trial of inhaled cyclosporine in lung-transplant recipients. N Engl J Med 2006;354:141–50.

237. Gerhardt SG, McDyer JF, Girgis RE, et al. Maintenance azithromycin therapy for bronchiolitis obliterans syndrome: results of a pilot study. Am J Respir Crit Care Med 2003;168:121–5.

238. Verleden GM, Dupont LJ. Azithromycin therapy for patients with bronchiolitis obliterans syndrome after lung transplantation. Transplantation 2004;77:1465–7.

239. Khalid M, Al Saghir A, Saleemi S, et al. Azithromycin in bronchiolitis obliterans complicating bone marrow transplantation: a preliminary study. Eur Respir J 2005;25:490–3.

240. Verleden GM, Vanaudenaerde BM, Dupont LJ, et al. Azithromycin reduces airway neutrophilia and interleukin-8 in patients with bronchiolitis obliterans syndrome. Am J Respir Crit Care Med 2006;174:566–70.
241. Miyake N, Chong Y, Nishida R, et al. Mycobacterium abscessus and massiliense lung infection during macrolide treatment for bronchiolitis obliterans after allogeneic hematopoietic stem cell transplantation. J Infect Chemother 2018; 24(1):78–81.
242. Yanik G, Hellerstedt B, Custer J, et al. Etanercept (Enbrel) administration for idiopathic pneumonia syndrome after allogeneic hematopoietic stem cell transplantation. Biol Blood Marrow Transplant 2002;8:395–400.
243. Fullmer JJ, Fan LL, Dishop MK, et al. Successful treatment of bronchiolitis obliterans in a bone marrow transplant patient with tumor necrosis factor-alpha blockade. Pediatrics 2005;116:767–70.
244. Couriel DR, Hosing C, Saliba R, et al. Extracorporeal photochemotherapy for the treatment of steroid-resistant chronic GVHD. Blood 2006;107:3074–80.
245. Oyan B, Koc Y, Emri S, et al. Improvement of chronic pulmonary graft-vs-host disease manifesting as bronchiolitis obliterans organizing pneumonia following extracorporeal photopheresis. Med Oncol 2006;23:125–9.
246. Heath JA, Kurland G, Spray TL, et al. Lung transplantation after allogeneic marrow transplantation in pediatric patients: the Memorial Sloan-Kettering experience. Transplantation 2001;72:1986–90.
247. Cordier JF. Bronchiolitis obliterans organizing pneumonia. Semin Respir Crit Care Med 2000;21:135–46.
248. Freudenberger TD, Madtes DK, Curtis JR, et al. Association between acute and chronic graft-versus-host disease and bronchiolitis obliterans organizing pneumonia in recipients of hematopoietic stem cell transplants. Blood 2003;102: 3822–8.
249. Palmas A, Tefferi A, Myers JL, et al. Late-onset noninfectious pulmonary complications after allogeneic bone marrow transplantation. Br J Haematol 1998;100: 680–7.
250. Patriarca F, Skert C, Sperotto A, et al. Incidence, outcome, and risk factors of late-onset noninfectious pulmonary complications after unrelated donor stem cell transplantation. Bone Marrow Transplant 2004;33:751–8.
251. Ishii T, Manabe A, Ebihara Y, et al. Improvement in bronchiolitis obliterans organizing pneumonia in a child after allogeneic bone marrow transplantation by a combination of oral prednisolone and low dose erythromycin. Bone Marrow Transplant 2000;26:907–10.

Antimicrobial Prophylaxis and Preemptive Approaches for the Prevention of Infections in the Stem Cell Transplant Recipient, with Analogies to the Hematologic Malignancy Patient

Dionysios Neofytos, MD, MPH

KEYWORDS

- Hematopoietic cell transplantation • Neutropenia • Antibiotic prophylaxis
- Empirical treatment • Preemptive treatment • Antibiotics • Infectious complications

KEY POINTS

- Routine antibacterial prophylaxis with a *Pseudomonas*-acting fluoroquinolone is currently recommended by most expert guidelines during prolonged and profound neutropenia.
- Antifungal prophylaxis is routinely administered after allogeneic hematopoietic cell transplant (HCT), against (predominately) *Candida* species pre-engraftment and with mold-active azoles postengraftment, during graft-versus-host disease.
- Anti–herpes simplex/varicella-zoster virus (VZV) prophylaxis is routinely administered in all allogeneic HCT recipients. VZV-prophylaxis may be continued for as long as 1-year after allogeneic HCT.
- Prevention of cytomegalovirus (CMV) disease can include routine CMV prophylaxis or preemptive treatment based on CMV viral activity monitoring.
- Hepatitis B–positive and hepatitis C–positive individuals should not be excluded from donors and recipients of allogeneic HCT transplant.

INTRODUCTION
General Concepts

Infectious complications represent one of the most common causes of morbidity and mortality in allogeneic hematopoietic cell transplant (HCT) recipients. The effect of conditioning chemotherapy during the pre-engraftment period, namely neutropenia

Disclosure Statement: Dr D. Neofytos has served as a consultant for Gilead, MSD, Pfizer and Roche Diagnostics and has received research grants by MSD.
Division of Infectious Diseases, University Hospital of Geneva, Rue Gabrielle-Perret-Gentil 4, Geneva CH-1211, Switzerland
E-mail address: dionysios.neofytos@hcuge.ch

Infect Dis Clin N Am 33 (2019) 361–380
https://doi.org/10.1016/j.idc.2019.02.002
0891-5520/19/© 2019 Elsevier Inc. All rights reserved.

id.theclinics.com

and gastrointestinal tract (GIT) mucositis, is similar to that in patients treated with intensive chemotherapy regimens, including patients with hematologic malignancies and/or autologous HCT recipients. Hence, most of the recommendations discussed in this article for allogeneic HCT recipients during the pre-engraftment period also may apply to most patients treated with intensive chemotherapy regimens with anticipated neutropenia for greater than 7 days.[1–4] Definitions important for the understanding of this article are summarized in **Table 1**. Prophylactic and preemptive strategies may vary from consensus guidelines and among different institutions, based on HCT practices and local epidemiology.

Infection risk and timing after hematopoietic cell transplantation
Risk factors for infectious complications heavily depend on the timing after an allogeneic HCT. Historically, 3 at-risk periods have been identified: (1) pre-engraftment: starting with conditioning initiation until engraftment; (2) early postengraftment: until day (D) 100 post-HCT; and (3) late postengraftment: after D100 post-HCT (**Fig. 1**). Furthermore, the presence of central venous catheters (CVCs) represents another major risk factor for infectious complications.

Pre-engraftment period
The main risk factors for infectious complications pre-engraftment include GIT mucositis and neutropenia. Mucositis represents the disruption of the GIT mucosa, allowing for gut flora to translocate and cause bloodstream infections (BSIs) due to gram-positive cocci (eg, viridans-group *Streptococcus* species, and Enterococci), gram-negative bacilli (ie, *Enterobacteriaceae* and *Pseudomonas aeruginosa*), and *Candida* species. Chemotherapy-induced neutropenia, the second major risk factor for infections during pre-engraftment, is associated with viral reactivation (ie, herpes simplex virus [HSV], HSV- I and HSV-II, and varicella-zoster virus [VZV]) and invasive fungal infections (IFIs) due to molds, mainly *Aspergillus* species.[5,6]

Table 1
Definitions of basic terms used in this article

Term	Definition
Neutropenia	Absolute neutrophil count <500 cells/mm^3
Neutropenic fever	A single episode of fever $\geq$38.3°C or 2 episodes of fever $\geq$38.0°C during neutropenia
Engraftment	Absolute neutrophil count >500 cells/mm^3 for 3 consecutive days
Pre-engraftment period	Time between infusion of stem cells until Absolute neutrophil count >500 cells/mm^3
Early postengraftment period	Time between engraftment and day +100 post-transplant
Late postengraftment period	Time after day +100 of infusion of stem cells until (usually) 1 y post-transplant
Antibiotic prophylaxis	Prophylaxis administered to prevent an infectious complication
Empirical treatment	Administration of an antibiotic agent to empirically treat a suspected infection, based on clinical suspicion
Preemptive treatment	Administration of antibiotic therapy at the onset of an infectious complication, as suggested by an early positive screening test

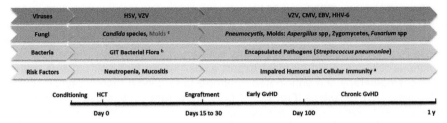

Fig. 1. Timing of risk factors and infectious complications in allogeneic HCT recipients, starting with conditioning until 1 year post-HCT. HCT, hematopoietic cell transplant. [a] Impaired humoral and cellular immunity may last for 6 months to 12 months. Diagnosis of GVHD in the early (acute) or late (chronic) postengraftment period and associated treatments may further delay cellular immune reconstitution. [b] GIT bacterial pathogens include, but are not limited to, the following: *S viridans* species, *Enterococcus* species, *Escherichia coli*, *Klebsiella* species, *Enterobacter* species, and *Pseudomonas aeruginosa*. [c] Molds are less commonly observed during pre-engraftment than postengraftment. Prolonged profound neutropenia pre-engraftment may be associated with more mold infections.[4–6] The most commonly identified molds include the following: *Aspergillus* species, Zygomycetes, *Fusarium* species, and *Scedosporium* species.

Early postengraftment period

Impaired cellular immunity due to acute graft-versus-host disease (GVHD) with associated treatments represents the major risk factor early postengraftment. Most common infections include viral infections (that is, VZV, cytomegalovirus [CMV], Epstein-Barr virus [EBV], and human herpes virus 6 [HHV-6]) and IFI, including *Pneumocystis jirovecii* and invasive mold infections (IMIs), with *Aspergillus* species the most commonly identified molds, followed by the Zygomycetes and *Fusarium* species.[5–7] Furthermore, acute GIT GVHD may lead to gut flora translocation.

Late postengraftment period

The main risk factor for infectious complications in the late postengraftment period is lack of adequate immune reconstitution, which may take between 6 months and 12 months. Furthermore, chronic GVHD and associated treatments further delay cellular immune reconstitution. Reactivation of viral infections (ie, CMV, EBV, and HHV-6) and IFI, including *P jirovecii* and IMI, represent the most frequently encountered infections during this stage. *Aspergillus* species remain the most commonly identified mold during this period as well, albeit the sum of other mold infections (due to the Zygomycetes, *Fusarium*, and *Scedosporium* species) are likely proportionally more frequent.[5–7] In addition, impaired humoral immunity increases the risk for infections due to encapsulated bacteria (ie, *Streptococcus pneumoniae*).

Antibacterial Prophylaxis

Antibacterial prophylaxis—pre-engraftment period

In a meta-analysis of more than 100 clinical trials of antibacterial prophylaxis during neutropenia, administration of fluoroquinolones was shown to significantly decrease infection-related mortality, febrile episodes, clinically and microbiologically documented infections, and BSI.[8] In a landmark clinical trial, 760 adult patients with cancer and chemotherapy-induced neutropenia were randomized to administration of levofloxacin and placebo.[9] Mortality and tolerability were similar in both groups, whereas patients in the levofloxacin arm were less likely to develop a microbiologically documented bacterial infection and BSI. In a recent meta-analysis of 2 randomized clinical trials and 12 observational studies performed between 2006 and 2014, primary antibacterial prophylaxis with a fluo-roquinolone was not associated with a survival benefit, although an association with lower rates of neutropenic fever and BSIs was demonstrated.[10] Based on these reports, administration of primary antibacterial prophylaxis with a fluoroqui-nolone is recommended by most expert guidelines for high-risk patients treated with chemotherapy and anticipated neutropenia for longer than 7 days, including allogeneic HCT recipients (**Fig. 2**).[1,3,4] Most transplant centers use a fluoroquino-lone with anti–*Pseudomonas aeruginosa* activity (ciprofloxacin or levofloxacin) for primary antibacterial prophylaxis. Levofloxacin has a broader antibacterial profile, to include gram-positive cocci, such as viridans-group *Streptococcus* species. Although breakthrough infections have been reported in patients who receive pro-phylaxis with fluoroquinolones, addition of an antibacterial agent (ie, amoxicillin or vancomycin) to a fluoroquinolone to improve gram-positive coverage is not recom-mended.[1] Antibacterial prophylaxis selection should be based on local epidemiology.[1,3,10]

Timing of antibacterial prophylaxis Timing of antibacterial prophylaxis initiation may vary, beginning anywhere from chemotherapy initiation to stem cell infusion to the first day of neutropenia, at different centers. A large meta-analysis of more than 100 clinical trials showed no difference in all-cause mortality when antibacterial prophylaxis was started at the time of chemotherapy initiation or with neutropenia.[8] Current guidelines suggest that initiation of antibacterial prophylaxis should be considered at the time of cell infusion and continued until neutropenia resolution or initiation of empirical broad-spectrum antibiotic therapy.[1,3]

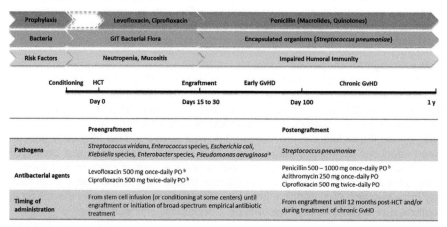

Fig. 2. Bacterial prophylaxis during the first year after an allogeneic hematopoietic cell transplant. PO, orally. [a] GIT bacterial pathogens include, but are not limited to, the listed pathogens. [b] Local epidemiology should be taken into account in terms of antibacterial pro-phylaxis agent selection. At centers where fluoroquinolones are routinely used for antibac-terial prophylaxis, regular monitoring of fluoroquinolone resistance should be applied. Local epidemiology of *Streptococcus pneumoniae* resistance patterns should be taken into account before selecting the appropriate prophylaxis. (*Data from* Tomblyn M, Chiller T, Einsele H, et al. Guidelines for preventing infectious complications among hematopoietic cell transplantation recipients: a global perspective. Biol Blood Marrow Transplant. 2009;15(10):1143–1238; and 2.2016 NGV. Prevention and treatment of Cancer-Related Infec-tions. National Comprehensive Cancer Network Clinical Practice Guidelines in Oncology (NCCN Guidelines) 2016; https://oralcancerfoundation.org/wp-content/uploads/2016/09/infections.pdf. Accessed September 30, 2018.)

Antibacterial resistance Concerns for increased rates of fluoroquinolone resistance have been raised with routine antibacterial prophylaxis with fluoroquinolones.[8] A recent prospective international study in allogeneic and autologous HCT recipients from 65 transplant centers in 25 countries identified fluoroquinolone prophylaxis as a significant risk factor for fluoroquinolone resistance.[11] Continuous vigilance and monitoring of resistance to fluoroquinolones is strongly advised for centers with routine use of these agents for antibacterial prophylaxis.[1,10]

Antibacterial prophylaxis—postengraftment period
Routine antibacterial prophylaxis against encapsulated bacterial pathogens, in particular *Streptococcus pneumoniae* is recommended until 1 year after HCT (see **Fig. 2**).[1,3] The selection of the appropriate agent depends on the local epidemiology and may include administration of penicillin, a macrolide, or a fluoroquinolone.[1,3] Gut flora translocation remains a major concern in patients with severe acute and/or chronic GIT GVHD. There are no formal recommendations as to the administration of antibacterial prophylaxis in such patients; however, some centers may select to initiate appropriate antibacterial prophylaxis in the setting.

Antifungal Prophylaxis

Antifungal prophylaxis—pre-engraftment
Fluconazole Fluconazole has been the mainstay of antifungal prophylaxis and is currently recommended as primary antifungal prophylaxis during the pre-engraftment period in allogeneic and autologous HCT recipients, based on a large number of data, ease of administration, predictable drug interactions, and a benign side-effect profile (**Fig. 3**).[1,3] In the pivotal prospective randomized clinical trials, administration of fluconazole prophylaxis was associated with significantly lower incidence of candidemia and improved overall survival in allogeneic (and autologous) HCT recipients.[12–14] In these clinical trials, fluconazole prophylaxis was started with or at the end of conditioning regimen and continued up to 75 days to 100 days post-transplant.[12–14] Administration of fluconazole for 75 days post-HCT has been associated with a lower incidence of GIT GVHD and a significant 8-year survival benefit compared with placebo.[13] Fluconazole has no activity against *C krusei* and molds, including *Aspergillus* species. Moreover, increasing resistance to fluconazole among *C glabrata* strains has been reported.[15] For patients at higher risk for IMI or colonized with fluconazole-resistant *Candida* species, alternative approaches, such as administration of mold-active azoles (discussed later) or echinocandins (discussed later) should be considered.[1]

Mold-active azoles Attempts to study itraconazole as a potential antifungal prophylactic agent failed, mainly due to poor tolerability, toxicities, and drug interactions.[16] Voriconazole was compared with fluconazole as antifungal prophylaxis in allogeneic transplant recipients between D0 and D100 post-HCT in a multicenter prospective randomized clinical trial.[17] Although there was a trend for fewer invasive aspergillosis (IA) infections in the voriconazole arm, there was no significant benefit in terms of fungal-free survival, IFI incidence, or empirical antifungal treatment.[17] Posaconazole and isavuconazole have not been studied as antifungal prophylaxis during the pre-engraftment period. Despite the lack of strong data, pre-engraftment antifungal prophylaxis with voriconazole or posaconazole is used in several transplant centers considering their extended spectrum of activity, particularly in patients at higher risk for mold infections, such as those with profound and prolonged neutropenia (eg, cord transplant recipients) or a diagnosis of an IMI prior to HCT.[1]

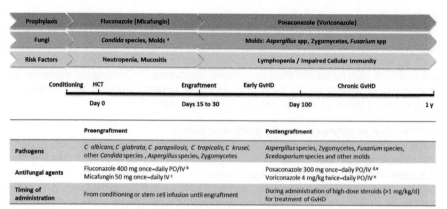

Fig. 3. Antifungal prophylaxis during the first year after an allogeneic hematopoietic cell transplant. IV, intravenously; PO, orally. [a] Molds are less commonly observed during pre-engraftment than postengraftment. Prolonged profound neutropenia pre-engraftment may be associated with more mold infections.[4–6] [b] Is occasionally used at certain institutions.[1] [c] Micafungin may be used in case of prolonged neutropenia and/or patients colonized with fluconazole-resistant *Candida* species. [d] Posaconazole is the only broad-spectrum azole validated for antifungal prophylaxis postengraftment.[18] Posaconazole delayed release tablets are preferred to posaconazole suspension for PO administration, due to better absorption. [e] Voriconazole and posaconazole prophylaxis may be used for pre-engraftment antifungal prophylaxis in patients at high risk for IMI or patients with a diagnosis of an IMI prior to HCT.[1] (*Data from* Tomblyn M, Chiller T, Einsele H, et al. Guidelines for preventing infectious complications among hematopoietic cell transplantation recipients: a global perspective. Biol Blood Marrow Transplant. 2009;15(10):1143–1238; and 2.2016 NGV. Prevention and treatment of Cancer-Related Infections. National Comprehensive Cancer Network Clinical Practice Guidelines in Oncology (NCCN Guidelines) 2016; https://oralcancerfoundation.org/wp-content/uploads/2016/09/infections.pdf. Accessed September 30, 2018)

Echinocandins Echinocandins have been considered for antifungal prophylaxis, based on their broad spectrum of activity, including fluconazole-resistant *Candida* species and *Aspergillus* species, benign side-effect profile and minimal drug interactions.[3,18] Micafungin was superior to fluconazole as antifungal prophylaxis during neutropenia in greater than 800 pediatric and adult HCT recipients in terms of absence of IFI by the end of antifungal prophylaxis and requirement for empirical antifungal therapy.[18] Although echinocandin use is limited due to requirement for IV administration and sometimes financial costs, micafungin prophylaxis may be considered in patients colonized with azole-resistant *Candida* species, during conditioning to avoid interactions between an azole and the administered chemotherapy, or in patients with abnormal liver function and/or at risk for QTc prolongation.[1,3]

Amphotericin B products Although variable doses of different amphotericin B formulations have been studied, prophylaxis with amphotericin B products is not currently recommended due to lack of beneficial outcomes and toxicity concerns.[1,19]

Antifungal prophylaxis—postengraftment
Current guidelines recommend posaconazole as antifungal prophylaxis in allogeneic HCT recipients with GVHD requiring treatment with high-dose (>1 mg/kg/d) corticosteroids.[1,3] This recommendation is based on the results of an international, double-blind clinical trial, where 600 allogeneic HCT recipients with GVHD were randomized

1:1 to posaconazole and fluconazole prophylaxis.[20] Posaconazole administration decreased the incidence of breakthrough IFI, IA, and IFI-related mortality but had no effect on overall survival.[20] In another study of patients with acute myeloid leukemia with prolonged neutropenia, administration of posaconazole versus fluconazole/itraconazole was associated with a lower incidence of proved and probable IFI and IA and improved overall survival.[21] These studies have led to the widespread use of posaconazole as antimold prophylaxis in high-risk patients. Multiple concerns have been raised on the generalizability of this approach, considering the (1) high numbers of patients that need to be treated, particularly at centers with low incidence of IA and IMI; (2) unnecessary exposure to potential drug-associated toxicities and interactions; (3) associated costs; and (4) antibiotic pressure for breakthrough IFI with resistant pathogens.[22] Ultimately, the selection of mold-active prophylaxis in high-risk allogeneic HCT recipients after engraftment remains a decision based on the interpretation of the existing body of literature, local epidemiology and economic considerations at each institution.

Pneumocystis jirovecii prophylaxis

Allogeneic HCT recipients should receive routine prophylaxis against *P jirovecii*.[1,3] Prophylaxis can be started at the time of transplantation or postengraftment and is continued for a minimum of 6 months to 12 months post-HCT.[1,3] A strong body of evidence supports the use of trimethoprim-sulfamethoxazole (TMP-SMX) as the preferred *Pneumocystis* prophylaxis, as a single-strength tablet once daily or a double-strength tablet 3 times weekly.[1,3] Due to potential myelosuppression, many centers do not initiate *Pneumocystis jirovecii* prophylaxis with TMP-SMX before engraftment.[1,3] A potentially additional benefit of TMP-SMX is its broad-spectrum of activity to include *Nocardia* and *Toxoplasma* species and common respiratory, urinary tract, and GIT pathogens. For patients allergic to TMP-SMX, desensitization should be strongly considered.[1,3] Alternatively, albeit inferior to TMP-SMX, options include administration of atovaquone, once-monthly aerosolized pentamidine, and dapsone. Administration of dapsone should be avoided in patients with severe allergy to TMP-SMX and deficient for glucose-6-phosphate dehydrogenase and aerosolized pentamidine has been associated with bronchospasm.

Antiviral Prophylaxis

Herpes simplex virus

Up to 60% to 80% of HSV-seropositive HCT recipients or patients with acute leukemia can reactivate HSV.[1,3] Anti-HSV prophylaxis with oral acyclovir or valacyclovir is recommended for HCT recipients and patients with acute leukemia (**Fig. 4**).[1,3] Valacyclovir is a valyl ester of acyclovir, with the same spectrum of activity but significantly higher (up to 50%–55%) bioavailability. In patients with severe mucositis and/or GIT GVHD who are not able to absorb oral medications, acyclovir can be administered intravenously. Although not approved for prophylaxis in allogeneic HCT recipients in the United States, valacyclovir is used frequently based on its half-life, allowing less frequent dosing, high bioavailability, and safety profile.[1,3] Antiviral prophylaxis should be initiated with chemotherapy or conditioning regimen initiation and continued until resolution of neutropenia.[1,3] For patients with frequent episodes of HSV reactivation or allogeneic HCT recipients with GVHD, longer courses of prophylaxis are recommended.[1,3]

Varicella-zoster virus

Up to 30% of VZV-seropositive HCT recipients may reactivate VZV, if antiviral prophylaxis is not administered.[23] Antiviral prophylaxis with oral acyclovir or valacyclovir

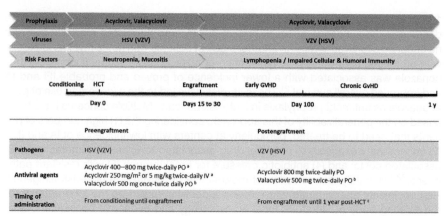

Prophylaxis	Acyclovir, Valacyclovir		Acyclovir, Valacyclovir	
Viruses	HSV (VZV)		VZV (HSV)	
Risk Factors	Neutropenia, Mucositis		Lymphopenia / Impaired Cellular & Humoral Immunity	

| Conditioning | HCT | Engraftment | Early GVHD | Chronic GvHD |
| | Day 0 | Days 15 to 30 | Day 100 | 1 y |

	Preengraftment	Postengraftment
Pathogens	HSV (VZV)	VZV (HSV)
Antiviral agents	Acyclovir 400–800 mg twice-daily PO ᵃ Acyclovir 250 mg/m² or 5 mg/kg twice-daily IV ᵃ Valacyclovir 500 mg once-twice daily PO ᵇ	Acyclovir 800 mg twice-daily PO Valacyclovir 500 mg twice-daily PO ᵇ
Timing of administration	From conditioning until engraftment	From engraftment until 1 year post-HCT ᶜ

Fig. 4. Antiherpetic prophylaxis during the first year after an allogeneic HCT. IV, intravenously; PO, orally. [a] Acyclovir pre-engraftment can be used either PO or IV, depending on the severity of mucositis and ability for oral intake. [b] Valacyclovir can be used instead of acyclovir, although it is not approved in the United States for prophylaxis in allogeneic HCT recipients. [c] Longer courses of prophylaxis should be considered in allogeneic HCT recipients with chronic GVHD requiring continued immunosuppressive treatments. (*Data from* Tomblyn M, Chiller T, Einsele H, et al. Guidelines for preventing infectious complications among hematopoietic cell transplantation recipients: a global perspective. Biol Blood Marrow Transplant. 2009;15(10):1143–1238; and 2.2016 NGV. Prevention and treatment of Cancer-Related Infections. National Comprehensive Cancer Network Clinical Practice Guidelines in Oncology (NCCN Guidelines) 2016; https://oralcancerfoundation.org/wp-content/uploads/2016/09/infections.pdf. Accessed September 30, 2018.)

should be administered in all VZV-seropositive HCT recipients, starting at the time of conditioning administration and until at least 1-year post-HCT (see **Fig. 4**).[1,3,23,24] Continuation of antiviral prophylaxis for 1 year post-HCT has been associated with significant reduction in VZV reactivation and overall mortality.[24] Recent data suggest that prolongation of prophylaxis, even beyond the first year post-HCT, may have a beneficial effect on VZV suppression, without preventing patients to develop protective VZV immunity.[23,24] Longer duration of anti-VZV prophylaxis should be considered in patients with continued immunosuppression, such as patients with chronic GVHD requiring treatment with high-dose corticosteroids.[1,3]

Cytomegalovirus

CMV infection is one of the most frequent complications after an allogeneic HCT, associated with significant morbidity and mortality.[25–28] CMV infection/reactivation is defined as the detection of the virus or viral particles in any body fluid or tissue.[29] CMV disease is defined as a viral syndrome and/or end-organ disease due to CMV.[29] CMV infection, as documented by a positive pp65 antigenemia and/or (almost exclusively today) with a CMV quantitative (q) polymerase chain reaction (PCR) assay, can develop into CMV disease if not treated.[25,26,28] Due to the devastating and complex consequences of CMV infection and disease in allogeneic HCT recipients, prevention of CMV infection has become standard in the management of these patients.[25–28]

CMV-seronegative recipients who receive a graft from CMV-seronegative donors have the lowest risk of developing CMV infection. It is strongly recommended that CMV-seronegative recipients receive grafts from CMV-seronegative donors and transfusions of CMV-seronegative and/or leukocyte-depleted blood products.[1]

CMV-seropositive recipients from a CMV-seronegative donor are at highest risk for CMV reactivation, followed by HCT recipients of CMV-seropositive donors.[28] CMV-seropositive recipients of cord blood grafts are at particularly high risk for CMV reactivation.[28] For CMV-seropositive HCT recipients and/or donors, there are 2 major approaches to prevent CMV disease: administration of primary anti-CMV prophylaxis and preemptive anti-CMV treatment (**Fig. 5**). There have been multiple clinical trials to evaluate the efficacy and safety of both approaches.[25,30–34] Current recommendations and pertinent data on both clinical approaches are discussed briefly.

Primary cytomegalovirus prophylaxis A large number of antivirals have been studied as primary CMV prophylaxis in allogeneic HCT recipients, including acyclovir, valacyclovir, ganciclovir, foscarnet, and valganciclovir.[25] Considering the associated

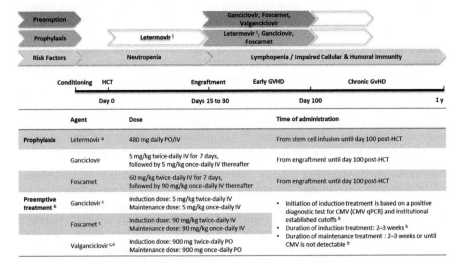

Fig. 5. CMV prophylaxis and preemptive treatment during the first year after an allogeneic HCT. IV, intravenously; PO, orally. [a] Letermovir was approved by the Food and Drug Administration for CMV prophylaxis in high-risk allogeneic HCT recipients, based on the results of a prospective randomized clinical trial.[28] It is not included in current US guidelines. It has been endorsed by the ECIL 2017 guidelines for CMV prophylaxis. Letermovir has no activity against HSV and VZV; hence, additional prophylaxis for these viruses is required. [b] Preemptive CMV treatment consists of regular monitoring of CMV reactivation with a CMV qPCR assay. Weekly CMV qPCR monitoring is recommended between the day of HCT or engraftment and until D100 post-HCT. More frequent monitoring should be applied in high-risk patients (recipients of umbilical cord blood or T-cell–depleted allografts) and continued beyond D100 in patients with GVHD requiring immunosuppressive treatment. There are no definitive CMV viral load cutoffs above which preemptive treatment should be started. Historically CMV PCR greater than 500 IU/mL to 1,000 IU/mL are used for preemptive treatment initiation. CMV viral load cutoffs to initiate preemptive therapy, duration of induction and maintenance treatment may vary across institutions. [c] Doses need to be adjusted based on renal function. [d] Valganciclovir can be used instead of intravenous ganciclovir if there are no concerns about absorption, particularly in patients with GVHD. (*Data from* Tomblyn M, Chiller T, Einsele H, et al. Guidelines for preventing infectious complications among hematopoietic cell transplantation recipients: a global perspective. Biol Blood Marrow Transplant. 2009;15(10):1143–1238; and 2.2016 NGV. Prevention and treatment of Cancer-Related Infections. National Comprehensive Cancer Network Clinical Practice Guidelines in Oncology (NCCN Guidelines) 2016; https://oralcancerfoundation.org/wp-content/uploads/2016/09/infections.pdf. Accessed September 30, 2018.)

toxicities and costs, CMV prophylaxis is predominately considered in high-risk patients, such as recipients of cord blood or T-cell–depleted grafts.[1] The concept of using high doses of acyclovir/valacyclovir for CMV suppression is used infrequently, due to the indirect activity/low efficacy of these agents against CMV. They may provide enough coverage of CMV, however, that several minor CMV blood viremia reactivations are blocked. The administration of CMV-active agents, such as ganciclovir/valganciclovir or foscarnet, for CMV prophylaxis has been hindered by several important associated drug-toxicities: cytopenias for ganciclovir/valganciclovir and nephrotoxicity for foscarnet. Recently, 3 new agents with activity against CMV and better side-effect profile have been considered for primary CMV prophylaxis in allogeneic HCT recipients, including letermovir, brincidofovir, and maribavir.[35–38] Although initially promising, clinical trial results have failed to show a benefit associated with brincidofovir and maribavir, due to dosing and toxicity issues.[36–38] More recently, letermovir for CMV prophylaxis during the first 100 days in adult CMV-seropositive allogeneic HCT recipients was compared with a placebo-based preemptive approach in a large prospective randomized multicenter phase-3 clinical trial.[35] By week 24, clinically significant CMV disease, defined as CMV disease and infection requiring initiation of CMV treatment, and mortality were significantly lower in the letermovir arm versus placebo. Letermovir has no activity against HSV and VZV; hence, additional antiherpetic prophylaxis is required. Based on the results of this study, the European Conference on Infections in Leukemia (ECIL) has endorsed letermovir for CMV prophylaxis in allogeneic HCT recipients.[39] US guidelines have not included letermovir as yet, because they were published before relevant data were available.

Preemptive cytomegalovirus therapy Due to potential drug toxicities and costs associated with universal primary CMV prophylaxis, most transplant centers today practice a preemptive approach for CMV prevention. Preemptive therapy with ganciclovir, valganciclovir, and foscarnet has been validated by several clinical trials.[30–34] A preemptive approach consists of regular monitoring of CMV reactivation with a CMV qPCR assay.[1,39] Weekly CMV qPCR monitoring is usually performed, starting on the day of engraftment and continued until D100 after HCT.[1,39] More frequent monitoring should be applied in high-risk patients, such as recipients of umbilical cord blood or T-cell–depleted allografts.[1,39] CMV qPCR monitoring should be continued beyond D100 in patients with GVHD requiring immunosuppressive treatment with corticosteroids.[1,39]

Cytomegalovirus threshold for preemptive treatment initiation There are no definitive CMV viral load cutoffs above which preemptive treatment should be started. At most centers, preemptive therapy is started when a CMV qPCR is greater than 500 IU/mL to 1000 IU/mL. Cutoffs as low as 150 IU/mL have been used, based on local guidelines and standard operating procedures at each center. In a recently published retrospective study, initiation of preemptive treatment at CMV PCR titers of 135 IU/mL to 440 IU/mL was associated with faster viremia resolution and lower rates of prolonged viremia and duration of antiviral treatment.[40]

Preemptive treatment agent selection Preemptive therapy can include ganciclovir, valganciclovir, or foscarnet.[1,3,39] The agent selection depends on the time of CMV infection post-HCT for an individual patient and on institutional protocols. Due to potential myelosuppression, ganciclovir/valganciclovir are generally avoided in the pre-engraftment and early postengraftment periods, during which foscarnet is usually favored by most transplant centers.[1] Administration of valganciclovir should be avoided in patients with GIT GVHD, due to potential poor absorption in the setting of almost any amount of diarrhea.[39] Foscarnet is avoided in patients with renal function impairment or in case of coadministration with other potentially nephrotoxic agents. Cidofovir may be considered as secondary preemptive treatment approach in specific cases, such as in patients treated with foscarnet for transition to outpatient treatment based on its convenient once-weekly dosing, albeit limited data are available.[39]

Preemptive treatment dosing and duration Induction dose of CMV preemptive therapy is usually administered for 2 weeks to 3 weeks with transition to maintenance-dose treatment of 2 to weeks 3 weeks and/or until an undetectable CMV viral load is documented by CMV qPCR.[1,39] Approaches may differ at different centers, according to the standard operating procedures at each institution.

Additional concepts There are no adequate data to support the use of intravenous administered immunoglobulin or CMV vaccines for the prevention of CMV infection in allogeneic HCT recipients. Similarly, there are not adequate data on the use of CMV-specific interferon-gamma–producing T cells for the management of CMV infection.[1,39]

Epstein-Barr virus

Frequent EBV monitoring with an EBV qPCR assay is recommended during the first 100 days post–allogeneic HCT, particularly for patients at higher risk for post-transplant lymphoproliferative disease, such as pediatric patients and cord blood, haploidentical, and T-cell–depleted graft recipients.[1] Monitoring of EBV reactivation should be continued beyond D100, in cases of GVHD and associated treatment.[1] The major concern about EBV reactivation is the development of post-transplant lymphoproliferative disorder, associated with the graft type and GVHD prophylaxis regimen selection.[1,41] A preemptive approach for the management of EBV reactivation is applied in most transplant centers. Although EBV viral load thresholds for preemptive treatment initiation are not as well defined, interventions, including reduction of immunosuppression and/or administration of rituximab, are applied for greater than 1000 copies/mL.[1]

Hepatitis B virus

Routine pretransplant and prechemotherapy hepatitis B virus (HBV) testing for all HCT donors and recipients is recommended, including HBV surface antigen (HBsAg), HBV surface antibody (HBsAb), HBV core antibody (HBcAb), and HBV DNA (**Fig. 6**).[1] Hepatitis B vaccination is recommended in all HBV-naive patients who undergo chemotherapy and/or HCT.[1] If HBV vaccination cannot be initiated or completed before initiation of chemotherapy or stem cell infusion, HCT-naive recipients should be vaccinated or complete their vaccination as soon as their immunity is restored post-HCT.[1] Patients at risk for HBV primary infection or reactivation should receive prophylaxis with an anti-HBV active agent at the time of conditioning and at least for another 6 months after discontinuation of all immunosuppression.[1] Entecavir and tenofovir are preferred over lamivudine, due to their higher efficacy and resistance barrier.[42] Appropriate antiviral treatment, preferably with entecavir, should be immediately initiated in patients with active HBV viremia at the time of chemotherapy or transplant and close monitoring of liver function and HBV viral load should apply.

Hematopoietic cell transplant donor and hepatitis B virus HBV-naive recipients should preferably receive a graft from HBsAg-negative donors.[1] HBV serostatus, however, should not exclude potential HCT donors and HBsAg-positive and/or HBV DNA–positive individuals can be considered potential HCT donors.[1] Specific

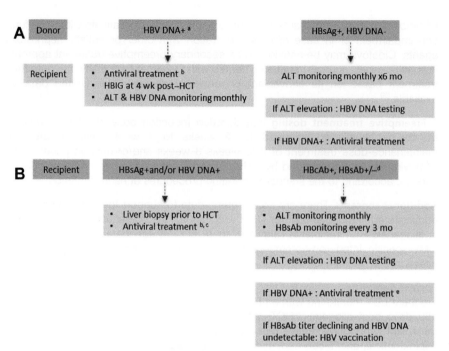

Fig. 6. Management of HBV infection in allogeneic HCT recipients: (*A*) in cases of HBV DNA/HBsAg–positive HCT donors and (*B*) HBsAg/HBcAb-positive HCT recipients. ALT, alanine aminotransferase. [a] Donor: if a donor is HBV DNA positive prior to stem cell harvest, treatment for 4 weeks should be administered, or until HBV DNA is undetectable. Recipient: in cases of a recipient not vaccinated for HBV, HBV vaccination should be administered, if feasible before HCT. If vaccination is not feasible or complete prior to HCT or HBsAb titer less than 10 IU/L, hepatitis B immunoglolulin should be administered with stem cell infusion. [b] Entecavir and tenofovir are preferred over lamivudine. [c] Antiviral treatment should be initiated before conditioning regimen. [d] HCT recipients who are HBcAb+/HBsAb− should receive HBV vaccination prior to HCT, if their HBV DNA is undetectable. [e] Antiviral treatment should be administered for a minimum of 6 months post discontinuation of immunosuppressive treatment. (*Data from* Tomblyn M, Chiller T, Einsele H, et al. Guidelines for preventing infectious complications among hematopoietic cell transplantation recipients: a global perspective. Biol Blood Marrow Transplant. 2009;15(10):1143–1238; and 2.2016 NGV. Prevention and treatment of Cancer-Related Infections. National Comprehensive Cancer Network Clinical Practice Guidelines in Oncology (NCCN Guidelines) 2016; https://oralcancerfoundation.org/wp-content/uploads/2016/09/infections.pdf. Accessed September 30, 2018.)

treatment and monitoring approaches are in place for HBsAg-positive donors and recipients to limit HBV transmission (see **Fig. 6**A).[1,43]

Hematopoietic cell transplant recipient and hepatitis B virus HBV recipients can be high risk, moderate risk, and low risk based on their HBV serology constellation: (1) high risk: HBsAg-positive and/or HBV DNA–positive patients; (2) moderate risk: HBcAb-positive and HBsAg-positive and HBsAb-negative patients, in particular those who are HBV DNA positive; and (3) low-risk: HBsAb-positive and/or HBcAb-positive patients. All high-risk HCT recipients should have a liver biopsy prior to their HCT and receive anti-HBV prophylaxis starting before conditioning.[1,43] For moderate-risk HCT recipients, HBV DNA should be monitored, and if negative HBV vaccine should be administered. If HBV DNA is positive, patients should receive antiviral prophylaxis. Low-risk patients should have ALT and HBsAb levels monitored once every month and every 3 months, respectively, as detailed in **Fig. 6B**.[1] HBcAb-positive and HBsAb-positive recipients with GVHD requiring prolonged steroid treatment courses are at higher risk for HBV reactivation and thus should receive antiviral prophylaxis.[1] Due to ease of administration, benign adverse event profile, and few drug interactions, most centers administer HBV prophylaxis in low risk patients as well.

Hepatitis C virus

Based on current guidelines, HCV seropositivity for the donor or the recipient is not an absolute contraindication for an allogeneic HCT.[1] Close monitoring of these patients and all efforts possible to decrease the risk of transmission and/or progression of HCV infection post-HCT is highly recommended.[1] HCV-seropositive, HCV RNA–positive donors should receive direct-acting antiviral (DAA) HCV-specific treatment, with the ultimate goal of achieving undetectable HCV viral load at the time of harvest.[44] HCV-seropositive, HCV RNA–positive recipients should receive treatment with a DAA agent, when possible.[1,44] There are no definitive data to suggest what time post-HCT DAA HCV–specific treatment should be initiated, but most experts agree to treatment initiation in approximately 6 months post-HCT or after all immuno-suppressive therapy is tapered.[44] HCV-seropositive recipients with fibrosis, cirrhosis, or HCV-associated lymphoproliferative disorder should be treated as soon as possible.[44] HCV-seropositive recipients should be carefully monitored for HCV progression and long-term complications.[1,44] Myeloablative conditioning regimens, in particular those containing cyclophosphamide and total body irradiation, should be avoided due to increased risk of post-HCT complications, including sinusoidal obstruction syndrome.[1]

Parasitic Prophylaxis

Toxoplasma gondii prophylaxis

Toxoplasmosis remains an uncommon complication after an allogeneic HCT, due to reactivation of an old infection in the vast majority of cases.[1,3] HCT recipients of T-cell–depleted or cord blood grafts and/or with GVHD are at higher risk for *Toxoplasma* reactivation.[1] Administration of TMP-SMX for *Pneumocystis jirovecii* prophylaxis also can be protective for toxoplasmosis, although dosing of TMP-SMX for prevention of toxoplasmosis has not, as yet, been well defined.[1,3] In patients at high risk for toxoplasmosis not receiving prophylaxis with TMP-SMX, screening by a qPCR for *Toxoplasma* species should be performed, albeit frequency of monitoring has not been established. This is discussed further in Driele Peixoto and Daniel P. Prestes's article, "Parasitic Infections of the Stem Cell Transplant Recipient and the Hematologic Malignancy Patient, Including Toxoplasmosis and Strongyloidiasis," in this issue.

Empirical Antibacterial and Antifungal Treatment for Neutropenic Fever

General concepts of neutropenic fever management

Neutropenic fever represents the most common complication of neutropenic patients, but a definitive bacterial infection is diagnosed in less than 25% of these patients.[1,2] Due to the inability of neutropenic patients to generate an adequate immune response and rapid progression to sepsis, prompt initiation of appropriate antibiotic therapy has become the standard of care since decades. Empirical antibacterial treatment should include a bactericidal, well-tolerated and broad-spectrum agent, with activity against gram-positive and gram-negative organisms, including *Pseudomonas aeruginosa*.[2] In this review, neutropenic fever management is discussed only for high-risk patients. All high-risk patients with neutropenic fever should be admitted to the hospital for prompt initiation of a detailed and comprehensive diagnostic work-up, parallel to antibiotic treatment initiation. Details on the diagnostic work-up of neutropenic fever are presented in Gowri Satyanarayana's article, "Work Up for Fever during Neutropenia for both the Stem Cell Transplant Recipient and the Hematologic Malignancy Patient," in this issue: Work-up for fever during neutropenia.

Antibacterial empirical treatment—initial neutropenic fever

In high-risk patients with neutropenic fever, intravenous administration of an appropriately dosed β-lactam with antipseudomonal activity (piperacillin-tazobactam, cefepime, imipenem-cilastatin, or meropenem) should be promptly initiated.[2] Concerns due to increased 30-day mortality associated with cefepime were raised, based on the results of a meta-analysis.[45] A new meta-analysis initiated by the Food and Drug Administration, however, in which more studies of cefepime in patients with febrile neutropenia were included, did not corroborate the findings of the prior study and hence cefepime remains a first-line agent for the management of febrile neutropenia.[2] Additional concepts considered in the selection of initial antibiotic treatment of neutropenic fever are presented in **Table 2**.

Antibacterial empirical treatment—persistent neutropenic fever

Persistent neutropenic fever, defined as neutropenic fever after 3 days to 5 days of empirical antibiotic treatment, is a frequent occurrence in allogeneic HCT recipients and leukemia patients receiving induction chemotherapy. High-risk patients with neutropenic fever may remain febrile for an average of 5 days, despite administration of empirical treatment.[2] In most cases, patients defervesce with resolution of neutropenia without an identified infectious etiology.[2] Persistent neutropenic fever in hemodynamically stable patients should not always generate additional antibiotic changes.[2] Antibiotic escalation is frequently applied, however, particularly in unstable patients or patients with persistent profound neutropenia (**Box 1**).[2]

Duration of empirical antibacterial treatment for neutropenic fever

Historically, neutropenic patients started on empirical antibiotic treatment of neutropenic fever remain on broad-spectrum empirical antibiotic therapy until both fever and neutropenia are resolved.[2,46] This approach has been recently challenged, considering the lack of robust data and significant improvements in the diagnosis and treatment of infectious complications and in the management of neutropenic patients achieved during the past 4 decades.[47,48] De-escalation to a fluoroquinolone has been suggested for low-risk patients and in cases of completion of a recommended antibiotic treatment course for a specific infection in an afebrile patient who remains neutropenic.[2] The recently revised ECIL recommendations for the management of patients with febrile neutropenia suggest that empirical antibiotic treatment can be discontinued after greater than or equal to 72 hours in neutropenic patients who remain afebrile for greater than or equal to 48 hours.[47] Secondary prophylaxis with a narrower-spectrum agent, such as a fluoroquinolone, may be used, depending on local epidemiology.[47,48] In a recent superiority open-label prospective randomized clinical trial, 158 hematologic malignancy patients or HCT recipients with high-risk febrile neutropenia were randomized 1:1 to 2 arms: an experimental arm, in which empirical treatment was discontinued greater than or equal to 72 hours after fever resolution, and a control arm, with empirical treatment continued until neutropenia resolution.[49] Fewer total days of empirical antibiotic treatment and side effects were observed in the experimental group, whereas days of fever, recurrent fever, and

Table 2
Considerations for initial empirical antibiotic treatment of neutropenic fever

Antibiotic	Indication
Aminoglycosides	• Routine inclusion of an aminoglycoside in the initial antibiotic regimen is not recommended. • In cases of hemodynamic instability, an aminoglycoside should be added, until more microbiological and clinical data are available. • Meta-analysis showed that addition of an aminoglycoside to a beta-lactam for the treatment of sepsis did not improve survival and was associated with more side effects than monotherapy.[58]

Antibiotics with activity against resistant gram-positive cocci (MRSA, VRE)	• Routine administration of antibiotics (vancomycin, daptomycin, and linezolid) with activity against resistant gram-positive cocci (MRSA, VRE) should not be included in the initial empirical treatment regimen.
	• Administration of agents with activity against resistant gram-positive cocci should be considered in case of
	  ○ Clinical suspicion for a CVC-associated, skin and soft tissue, or a positive blood culture for gram-positive cocci
	  ○ Patients with known colonization, prior infection or high clinical suspicion for resistant gram-positive organisms
	  ○ *Streptococcus viridans* bacteremia if the prevalence of penicillin-resistant *Streptococcus viridans* species is high
	• If blood cultures remain negative, treatment with these agents can be discontinued after 2–3 d

Agents with activity against MDR gram-negative organisms (ESBL, CPE)	• A carbapenem is preferred in patients with colonization, prior infection, or clinical suspicion for an ESBL-producing organism. • In patients with colonization, prior infection or clinical suspicion for CPE-producing organisms, empirical antibiotic therapy should be adjusted (ie, colistin, prolonged administration of a carbapenem) after discussion with the infectious disease consultation team and based on the local epidemiology and antibiotic susceptibility profile.
Ceftazidime	• Ceftazidime is not included in the list of preferred empirical treatments, due to its lack of activity against gram-positive pathogens.

Abbreviations: CPE, carbapenemase enzyme; ESBL, extended-spectrum β-lactamase; MDR, multidrug resistant; MRSA, methicillin-resistant *Staphylococcus aureus*; VRE, vancomycin-resistant *Enterococcus*.

Data from Freifeld AG, Bow EJ, Sepkowitz KA, et al. Clinical practice guideline for the use of antimicrobial agents in neutropenic patients with cancer: 2010 update by the infectious diseases society of America. Clin Infect Dis. 2011;52(4):e56–93.

mortality were similar in both arms. Although not definitive, the results of this study can reignite the discussion on the efficacy and safety of empirical treatment discontinuation in certain subsets of neutropenic patients.

Antifungal empirical treatment

Empirical antifungal treatment is defined as the initiation of a broad-spectrum antifungal agent in the setting of neutropenic fever that persists after 4 days to 7 days of empirical antibacterial treatment based on high clinical suspicion for an IFI.[2] The concept of empirical antifungal treatment was introduced in the early 1980s with the landmark study by Pizzo and colleagues,[50] showing decreased mortality after the introduction of empirical treatment with conventional amphotericin B in patients with neutropenic fever. Empirical antifungal treatment has been widely practiced

---

Box 1
Considerations for empirical antibiotic treatment of persistent neutropenic fever

In cases of empirical treatment with cefepime or piperacillin-tazobactam and/or ESBL-producing gram-negative organism colonization, treatment should be broadened to either imipenem-cilastatin or meropenem, to include coverage against ESBL-producing pathogens.

In cases of MRSA and/or VRE or penicillin-resistant *S viridans* colonization/infection, treatment with vancomycin (daptomycin or linezolid) should be instituted.

In cases of CPE-producing gram-negative organism colonization/infection, antibiotic treatment should be adjusted based on antibiogram results and after consultation with the infectious disease consultation team.

In patients with persistent neutropenic fever despite broad-spectrum antibacterial treatment, less common bacterial pathogens should be considered, including *Streptococcus pneumoniae* or *Nocardia* species.

In patients with a definitive diagnosis of a specific infection, antibiotic treatment should be tailored based on culture and antibiotic susceptibility results.

In patients with hemodynamic instability, addition of an aminoglycoside (ie, amikacin) should be considered.

Abbreviations: CPE, carbapenemase enzyme; ESBL, extended-spectrum β-lactamase; MRSA, methicillin-resistant *Staphylococcus aureus*; VRE, vancomycin resistant *Enterococcus*.
   Data from Freifeld AG, Bow EJ, Sepkowitz KA, et al. Clinical practice guideline for the use of antimicrobial agents in neutropenic patients with cancer: 2010 update by the infectious diseases society of america Clin Infect Dis 2011;52(4):e56–93.

---

ever since, with multiple clinical trials validating the use of amphotericin B lipid formulations, broad-spectrum azoles, and echinocandins.[1,51–53] The low incidence of IFI, treatment associated-toxicities, and costs and improved diagnostic modalities for the detection of IFI, however, have led to the investigation of other approaches, namely antifungal preemptive treatment.

Antifungal preemptive treatment

Antifungal preemptive treatment is defined as initiation of early antifungal treatment based on clinical, laboratory, and radiographic evidence of an early IFI. This approach has been possible, because of the significant progress attained in the field of IA diagnosis. Identification of the halo-sign, crescent-sign, and nodular lesions on chest CT as signs of IA has led to early diagnosis of IA and prompt initiation of appropriate treatment, leading to improved survival outcomes.[54–56] In addition, fungal biomarkers, such as the galactomannan GM enzyme immunoassay (EIA) and β-d glucan, have been introduced in clinical practice in the past 2 decades and may lead to earlier diagnosis of IMI. Maertens and colleagues[56] were the first to assess the feasibility of a preemptive antifungal approach in a cohort of neutropenic patients receiving fluconazole prophylaxis. Initiation of treatment with liposomal amphotericin B was based on predefined chest CT findings and positive microbiologic evidence, including a positive GM EIA (2 consecutive GM EIA tests with an optical density index [ODI] >0.5). A 78% reduction in antifungal treatment administration was observed, when compared with empirical antifungal treatment based on predefined criteria. This study was followed by a multicenter, open-label, randomized, noninferiority clinical trial comparing empirical and preemptive antifungal treatment in hematologic malignancy patients with neutropenia; no allogeneic HCT recipients were included in this trial.[57] An ODI greater than or equal to 1.5 was considered for GM EIA positivity. Overall survival at 14-days post–neutropenia recovery, IFI-associated mortality, duration of neutropenic fever, and length of hospital stay were similar between the 2 arms. Preemptive anti-fungal treatment was associated with decreased costs of antifungal therapy by 35% but more proven and probable IFI (IA and *Candida* infections) compared with empirical antifungal treatment. Approximately half patients did not receive any anti-fungal prophylaxis, which could have contributed to more candidal infections. Although not studied in allogeneic HCT recipients, most centers follow a preemptive antifungal treatment approach in the pre-engraftment period in cases of persistent neutropenic fever.

REFERENCES

1. Tomblyn M, Chiller T, Einsele H, et al. Guidelines for preventing infectious compli-cations among hematopoietic cell transplantation recipients: a global perspec-tive. Biol Blood Marrow Transplant 2009;15(10):1143–238.
2. Freifeld AG, Bow EJ, Sepkowitz KA, et al. Clinical practice guideline for the use of antimicrobial agents in neutropenic patients with cancer: 2010 update by the in-fectious diseases society of america. Clin Infect Dis 2011;52(4):e56–93.
3. 2.2016 NGV. Prevention and treatment of cancer-related infections. National Comprehensive Cancer Network clinical practice guidelines in oncology (NCCN guidelines). 2016. Available at: https://oralcancerfoundation.org/wp-content/uploads/2016/09/infections.pdf. Accessed September 30, 2018.
4. Taplitz RA, Kennedy EB, Bow EJ, et al. Antimicrobial prophylaxis for adult pa-tients with cancer-related immunosuppression: ASCO and IDSA clinical practice guideline update. J Clin Oncol 2018;36(30):3043–53.
5. Kontoyiannis DP, Marr KA, Park BJ, et al. Prospective surveillance for invasive fungal infections in hematopoietic stem cell transplant recipients, 2001-2006: overview of the Transplant-Associated Infection Surveillance Network (TRANS-NET) Database. Clin Infect Dis 2010;50(8):1091–100.
6. Marr KA, Carter RA, Crippa F, et al. Epidemiology and outcome of mould infec-tions in hematopoietic stem cell transplant recipients. Clin Infect Dis 2002; 34(7):909–17.
7. Kontoyiannis DP, Wessel VC, Bodey GP, et al. Zygomycosis in the 1990s in a tertiary-care cancer center. Clin Infect Dis 2000;30(6):851–6.
8. Gafter-Gvili A, Paul M, Fraser A, et al. Effect of quinolone prophylaxis in afebrile neutropenic patients on microbial resistance: systematic review and meta-anal-ysis. J Antimicrob Chemother 2007;59(1):5–22.
9. Bucaneve G, Micozzi A, Menichetti F, et al. Levofloxacin to prevent bacterial infection in patients with cancer and neutropenia. N Engl J Med 2005;353(10): 977–87.
10. Mikulska M, Averbuch D, Tissot F, et al. Fluoroquinolone prophylaxis in haemato-logical cancer patients with neutropenia: ECIL critical appraisal of previous guidelines. J Infect 2018;76(1):20–37.
11. Averbuch D, Tridello G, Hoek J, et al. Antimicrobial resistance in gram-negative rods causing bacteremia in hematopoietic stem cell transplant recipients: inter-continental prospective study of the infectious diseases working party of the European Bone Marrow Transplantation Group. Clin Infect Dis 2017;65(11): 1819–28.
12. Goodman JL, Winston DJ, Greenfield RA, et al. A controlled trial of fluconazole to prevent fungal infections in patients undergoing bone marrow transplantation. N Engl J Med 1992;326(13):845–51.

13. Marr KA, Seidel K, Slavin MA, et al. Prolonged fluconazole prophylaxis is associated with persistent protection against candidiasis-related death in allogeneic marrow transplant recipients: long-term follow-up of a randomized, placebo-controlled trial. Blood 2000;96(6):2055–61.

14. Slavin MA, Osborne B, Adams R, et al. Efficacy and safety of fluconazole prophylaxis for fungal infections after marrow transplantation–a prospective, randomized, double-blind study. J Infect Dis 1995;171(6):1545–52.

15. Pfaller MA, Diekema DJ, Gibbs DL, et al. Results from the ARTEMIS DISK Global Antifungal Surveillance study, 1997 to 2005: an 8.5-year analysis of susceptibilities of Candida species and other yeast species to fluconazole and voriconazole determined by CLSI standardized disk diffusion testing. J Clin Microbiol 2007; 45(6):1735–45.

16. Marr KA, Crippa F, Leisenring W, et al. Itraconazole versus fluconazole for prevention of fungal infections in patients receiving allogeneic stem cell transplants. Blood 2004;103(4):1527–33.

17. Wingard JR, Carter SL, Walsh TJ, et al. Randomized, double-blind trial of fluconazole versus voriconazole for prevention of invasive fungal infection after allogeneic hematopoietic cell transplantation. Blood 2010;116(24):5111–8.

18. van Burik JA, Ratanatharathorn V, Stepan DE, et al. Micafungin versus fluconazole for prophylaxis against invasive fungal infections during neutropenia in patients undergoing hematopoietic stem cell transplantation. Clin Infect Dis 2004; 39(10):1407–16.

19. Cordonnier C, Mohty M, Faucher C, et al. Safety of a weekly high dose of liposomal amphotericin B for prophylaxis of invasive fungal infection in immunocompromised patients: PROPHYSOME study. Int J Antimicrob Agents 2008;31(2): 135–41.

20. Ullmann AJ, Lipton JH, Vesole DH, et al. Posaconazole or fluconazole for prophylaxis in severe graft-versus-host disease. N Engl J Med 2007;356(4):335–47.

21. Cornely OA, Maertens J, Winston DJ, et al. Posaconazole vs. fluconazole or itraconazole prophylaxis in patients with neutropenia. N Engl J Med 2007;356(4): 348–59.

22. De Pauw BE, Donnelly JP. Prophylaxis and aspergillosis–has the principle been proven? N Engl J Med 2007;356(4):409–11.

23. Boeckh M, Kim HW, Flowers ME, et al. Long-term acyclovir for prevention of varicella zoster virus disease after allogeneic hematopoietic cell transplantation–a randomized double-blind placebo-controlled study. Blood 2006;107(5):1800–5.

24. Erard V, Guthrie KA, Varley C, et al. One-year acyclovir prophylaxis for preventing varicella-zoster virus disease after hematopoietic cell transplantation: no evidence of rebound varicella-zoster virus disease after drug discontinuation. Blood 2007;110(8):3071–7.

25. Chen K, Cheng MP, Hammond SP, et al. Antiviral prophylaxis for cytomegalovirus infection in allogeneic hematopoietic cell transplantation. Blood Adv 2018;2(16): 2159–75.

26. Green ML, Leisenring W, Xie H, et al. Cytomegalovirus viral load and mortality after haemopoietic stem cell transplantation in the era of pre-emptive therapy: a retrospective cohort study. Lancet Haematol 2016;3(3):e119–27.

27. Yong MK, Ananda-Rajah M, Cameron PU, et al. Cytomegalovirus reactivation is associated with increased risk of late-onset invasive fungal disease after allogeneic hematopoietic stem cell transplantation: a multicenter study in the current era of viral load monitoring. Biol Blood Marrow Transplant 2017;23(11):1961–7.

28. Ljungman P. The role of cytomegalovirus serostatus on outcome of hematopoietic stem cell transplantation. Curr Opin Hematol 2014;21(6):466–9.

29. Ljungman P, Boeckh M, Hirsch HH, et al. Definitions of cytomegalovirus infection and disease in transplant patients for use in clinical trials. Clin Infect Dis 2017; 64(1):87–91.

30. Boeckh M, Gooley TA, Myerson D, et al. Cytomegalovirus pp65 antigenemia-guided early treatment with ganciclovir versus ganciclovir at engraftment after allogeneic marrow transplantation: a randomized double-blind study. Blood 1996;88(10):4063–71.

31. Einsele H, Reusser P, Bornhauser M, et al. Oral valganciclovir leads to higher exposure to ganciclovir than intravenous ganciclovir in patients following allogeneic stem cell transplantation. Blood 2006;107(7):3002–8.

32. van der Heiden PL, Kalpoe JS, Barge RM, et al. Oral valganciclovir as preemptive therapy has similar efficacy on cytomegalovirus DNA load reduction as intravenous ganciclovir in allogeneic stem cell transplantation recipients. Bone Marrow Transplant 2006;37(7):693–8.

33. Ayala E, Greene J, Sandin R, et al. Valganciclovir is safe and effective as preemptive therapy for CMV infection in allogeneic hematopoietic stem cell transplantation. Bone Marrow Transplant 2006;37(9):851–6.

34. Busca A, de Fabritiis P, Ghisetti V, et al. Oral valganciclovir as preemptive therapy for cytomegalovirus infection post allogeneic stem cell transplantation. Transpl Infect Dis 2007;9(2):102–7.

35. Marty FM, Ljungman P, Chemaly RF, et al. Letermovir prophylaxis for cytomegalovirus in hematopoietic-cell transplantation. N Engl J Med 2017;377(25): 2433–44.

36. Marty FM, Ljungman P, Papanicolaou GA, et al. Maribavir prophylaxis for prevention of cytomegalovirus disease in recipients of allogeneic stem-cell transplants: a phase 3, double-blind, placebo-controlled, randomised trial. Lancet Infect Dis 2011;11(4):284–92.

37. Marty FM, Winston DJ, Rowley SD, et al. CMX001 to prevent cytomegalovirus disease in hematopoietic-cell transplantation. N Engl J Med 2013;369(13):1227–36.

38. Marty FM, Winston DJ, Chemaly R. Brincidofovir for prevention of cytomegalovirus (CMV) after allogeneic hematopoietic cell transplantation (HCT) in CMV-seropositive patients: a randomized, double-blind, placebo-controlled, parallel-group phase 3 trial. Biol Blood Marrow Transplant 2016;22(3):369–81.

39. Update E-C. 7th European conference on infections in leukaemia. Antipolis, France, September 21-23, 2017. Available at: http://www.ecil-leukaemia.com/telechargements/ECIL%207%20CMV%20final%20slides.pdf. Accessed September 30, 2018.

40. Tan SK, Waggoner JJ, Pinsky BA. Cytomegalovirus load at treatment initiation is predictive of time to resolution of viremia and duration of therapy in hematopoietic cell transplant recipients. J Clin Virol 2015;69:179–83.

41. Kanakry JA, Kasamon YL, Bolanos-Meade J, et al. Absence of post-transplantation lymphoproliferative disorder after allogeneic blood or marrow transplantation using post-transplantation cyclophosphamide as graft-versus-host disease prophylaxis. Biol Blood Marrow Transplant 2013;19(10):1514–7.

42. Shang J, Wang H, Sun J, et al. A comparison of lamivudine vs entecavir for prophylaxis of hepatitis B virus reactivation in allogeneic hematopoietic stem cell transplantation recipients: a single-institutional experience. Bone Marrow Transplant 2016;51(4):581–6.

43. Lubel JS, Angus PW. Hepatitis B reactivation in patients receiving cytotoxic chemotherapy: diagnosis and management. J Gastroenterol Hepatol 2010; 25(5):864–71.

44. Torres HA, Chong PP, De Lima M, et al. Hepatitis C virus infection among hematopoietic cell transplant donors and recipients: American Society for Blood and Marrow Transplantation task force recommendations. Biol Blood Marrow Transplant 2015;21(11):1870–82.

45. Yahav D, Paul M, Fraser A, et al. Efficacy and safety of cefepime: a systematic review and meta-analysis. Lancet Infect Dis 2007;7(5):338–48.

46. Pizzo PA. Management of fever in patients with cancer and treatment-induced neutropenia. N Engl J Med 1993;328(18):1323–32.

47. Averbuch D, Orasch C, Cordonnier C, et al. European guidelines for empirical antibacterial therapy for febrile neutropenic patients in the era of growing resistance: summary of the 2011 4th European Conference on Infections in Leukemia. Haematologica 2013;98(12):1826–35.

48. Orasch C, Averbuch D, Mikulska M, et al. Discontinuation of empirical antibiotic therapy in neutropenic leukaemia patients with fever of unknown origin is ethical. Clin Microbiol Infect 2015;21(3):e25–7.

49. Aguilar-Guisado M, Espigado I, Martin-Pena A, et al. Optimisation of empirical antimicrobial therapy in patients with haematological malignancies and febrile neutropenia (How Long study): an open-label, randomised, controlled phase 4 trial. Lancet Haematol 2017;4(12):e573–83.

50. Pizzo PA, Robichaud KJ, Gill FA, et al. Empiric antibiotic and antifungal therapy for cancer patients with prolonged fever and granulocytopenia. Am J Med 1982;72(1):101–11.

51. Walsh TJ, Finberg RW, Arndt C, et al. Liposomal amphotericin B for empirical therapy in patients with persistent fever and neutropenia. National Institute of Allergy and Infectious Diseases Mycoses Study Group. N Engl J Med 1999;340(10): 764–71.

52. Walsh TJ, Pappas P, Winston DJ, et al. Voriconazole compared with liposomal amphotericin B for empirical antifungal therapy in patients with neutropenia and persistent fever. N Engl J Med 2002;346(4):225–34.

53. Walsh TJ, Teppler H, Donowitz GR, et al. Caspofungin versus liposomal amphotericin B for empirical antifungal therapy in patients with persistent fever and neutropenia. N Engl J Med 2004;351(14):1391–402.

54. Caillot D, Casasnovas O, Bernard A, et al. Improved management of invasive pulmonary aspergillosis in neutropenic patients using early thoracic computed tomographic scan and surgery. J Clin Oncol 1997;15(1):139–47.

55. Greene RE, Schlamm HT, Oestmann JW, et al. Imaging findings in acute invasive pulmonary aspergillosis: clinical significance of the halo sign. Clin Infect Dis 2007;44(3):373–9.

56. Maertens J, Theunissen K, Verhoef G, et al. Galactomannan and computed tomography-based preemptive antifungal therapy in neutropenic patients at high risk for invasive fungal infection: a prospective feasibility study. Clin Infect Dis 2005;41(9):1242–50.

57. Cordonnier C, Pautas C, Maury S, et al. Empirical versus preemptive antifungal therapy for high-risk, febrile, neutropenic patients: a randomized, controlled trial. Clin Infect Dis 2009;48(8):1042–51.

58. Paul M, Silbiger I, Grozinsky S, et al. Beta lactam antibiotic monotherapy versus beta lactam-aminoglycoside antibiotic combination therapy for sepsis. Cochrane Database Syst Rev 2006;(1):CD003344.

Work-up for Fever During Neutropenia for Both the Stem Cell Transplant Recipient and the Hematologic Malignancy Patient

Gowri Satyanarayana, MD

KEYWORDS

- Evaluation of fever and neutropenia • Empiric therapy of fever and neutropenia
- Typhlitis • Fungal antigen testing

KEY POINTS

- Fever is defined as a single temperature of 38.3°C or 38°C over a 1-hour period, and neutropenia is defined as an absolute neutrophil count less than 500 cells/mm^3.
- Fever in patients with neutropenia is associated with increased mortality, especially in those with acute myelogenous leukemia and have undergone hematopoietic cell transplant.
- Evaluation for specific infections, with a focus on bacterial and fungal etiologies, should be based on clinical sign/symptoms as well as duration of neutropenia.
- Microbiology and radiographic diagnostic testing may be useful when evaluation for infectious etiologies of fever and neutropenia.
- A center-based algorithm may guide initiation and de-escalation of empiric antimicrobial therapy in patients with fever and neutropenia.

INTRODUCTION
Fever and Neutropenia

Neutropenia is a common complication in cancer patients who receive cytotoxic chemotherapy and/or conditioning chemotherapy prior to hematopoietic cell transplantation (HCT). Neutropenia is defined as an absolute neutrophil count (ANC) less than 500 cells/mm^3 and profound neutropenia as an ANC less than 100 cells/mm^3.[1–3]

Fever often is the only sign of infection in a cancer patient who has received cytotoxic or conditioning chemotherapy and has a low ANC. The Infectious Diseases

Disclosure Statement: Merck honorarium Scientific Advisory Committee.
Division of Infectious Diseases, Vanderbilt University Medical Center, A2200 MCN, 1161 21st Avenue South, Nashville, TN 37232-2605, USA
E-mail addresses: gowri.satyanarayana@vumc.org; gowri_satyanarayana@yahoo.com

Infect Dis Clin N Am 33 (2019) 381–397
https://doi.org/10.1016/j.idc.2019.02.003
id.theclinics.com
0891-5520/19/© 2019 Elsevier Inc. All rights reserved.

Society of America and the National Comprehensive Cancer Network define fever as a single temperature of 38.3oC or higher orally or above 38.0oC orally over a 1-hour period.[1,3]

- Fever is a single temperature of 38.3oC or higher orally or above 38oC orally over a 1-hour period.

As the neutrophil count declines, the risk for infection increases.[1–3] Changes in cancer therapeutic techniques have not changed this basic concept. Patients with neutropenia are unable to mount an inflammatory response and, therefore, do not have typical signs or symptoms of infection. Fever in this clinical context requires careful evaluation and management. The risk of fever and infection is related to the type of chemotherapeutic agent administered as well as the underlying malignancy, both of which influence the depth and duration of neutropenia **Table 1**.[1] Patients with acute leukemia and those who have undergone allogeneic HCT are in the highest risk group for developing fever and neutropenia.

Clinical Outcomes in Neutropenic Patients

There is an increased risk of mortality in cancer patients who experience fever during neutropenia compared with those who do not.[4] The rates of fever and neutropenia in patients with hematologic malignancies and HCT have been reported to range from more than 20% to 70% to 100%, respectively.[5,6]

Several studies and collaborative groups have tried to identify clinical characteristics that predict clinical outcomes in patients with fever and neutropenia. Evidence of early bone marrow recovery, duration of neutropenia less than 7 days to 10 days, a short period of fever, and lack of comorbid conditions are features that are associated with a low risk for infectious complications during an episode of fever and neutropenia.[3,7–9]

The Study Section on Infections of the Multinational Association for Supportive Care in Cancer (MASCC) developed a risk score based on signs and symptoms of illness and comorbidities to identify those patients at low risk for complications related to fever and neutropenia (**Table 2**). A MASCC score of 21 or higher predicts low risk of complications, with a specificity of 68% and sensitivity of 71%.[10] The use of this type of scoring system can help guide the management of the febrile neutropenic patient.

FEVER AND NEUTROPENIA: INITIAL EVALUATION
Bacterial Infection

Bacteria are the most commonly identified infectious pathogens early in the course of fever and neutropenia, with gram-negative bloodstream infections occurring in up to 15% of patients with neutropenia.[11] The source of bacterial infection in a neutropenic

Table 1
Risk for fever during neutropenia based on underlying hematologic condition

High Risk	Moderate Risk	Low Risk
Acute leukemia	Autologous HCT	Solid tumor
Alemtuzumab treatment	Chronic lymphocytic leukemia	Neutropenia <7 d
Allogeneic HCT	Lymphoma	
GVHD treated with >20 mg/d steroids	Multiple myeloma	
Neutropenia >10 d	Neutropenia 7–10 d	
	Purine analog therapy	

Table 2 Multinational Association for Supportive Care in Cancer risk score	
Characteristic	**Weight**
Burden of illness: no or mild symptoms	5
No hypotension	5
No chronic obstructive pulmonary disease	4
Solid tumor or no previous fungal infection	4
No dehydration	3
Burden of illness: moderate symptoms	3
Outpatient status	3
Age <60 y	2

Note: points attributed to the variable "burden of illness" are not cumulative. The maximum theoretic score, therefore, is 26.

(From Klastersky J, Paesmans M, Rubenstein EB, et al. The multinational association for supportive care in cancer risk index: a multinational scoring system for identifying low-risk febrile neutropenic cancer patients. J Clin Oncol 2000;18(16):3046; with permnission.)

patient often is host endogenous flora from the gastrointestinal tract, mouth, and skin in the context of chemotherapy-induced gastrointestinal and oral mucositis and indwelling venous catheters. Common bacterial species isolated during neutropenia are demonstrated in **Table 3**.

- Bacteria are the most common pathogens early in the course of fever and neutropenia.

Historically, gram-negative bacteria were the most common type of bacteria isolated during febrile neutropenia, specifically *Pseudomonas aeruginosa*, which led to empiric treatment algorithms that include initial antibacterial therapy with an antipseudomonal agent. Over the past several decades, however, gram-positive organisms have become the most common cause of acute bacterial infection during febrile neutropenia. This shift has been attributed to a variety of factors, including the use of indwelling central venous catheters, use of antimicrobial prophylaxis, and changes in chemotherapeutic regimens.[12–14]

- Gram-negative or gram-positive bacteria may be the underlying bacterial pathogen during an episode of fever and neutropenia.

The initial evaluation of a patient with fever and neutropenia should include performing a detailed history and physical examination and obtaining 2 sets of blood cultures, defined as 2 aerobic blood cultures bottles and 2 anaerobic blood culture bottles.

Table 3 Common bacterial pathogens in fever during neutropenia	
Gram-negative Bacteria	**Gram-positive Bacteria**
Acinetobacter species	Coagulase-negative staphylococcus
Citrobacter species	*Enterococcus*
Escherichia coli	*Staphylococcus aureus*
Enterobacter species	*Streptococcus pneumoniae*
Klebsiella species	Viridans group streptococcus
P aeruginosa	
Stenotrophomonas maltophilia	

Sites may include 1 set of peripheral blood cultures and 1 set of central venous catheter blood cultures or 2 peripheral blood cultures or 2 sets of central venous catheter blood cultures. Subsequent blood culture evaluations may include only 1 set if a patient has limited intravenous (IV) access.

Initial Fever and Neutropenia: Traditional Management

The goal in the management of early febrile neutropenia is to start empiric antimicrobial therapy directed at bacterial pathogens that can cause serious morbidity and mortality, including P aeruginosa and the endogenous flora of the gastrointestinal tract.

Patients with underlying hematologic malignancy or those who have undergone HCT are at a higher risk of complications during episodes of fever during neutropenia, and empiric therapy with an IV β-lactam that has activity against P aeruginosa, such as ceftazidime, cefepime, piperacillin-tazobactam, imipenem-cilastin, or meropenem, should be initiated.[1,3] The initial empiric antibacterial agent should be a different agent from that used for prophylaxis. Gram-negative infections are associated with higher morbidity and mortality than gram-positive infections and, therefore, are the primary target of initial empiric therapy.

Review of prior microbiology data allows for identification of pathogens that may influence selection of antibacterial therapy, including multidrug-resistant (MDR) pathogens. An institution-specific febrile neutropenia algorithm may be beneficial because resistance patterns vary from center to center (**Fig. 1**).

If a patient has an immediate-type hypersensitivity reaction or a history of a severe drug reaction to penicillins, cephalosporins, and carbapenems, empiric therapy with ciprofloxacin and clindamycin or aztreonam with/without an aminoglycoside and vancomycin are other potential options (**Fig. 2**).

Addition of vancomycin to the initial antimicrobial regimen does not lead to a decrease in mortality[15]; therefore, empiric use of this agent during fever and neutropenia is not routinely recommend unless specific clinical or microbiologic risk factors are present, as outlined in **Box 1**.[1] If there is no evidence of a resistant gram-positive infection 48 hours after the addition of vancomycin, it can be stopped even if the patient remains neutropenic.

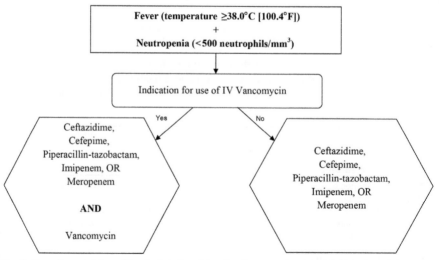

Fig. 1. Sample empiric antibacterial algorithm for fever and neutropenia.

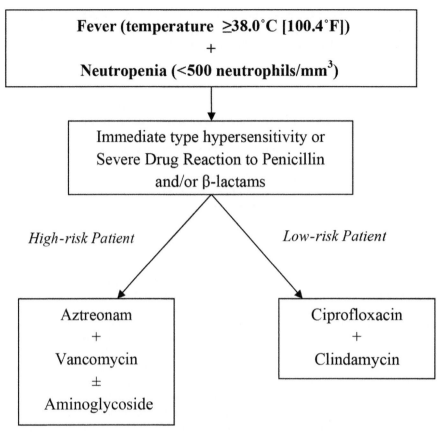

Fig. 2. Alternative empiric antibacterial algorithm for fever and neutropenia.

Broadening of antimicrobial therapy may be necessary to target resistant gram-negative and gram-positive bacteria, anaerobic bacteria, and fungi in those patients with persistent fever and continued hemodynamic instability despite treatment with an antipseudomonal β-lactam with or without vancomycin.

For those patients with ongoing fever and/or clinical instability despite escalation of antibacterial therapy, consideration should be given to escalation of empiric antifungal therapy and evaluation for fungal disease (discussed later).

Box 1
Indications for addition of intravenous vancomycin to the empiric therapy for fever during neutropenia
Clinically suspected catheter-related infection
Gram-positive bacteria growing in blood culture/s, before final susceptibilities available
Hemodynamic instability
Severe mucositis
Skin of soft tissue infection
Pneumonia

Current US guidelines recommend empiric antipseudomonal therapy be continued until the ANC is greater than 500 cells/mm^3 in patients who experience resolution of fever without identification of a specific infection.[1,3]

De-escalation of Empiric Antimicrobial Therapy: Culture-negative Fever and Neutropenia

In the era of growing antimicrobial resistance, investigators have begun to study de-escalation of antipseudomonal therapy in neutropenic patients with fever. Support for adopting this strategy includes antimicrobial stewardship efforts at decreasing rates of MDR infections and the limited pipeline of new gram-negative antibiotics effective against MDR isolates.

Aguilar-Guisado and colleagues[16] performed an open-label randomized trial to evaluate outcomes of de-escalation of empiric antibacterial therapy in neutropenic patients with fevers. In this study, adult febrile neutropenic patients with hematologic malignancies or HCT with no identified microbiologic source of fever were randomized to receive antipseudomonal therapy until the ANC was 500 cells/mm^3 versus early discontinuation of antipseudomonal therapy after 72 hours or more of being afebrile with clinical improvement, despite having an ANC less than 500 cells/mm^3. Patients in the early discontinuation group had fewer days of empiric antimicrobial therapy administration and no significant increase in mortality or days of fever compared with the standard-of-care group. Although patients in the early discontinuation group experienced more adverse events, a majority were mild to moderate and included mucositis, diarrhea, nausea, and vomiting.

This study provides data supporting the 2011 European Conference on Infections in Leukaemia (ECIL) guideline recommendation of antibacterial discontinuation at 72 hours of more for patients with initial fever and neutropenia with no documented bacterial infection and no fever for 48 hours or more.[17] The changes in practice outlined by the ECIL have yet to be adopted by US guideline committees.[1,3]

NEUTROPENIA-SPECIFIC BACTERIAL SYNDROMES
Ecthyma Gangrenosum

Etiology
Ecthyma gangrenosum (EG) is a necrotic cutaneous lesion that forms in patients with underlying neutropenia.[18] The pathogenesis of EG involves bacteremia causing occlusive vasculitis and local infarction, leading to the development of EG (**Fig. 3**).[19,20]

P aeruginosa is the most frequently implicated pathogen, but infection with other bacteria, such as Staphylococcus aureus or other gram-negative bacteria, also may lead to the development of EG lesions.[20–22] EG skin lesions most often involve the perineum or lower extremities but have also involved areas above the diaphragm.[22]

Diagnosis
A skin biopsy of the necrotic lesion, with tissue sent for culture, may have the highest microbiologic yield because blood cultures are positive in fewer than 50% of cases of Pseudomonas-related EG and even less during infection with other bacterial etiologies.[22]

Management
Treatment of EG includes antibiotic therapy directed at the underlying bacterial etiology and surgical débridement for removal of dead tissue.[22]

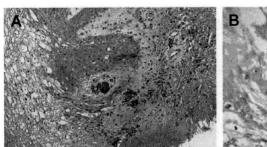
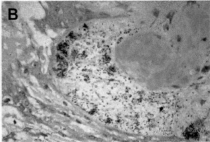

Fig. 3. Pathogenesis of EG. (*A*), Skin biopsy specimen showing epidermal necrosis and perivascular bacterial colonies in papillary dermis (hematoxylin-eosin stain; original magnification ×150). (*B*), Numerous gram-negative bacilli surround papillary dermal vessels (Gram stain; original magnification ×100.). (*From* Reich HL, Williams Fadeyi D, Naik NS, et al. Nonpseudomonal ecthyma gangrenosum. J Am Acad Dermatol 2004;50(5 Suppl):S115; with permission.)

Neutropenic Enterocolitis

Etiology

Chemotherapy and total body radiation can lead to mucosal barrier injury (MBI), predisposing patients to severe gut MBI, which may manifest as neutropenic enterocolitis (NEC). The pathogenesis of NEC involves decreased immune responses in the setting of neutropenia, MBI, and a shift in the intestinal microbiome from normal flora to pathogenic bacteria, leading to bowel damage and most significantly, perforation in 5% to 10% of cases.[23,24]

Typhlitis is gut MBI that specifically involves the ileocecal region of the small bowel.[25] Patients at highest risk for developing NEC are those with acute myelogenous leukemia who have received cytotoxic chemotherapy, with a reported pooled incidence of 5.6%.[24]

Diagnosis

Fever and abdominal pain in a neutropenic patient may indicate abdominal pathology and bowel wall abnormalities may be identified on ultrasound or computed tomography of the abdomen. Suggested diagnostic criteria for NEC are outlined in **Box 2**.[23–25]

Management

Initial medical management includes bowel rest and administration of antibacterial therapy targeting enteric gram-negative bacteria, enterococci, and anaerobes, with piperacillin-tazobactam, cefepime and metronidazole, imipenem-cilastin, or meropenem. Empiric antifungal therapy is not indicated.[23–25]

Box 2
Neutropenic enterocolitis criteria
Fever >38.3
ANC <500
Abdominal pain
Bowel wall thickening >4 mm for more than 30 mm in length

Consideration should be given to local antimicrobial resistance patterns. Surgical evaluation may be necessary if a patient develops an acute abdomen or there is concern for perforation.[23,25]

VIRAL INFECTIONS DURING NEUTROPENIA
Acyclovir-resistant Herpes Simplex Virus Infection

The prevalence of acyclovir-resistant herpes simplex virus (HSV) infection has been reported to range from 4% to 11% in HCT patients.[26–28] Extensive exposure to acyclovir in patients with prolonged HSV shedding can lead to the emergence of an acyclovir-resistant HSV isolate.[29,30] This may manifest clinically as new or persistent HSV-positive lesions in patients on acyclovir therapy.[29] In the correct clinical setting, testing for acyclovir resistance should be done and consideration should be given to change to alternate antiviral therapy, such as foscarnet or cidofovir.

Human herpesvirus 6 infection

Human herpesvirus 6 (HHV6) is a member of the β-herpesvirus family, replicates in activated $CD4^+$ T lymphocytes, and establishes latency in $CD34^+$ cells, monocytes, and macrophages.[31,32] HHV6 reactivation may occur after allogeneic HCT, with DNA detected in the blood of 40% to 60% of patients.[33–36] Development of HHV6 viremia may be associated with fever in a neutropenic patient after allogeneic HCT but also may lead to rash, bone marrow suppression, pneumonitis, hepatitis, or encephalitis.[33–35,37–41] Ganciclovir, foscarnet, and cidofovir have been used to treat HHV6 infection. Routine surveillance for HHV6 DNA with targeted treatment after HCT has not shown to decrease mortality.[42]

ADDITIONAL EVALUATION

A thorough history and examination are important and should include questions about exposures, medications, and focal symptoms that may help identify other specific sites of infection. Further assessments should be based on clinical signs and symptoms, as outlined in **Table 4**.

INVASIVE FUNGAL DISEASE DURING NEUTROPENIA

Patients with neutropenia lasting for 7 days or more are at risk for developing invasive fungal disease (IFD).[1,3]

Epidemiology
Candida
Candida species have been the most common cause of IFD in patients with underlying hematologic malignancies and HCT. Colonization of the gastrointestinal tract with Candida followed by administration of cytotoxic chemotherapy leading to injury of the gastrointestinal mucosal barrier is 1 of the most important risk factors for invasive candidiasis during neutropenia.[43,44]

Widespread use of antifungal prophylaxis in the United States, and less so in Europe, targeting Candida has led to a decrease in overall rates of Candida infections,[45] with an increase in infections caused by more resistant species, such as C glabrata and C krusei.[45–47]

Invasive Candida infection during febrile neutropenia typically manifests as a bloodstream infection, cutaneous nodules, or hepatosplenic disease, in which microabscesses form in the liver and spleen.[45]

Table 4	
Signs and symptoms in fever during neutropenia	
Sign/Symptom	**Evaluation**
Abdominal pain	Abdominal examination Radiograph of the abdomen Abdomen CT
Rectal pain	Examination of rectal mucosa Pelvis CT
Diarrhea	Clostridium difficile testing Testing for other stool pathogens
Dysuria, urgency, frequency	Urinalysis and urine culture Prostate
Hypoxia/cough	Chest radiograph Chest CT Bronchoscopy
Mouth pain or oral mucosal lesions	Virus testing of vesicular lesions Rule out thrush Biopsy of necrotic lesion/s
Nasal or sinus pain	Sinus CT Direct visualization of sinuses by otolaryngology
Headache	Neurologic status assessment Head CT Lumbar puncture for cerebrospinal fluid assessment

Molds

Over the past 2 decades, IFD secondary to opportunistic molds has become more prevalent than Candida in patients with hematologic malignancies and HCT recipients. Infection secondary to Aspergillus species is the most common, followed by Mucorales and Fusarium species.[48–53]

The degree and duration of neutropenia during treatment of acute myelogenous leukemia and immediately after HCT are important risk factors for the development of opportunistic mold infection.[49,54–56]

Invasive mold infections, which occur in patients with underlying neutropenia, have varied symptoms, depending on the site/s of infection. The lungs are the most common site of invasive fungal disease during neutropenia, and the symptoms of invasive pulmonary mold infection during neutropenia can range from isolated fever with no respiratory symptoms to pleuritic chest pain with or without cough.

Once a diagnosis of IFD is made, careful examination of the patient for other foci of infection is important because dissemination of mold infections can occur during neutropenia.

Laboratory Evaluation

Blood cultures

In many cases, initial fungal blood cultures may be negative, with reports of sensitivity as low as 30% for the diagnosis of invasive candidiasis in neutropenic patients and missed diagnoses of disseminated candidiasis in more than 50% of patients.[57–59]

Invasive Candida infections often have no localizing symptoms and can cause fevers that persist for days even after the appropriate antifungal therapy has been started.

Nanodiagnostics

Magnetic resonance technology has been used to create a panel that detects the DNA of 5 different species of Candida, including C albicans, C tropicalis, C parapsilosis,

C krusei, and *C glabrata*, in the blood. The Food and Drug Administration–approved T2Candida Panel (T2 Biosystems) has a sensitivity of 90% and specificity of 98% for candidemia.[60] A 98% negative predictive value of the T2Candida panel for candidemia in neutropenic patients has been reported.[60]

The T2Candida Panel may be more useful than standard blood cultures when deescalating empiric antifungal therapy, with reports of patients receiving fewer days of antifungal therapy when using the T2Candida Panel.[61–63]

Further studies using this technology in the neutropenic patient population are needed.

Fungal antigen testing

Serologic assays that detect polysaccharides found in the fungal cell wall may be useful for the evaluation and diagnosis of IFD in neutropenic patients with prolonged or recurrent fevers.

Serum (1→3)-β-ᴅ-glucan

(1→3)-β-ᴅ-glucan (BG) is a polysaccharide in the cell wall of most fungi, with the exception of Mucorales and *Cryptococcus*.[64] Commercially available tests rely on activation of the coagulation cascade of the horseshoe crab in the presence of BG, with a positive test detecting concentrations of BG in the picogram per milliliter range. The Fungitell assay (Associates of Cape Cod, East Falmouth, MA), which is Food and Drug Administration approved, reports a positive result as a concentration greater than 80 pg/mL.[65]

The reported pooled sensitivity and specificity of 1 positive BG test in the setting of proved or probable IFD are 76.8% and 85.3%, respectively,[64] whereas 2 consecutive positive BG tests had a sensitivity of 49.6% and specificity of 98.9% in a cohort of hematology-oncology patients with proved or probable IFD.[66]

Invasive fungal disease due to *Candida* or *Aspergillus* species, 2 of the most common fungal pathogens that cause invasive infection during febrile neutropenia, can produce a positive glucan, so a positive result does not help identify the exact species of fungus causing infection.

False-positive test results can occur in patients who have been treated with IV albumin, IV immunoglobulin, and hemodialysis with a cellulose-containing membrane.[67]

Galactomannan

Galactomannan (GM) is a polysaccharide found in the cell walls of *Aspergillus* and *Penicillium* species and is released into the blood during fungal growth. The detection of GM in serum and/or bronchoalveolar lavage fluid (BAL) is a diagnostic tool for invasive aspergillosis (IA).

The Platelia assay, an enzyme immunoassay, can be used to measure GM in serum and BAL. A large meta-analysis found an overall sensitivity of 71% and specificity of 89% when using serum GM in cases of proved IA.[68] Biweekly GM testing has been found to increase the diagnostic sensitivity for IA in high-risk HCT patients but may be associated with higher costs and fewer additional diagnoses of IA.[69–71] Two large meta-analyses evaluating BAL GM reported a pooled sensitivity of 86% to 87% and specificity of 89% in cases of proved or probable IA infection.[72,73]

The sensitivity of the test decreases in patients receiving antimold therapy. Several published reports described false-positive GM results in patients receiving piperacillin-tazobactam,[74–77] although this problem has been attributed to contamination of the drug lot.[77,78] False-positive serum GM test results also have been reported in patients with underlying *Histoplasma* infection due to cross-reactivity in the assay.[79]

Radiographic Studies

CT of the chest may be useful in diagnosing IFD in neutropenic patients due to molds, such as *Aspergillus* species or Mucorales. The radiographic morphology of a pulmonary opacity on a CT scan of the chest can be suggestive of a potential fungal etiology.

Pulmonary IA classically manifests radiographically as a halo sign (**Fig. 4**), which is a masslike infiltrate with a surrounding halo of ground-glass attenuation.[80–82] Other radiographic findings in the setting of pulmonary IA at various stages of evolution include cavitary lesions, infarct-shaped nodules or consolidations, and air-crescent signs.[83]

Invasive pulmonary mucormycosis has been linked to a different radiographic sign, the reversed halo sign (**Fig. 5**), which is a central ground-glass opacity surrounded by a denser airspace consolidation.[84]

Empiric Antifungal Therapy

Current guidelines recommend the addition of an empiric antifungal agent if fever persists or recurs after 4 days to 7 days of initiation of antibacterial therapy during an episode of neutropenia.[1,3,85,86] The choice of empiric antifungal agent varies based on administration of antifungal prophylaxis. An echinocandin might be an appropriate empiric antifungal agent if no antifungal prophylaxis or if fluconazole or posaconazole were used for antifungal prophylaxis. If an echinocandin was used for antifungal prophylaxis, either voriconazole or amphotericin formulations might be potential empirical antifungal therapies.[1,3,85,86] Amphotericin formulations might be another option for empiric antifungal therapy if posaconazole was used for prophylaxis.[1,3]

Current guidelines do not provide guidance regarding duration of empiric antifungal therapy, but this treatment is often continued until the ANC is greater than or equal to 500 mm^3 if resolution of fever is achieved after addition of the antifungal agent.[1,3]

Preemptive Antifungal Therapy

Preemptive antifungal strategies, which include utilization of radiographic studies and serum fungal antigen tests before starting antifungal therapy, provide an alternative to empiric antifungal therapy in persistently febrile neutropenic patients. Proponents of this strategy argue that that preemptive therapy decreases unnecessary use of antifungal therapy and may have a place in fever and neutropenia algorithms.[71]

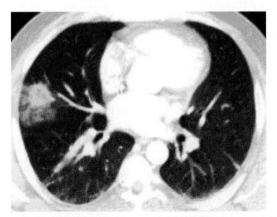

Fig. 4. Halo sign on chest CT. (*From* Raveendran S, Lu Z. CT findings and differential diagnosis in adults with invasive pulmonary aspergillosis. Radiol Infect Dis 2018;5(1):18; with permission.)

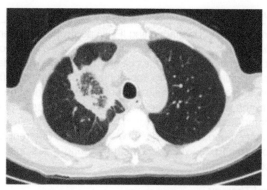

Fig. 5. Reversed halo sign. (*From* Cornely OA, Arikan-Akdagli S, Dannaoui E, et al. ESCMID and ECMM joint clinical guidelines for the diagnosis and management of mucormycosis 2013. Clin Microbiol Infect 2014;20 Suppl 3:12; with permission.)

A preemptive approach to antifungal therapy in febrile neutropenic patients is not currently recommended in either the Infectious Diseases Society of America or National Comprehensive Cancer Networksguidelines.[1,3]

SUMMARY

The approach to fever in a neutropenic patient with underlying hematologic malignancy or HCT should take into consideration the depth and duration of neutropenia, with a subsequent stepwise evaluation and empiric or directed therapies for bacterial and fungal infections. Use of center-specific algorithms may aid in appropriate escalation or de-escalation strategies in this patient population. In the era of growing antimicrobial resistance, newer de-escalation strategies based on diagnostic testing or clinical improvement may prove useful.

REFERENCES

1. Baden LR, Swaminathan S, Angarone M, et al. Prevention and treatment of cancer-related infections, version 2.2016, NCCN Clinical Practice Guidelines in Oncology. J Natl Compr Canc Netw 2016;14(7):882–913.
2. Bodey GP, Buckley M, Sathe YS, et al. Quantitative relationships between circulating leukocytes and infection in patients with acute leukemia. Ann Intern Med 1966;64(2):328–40.
3. Freifeld AG, Bow EJ, Sepkowitz KA, et al. Clinical practice guideline for the use of antimicrobial agents in neutropenic patients with cancer: 2010 update by the infectious diseases society of america. Clin Infect Dis 2011;52(4):e56–93.
4. Lyman GH, Michels SL, Reynolds MW, et al. Risk of mortality in patients with cancer who experience febrile neutropenia. Cancer 2010;116(23):5555–63.
5. Penack O, Buchheidt D, Christopeit M, et al. Management of sepsis in neutropenic patients: guidelines from the infectious diseases working party of the German Society of Hematology and Oncology. Ann Oncol 2011;22(5):1019–29.
6. Pettengell R, Schwenkglenks M, Leonard R, et al. Neutropenia occurrence and predictors of reduced chemotherapy delivery: results from the INC-EU prospective observational European neutropenia study. Support Care Cancer 2008; 16(11):1299–309.

7. Aquino VM, Herrera L, Sandler ES, et al. Feasibility of oral ciprofloxacin for the outpatient management of febrile neutropenia in selected children with cancer. Cancer 2000;88(7):1710–4.
8. Buchanan GR. Approach to treatment of the febrile cancer patient with low-risk neutropenia. Hematol Oncol Clin North Am 1993;7(5):919–35.
9. Paganini H, Rodriguez-Brieshcke T, Zubizarreta P, et al. Oral ciprofloxacin in the management of children with cancer with lower risk febrile neutropenia. Cancer 2001;91(8):1563–7.
10. Klastersky J, Paesmans M, Rubenstein EB, et al. The multinational association for supportive care in cancer risk index: a multinational scoring system for identifying low-risk febrile neutropenic cancer patients. J Clin Oncol 2000;18(16):3038–51.
11. Schimpff SC. Empiric antibiotic therapy for granulocytopenic cancer patients. Am J Med 1986;80(5C):13–20.
12. Gonzalez-Barca E, Fernandez-Sevilla A, Carratala J, et al. Prospective study of 288 episodes of bacteremia in neutropenic cancer patients in a single institution. Eur J Clin Microbiol Infect Dis 1996;15(4):291–6.
13. Ramphal R. Changes in the etiology of bacteremia in febrile neutropenic patients and the susceptibilities of the currently isolated pathogens. Clin Infect Dis 2004; 39(Suppl 1):S25–31.
14. Wisplinghoff H, Seifert H, Wenzel RP, et al. Current trends in the epidemiology of nosocomial bloodstream infections in patients with hematological malignancies and solid neoplasms in hospitals in the United States. Clin Infect Dis 2003; 36(9):1103–10.
15. Paul M, Borok S, Fraser A, et al. Additional anti-Gram-positive antibiotic treatment for febrile neutropenic cancer patients. Cochrane Database Syst Rev 2005;(3):CD003914.
16. Aguilar-Guisado M, Espigado I, Martin-Pena A, et al. Optimisation of empirical antimicrobial therapy in patients with haematological malignancies and febrile neutropenia (How Long study): an open-label, randomised, controlled phase 4 trial. Lancet Haematol 2017;4(12):e573–83.
17. Averbuch D, Orasch C, Cordonnier C, et al. European guidelines for empirical antibacterial therapy for febrile neutropenic patients in the era of growing resistance: summary of the 2011 4th European Conference on Infections in Leukemia. Haematologica 2013;98(12):1826–35.
18. Karimi K, Odhav A, Kollipara R, et al. Acute cutaneous necrosis: a guide to early diagnosis and treatment. J Cutan Med Surg 2017;21(5):425–37.
19. O'Sullivan GM, Worsnop F, Natkunarajah J. Ecthyma gangrenosum, an important cutaneous infection to recognize in the immunosuppressed patient. Clin Exp Dermatol 2018;43(1):67–9.
20. Reich HL, Williams Fadeyi D, Naik NS, et al. Nonpseudomonal ecthyma gangrenosum. J Am Acad Dermatol 2004;50(5 Suppl):S114–7.
21. Chang AY, Carlos CA, Schuster M, et al. Nonpseudomonal ecthyma gangrenosum associated with methicillin-resistant staphylococcus aureus infection: a case report and review of the literature. Cutis 2012;90(2):67–9.
22. Vaiman M, Lazarovitch T, Heller L, et al. Ecthyma gangrenosum and ecthyma-like lesions: review article. Eur J Clin Microbiol Infect Dis 2015;34(4):633–9.
23. Blijlevens NM, Donnelly JP, De Pauw BE. Mucosal barrier injury: biology, pathology, clinical counterparts and consequences of intensive treatment for haematological malignancy: an overview. Bone Marrow Transplant 2000;25(12):1269–78.
24. Gorschluter M, Mey U, Strehl J, et al. Neutropenic enterocolitis in adults: systematic analysis of evidence quality. Eur J Haematol 2005;75(1):1–13.

25. Nesher L, Rolston KV. Neutropenic enterocolitis, a growing concern in the era of widespread use of aggressive chemotherapy. Clin Infect Dis 2013;56(5):711–7.

26. Chakrabarti S, Pillay D, Ratcliffe D, et al. Resistance to antiviral drugs in herpes simplex virus infections among allogeneic stem cell transplant recipients: risk factors and prognostic significance. J Infect Dis 2000;181(6):2055–8.

27. Danve-Szatanek C, Aymard M, Thouvenot D, et al. Surveillance network for herpes simplex virus resistance to antiviral drugs: 3-year follow-up. J Clin Microbiol 2004;42(1):242–9.

28. Stranska R, Schuurman R, Nienhuis E, et al. Survey of acyclovir-resistant herpes simplex virus in the Netherlands: prevalence and characterization. J Clin Virol 2005;32(1):7–18.

29. Englund JA, Zimmerman ME, Swierkosz EM, et al. Herpes simplex virus resistant to acyclovir. A study in a tertiary care center. Ann Intern Med 1990;112(6):416–22.

30. Kimberlin DW, Crumpacker CS, Straus SE, et al. Antiviral resistance in clinical practice. Antiviral Res 1995;26(4):423–38.

31. Agut H, Bonnafous P, Gautheret-Dejean A. Laboratory and clinical aspects of human herpesvirus 6 infections. Clin Microbiol Rev 2015;28(2):313–35.

32. Salahuddin SZ, Ablashi DV, Markham PD, et al. Isolation of a new virus, HBLV, in patients with lymphoproliferative disorders. Science 1986;234(4776):596–601.

33. Hentrich M, Oruzio D, Jager G, et al. Impact of human herpesvirus-6 after haematopoietic stem cell transplantation. Br J Haematol 2005;128(1):66–72.

34. Ihira M, Yoshikawa T, Suzuki K, et al. Monitoring of active HHV-6 infection in bone marrow transplant recipients by real time PCR; comparison to detection of viral DNA in plasma by qualitative PCR. Microbiol Immunol 2002;46(10):701–5.

35. Imbert-Marcille BM, Tang XW, Lepelletier D, et al. Human herpesvirus 6 infection after autologous or allogeneic stem cell transplantation: a single-center prospective longitudinal study of 92 patients. Clin Infect Dis 2000;31(4):881–6.

36. Yoshikawa T, Asano Y, Ihira M, et al. Human herpesvirus 6 viremia in bone marrow transplant recipients: clinical features and risk factors. J Infect Dis 2002;185(7):847–53.

37. Cone RW, Huang ML, Corey L, et al. Human herpesvirus 6 infections after bone marrow transplantation: clinical and virologic manifestations. J Infect Dis 1999;179(2):311–8.

38. Ogata M, Kikuchi H, Satou T, et al. Human herpesvirus 6 DNA in plasma after allogeneic stem cell transplantation: incidence and clinical significance. J Infect Dis 2006;193(1):68–79.

39. Sashihara J, Tanaka-Taya K, Tanaka S, et al. High incidence of human herpesvirus 6 infection with a high viral load in cord blood stem cell transplant recipients. Blood 2002;100(6):2005–11.

40. Tomonari A, Takahashi S, Ooi J, et al. Human herpesvirus 6 variant A infection with fever, skin rash, and liver dysfunction in a patient after unrelated cord blood transplantation. Bone Marrow Transplant 2005;36(12):1109–10.

41. Zerr DM, Corey L, Kim HW. Clinical outcomes of human herpesvirus 6 reactivation after hematopoietic stem cell transplantation. Clin Infect Dis 2005;40(7):932–40.

42. Betts BC, Young JA, Ustun C, et al. Human herpesvirus 6 infection after hematopoietic cell transplantation: is routine surveillance necessary? Biol Blood Marrow Transplant 2011;17(10):1562–8.

43. Blijlevens NM, Donnelly JP, de Pauw BE. Impaired gut function as risk factor for invasive candidiasis in neutropenic patients. Br J Haematol 2002;117(2):259–64.

44. Bow EJ. Considerations in the approach to invasive fungal infection in patients with haematological malignancies. Br J Haematol 2008;140(2):133–52.

45. Van Burik JA, Leisenring W, Myerson D, et al. The effect of prophylactic flucona-zole on the clinical spectrum of fungal diseases in bone marrow transplant recip-ients with special attention to hepatic candidiasis: an autopsy study of 355 patients. Medicine 1998;77(4):246–54.

46. Hachem R, Hanna H, Kontoyiannis D, et al. The changing epidemiology of inva-sive candidiasis: Candida glabrata and Candida krusei as the leading causes of candidemia in hematologic malignancy. Cancer 2008;112(11):2493–9.

47. Robenshtok E, Gafter-Gvili A, Goldberg E, et al. Antifungal prophylaxis in cancer patients after chemotherapy or hematopoietic stem-cell transplantation: system-atic review and meta-analysis. J Clin Oncol 2007;25(34):5471–89.

48. Chamilos G, Luna M, Lewis RE, et al. Invasive fungal infections in patients with hematologic malignancies in a tertiary care cancer center: an autopsy study over a 15-year period (1989-2003). Haematologica 2006;91(7):986–9.

49. Marr KA, Carter RA, Boeckh M, et al. Invasive aspergillosis in allogeneic stem cell transplant recipients: changes in epidemiology and risk factors. Blood 2002; 100(13):4358–66.

50. Marr KA, Carter RA, Crippa F, et al. Epidemiology and outcome of mould infec-tions in hematopoietic stem cell transplant recipients. Clin Infect Dis 2002; 34(7):909–17.

51. Pagano L, Caira M, Candoni A, et al. The epidemiology of fungal infections in pa-tients with hematologic malignancies: the SEIFEM-2004 study. Haematologica 2006;91(8):1068–75.

52. Pagano L, Caira M, Nosari A, et al. Fungal infections in recipients of hematopoi-etic stem cell transplants: results of the SEIFEM B-2004 study–Sorveglianza Epi-demiologica Infezioni Fungine Nelle Emopatie Maligne. Clin Infect Dis 2007; 45(9):1161–70.

53. Wingard JR, Hsu J, Hiemenz JW. Hematopoietic stem cell transplantation: an overview of infection risks and epidemiology. Hematol Oncol Clin North Am 2011;25(1):101–16.

54. Gerson SL, Talbot GH, Hurwitz S, et al. Prolonged granulocytopenia: the major risk factor for invasive pulmonary aspergillosis in patients with acute leukemia. Ann Intern Med 1984;100(3):345–51.

55. Prentice HG, Kibbler CC, Prentice AG. Towards a targeted, risk-based, antifungal strategy in neutropenic patients. Br J Haematol 2000;110(2):273–84.

56. Segal BH. Aspergillosis. N Engl J Med 2009;360(18):1870–84.

57. Kozel TR, Wickes B. Fungal diagnostics. Cold Spring Harb Perspect Med 2014; 4(4):a019299.

58. Ostrosky-Zeichner L, Pappas PG. Invasive candidiasis in the intensive care unit. Crit Care Med 2006;34(3):857–63.

59. Stevens DA. Diagnosis of fungal infections: current status. J Antimicrob Chemo-ther 2002;49(Suppl 1):11–9.

60. Clancy CJ, Nguyen MH. T2 magnetic resonance for the diagnosis of bloodstream infections: charting a path forward. J Antimicrob Chemother 2018;73(suppl_4): iv2–5.

61. Munoz P, Vena A, Machado M, et al. T2Candida MR as a predictor of outcome in patients with suspected invasive candidiasis starting empirical antifungal treat-ment: a prospective pilot study. J Antimicrob Chemother 2018;73(suppl_4): iv6–12.

62. Munoz P, Vena A, Machado M, et al. T2MR contributes to the very early diagnosis of complicated candidaemia. A prospective study. J Antimicrob Chemother 2018; 73(suppl_4):iv13–9.

63. Patch ME, Weisz E, Cubillos A, et al. Impact of rapid, culture-independent diagnosis of candidaemia and invasive candidiasis in a community health system. J Antimicrob Chemother 2018;73(suppl_4):iv27–30.

64. Karageorgopoulos DE, Vouloumanou EK, Ntziora F, et al. beta-D-glucan assay for the diagnosis of invasive fungal infections: a meta-analysis. Clin Infect Dis 2011; 52(6):750–70.

65. Persat F, Ranque S, Derouin F, et al. Contribution of the (1–>3)-beta-D-glucan assay for diagnosis of invasive fungal infections. J Clin Microbiol 2008;46(3): 1009–13.

66. Lamoth F, Cruciani M, Mengoli C, et al. beta-Glucan antigenemia assay for the diagnosis of invasive fungal infections in patients with hematological malignancies: a systematic review and meta-analysis of cohort studies from the Third European Conference on Infections in Leukemia (ECIL-3). Clin Infect Dis 2012; 54(5):633–43.

67. Koo S, Bryar JM, Page JH, et al. Diagnostic performance of the (1–>3)-beta-D-glucan assay for invasive fungal disease. Clin Infect Dis 2009;49(11):1650–9.

68. Pfeiffer CD, Fine JP, Safdar N. Diagnosis of invasive aspergillosis using a galactomannan assay: a meta-analysis. Clin Infect Dis 2006;42(10):1417–27.

69. Foy PC, van Burik JA, Weisdorf DJ. Galactomannan antigen enzyme-linked immunosorbent assay for diagnosis of invasive aspergillosis after hematopoietic stem cell transplantation. Biol Blood Marrow Transplant 2007;13(4):440–3.

70. Ji Y, Xu LP, Liu DH, et al. Positive results of serum galactomannan assays and pulmonary computed tomography predict the higher response rate of empirical antifungal therapy in patients undergoing allogeneic hematopoietic stem cell transplantation. Biol Blood Marrow Transplant 2011;17(5):759–64.

71. Maertens J, Theunissen K, Verhoef G, et al. Galactomannan and computed tomography-based preemptive antifungal therapy in neutropenic patients at high risk for invasive fungal infection: a prospective feasibility study. Clin Infect Dis 2005;41(9):1242–50.

72. Guo YL, Chen YQ, Wang K, et al. Accuracy of BAL galactomannan in diagnosing invasive aspergillosis: a bivariate metaanalysis and systematic review. Chest 2010;138(4):817–24.

73. Zou M, Tang L, Zhao S, et al. Systematic review and meta-analysis of detecting galactomannan in bronchoalveolar lavage fluid for diagnosing invasive aspergillosis. PLoS One 2012;7(8):e43347.

74. Adam O, Auperin A, Wilquin F, et al. Treatment with piperacillin-tazobactam and false-positive Aspergillus galactomannan antigen test results for patients with hematological malignancies. Clin Infect Dis 2004;38(6):917–20.

75. Aubry A, Porcher R, Bottero J, et al. Occurrence and kinetics of false-positive Aspergillus galactomannan test results following treatment with beta-lactam antibiotics in patients with hematological disorders. J Clin Microbiol 2006;44(2): 389–94.

76. Sulahian A, Touratier S, Ribaud P. False positive test for aspergillus antigenemia related to concomitant administration of piperacillin and tazobactam. N Engl J Med 2003;349(24):2366–7.

77. Viscoli C, Machetti M, Cappellano P, et al. False-positive galactomannan platelia Aspergillus test results for patients receiving piperacillin-tazobactam. Clin Infect Dis 2004;38(6):913–6.

78. Mikulska M, Furfaro E, Del Bono V, et al. Piperacillin/tazobactam (Tazocin) seems to be no longer responsible for false-positive results of the galactomannan assay. J Antimicrob Chemother 2012;67(7):1746–8.

79. Wheat LJ, Hackett E, Durkin M, et al. Histoplasmosis-associated cross-reactivity in the BioRad Platelia Aspergillus enzyme immunoassay. Clin Vaccine Immunol 2007;14(5):638–40.
80. Kuhlman JE, Fishman EK, Siegelman SS. Invasive pulmonary aspergillosis in acute leukemia: characteristic findings on CT, the CT halo sign, and the role of CT in early diagnosis. Radiology 1985;157(3):611–4.
81. Orr DP, Myerowitz RL, Dubois PJ. Patho-radiologic correlation of invasive pulmonary aspergillosis in the compromised host. Cancer 1978;41(5):2028–39.
82. Primack SL, Hartman TE, Lee KS, et al. Pulmonary nodules and the CT halo sign. Radiology 1994;190(2):513–5.
83. Greene RE, Schlamm HT, Oestmann JW, et al. Imaging findings in acute invasive pulmonary aspergillosis: clinical significance of the halo sign. Clin Infect Dis 2007;44(3):373–9.
84. Wahba H, Truong MT, Lei X, et al. Reversed halo sign in invasive pulmonary fungal infections. Clin Infect Dis 2008;46(11):1733–7.
85. Freifeld A, Marchigiani D, Walsh T, et al. A double-blind comparison of empirical oral and intravenous antibiotic therapy for low-risk febrile patients with neutropenia during cancer chemotherapy. N Engl J Med 1999;341(5):305–11.
86. van Burik JA, Ratanatharathorn V, Stepan DE, et al. Micafungin versus fluconazole for prophylaxis against invasive fungal infections during neutropenia in patients undergoing hematopoietic stem cell transplantation. Clin Infect Dis 2004; 39(10):1407–16.

Bacterial Infections in the Stem Cell Transplant Recipient and Hematologic Malignancy Patient

Elizabeth Ann Misch, MD*, David R. Andes, MD

KEYWORDS

- Stem cell transplantation • Resistance • Gram negative • Gram positive
- Bacteremia • KPC-Kp • Vancomycin-resistant *enterococcus*

KEY POINTS

- Bacteremia (bloodstream infection [BSI]) is frequent in the stem cell transplant and hematologic malignancy population (20%–30% incidence) and often occurs in the early post-transplant engraftment period.
- In most studies, gram-positive bacteria (GPB) occur at greater frequency than gram-negative bacteria (GNB), although some centers report that rates of gram-negative BSI have recently increased.
- In many centers, resistance rates among *Enterococci* and GNB, especially the *Enterobacteriaceae*, are extensive and associated with increased mortality.
- *Pseudomonas aeruginosa* and *Acinetobacter baumannii* are less frequent causes of BSI but are often highly resistant.
- Better prediction tools, enhanced infection control, and new anti-infective agents hold promise for the treatment of highly resistant pathogens in this population.

INTRODUCTION

Patients with hematologic malignancy (HM) and individuals undergoing stem cell transplantation (SCT) are particularly vulnerable to bacterial infections for several reasons. This extra susceptibility stems from features of the underlying diseases in this population (acute myeloid leukemia [AML] and myelodysplastic syndrome are high risk), cytotoxic treatment regimens, immunologic incompatibility between donor and recipient, exposure to the health care environment, the presence

Disclosure: Each author reports no disclosures.
Department of Medicine, Division of Infectious Disease, University of Wisconsin School of Medicine and Public Health, 1685 Highland Drive, Centennial Building, 5th Floor, Madison, WI 53705, USA
* Corresponding author.
E-mail address: eamisch@medicine.wisc.edu

Infect Dis Clin N Am 33 (2019) 399–445
https://doi.org/10.1016/j.idc.2019.02.011
0891-5520/19/© 2019 Elsevier Inc. All rights reserved.

id.theclinics.com

of colonizing bacteria, and reliance on invasive devices (urinary and central venous catheters). The period of greatest vulnerability is generally within the first 30 days after transplant (**Fig. 1**). During this period, known as the pre-engraftment phase, myeloid and lymphoid cell lines may be entirely absent. Furthermore, SCT conditioning and cancer chemotherapy may cause epithelial cell injury (mucositis). Mucositis disrupts the usual barriers against incursions by endogenous flora. Individuals are generally hospitalized during this phase and highly exposed to nosocomial pathogens and invasive devices (see **Fig. 1**). An indicator of this vulnerability, febrile neutropenia, occurs in as many as 80% of patients undergoing chemotherapy or SCT.[1] Fever during neutropenia signals both immune perturbation and an encounter with microbes, often a host's own endogenous flora.

Bacteria are the most important pathogens during febrile neutropenia and the pre-engraftment phase, and bloodstream infection (BSI) is the most common infection event.[2,8,9] Central venous catheters allow easy access of skin-commensal organisms to the bloodstream. Central line–associated BSIs (CLABSIs) are especially frequent in the early postengraftment period and are most often due to gram-positive (GP)

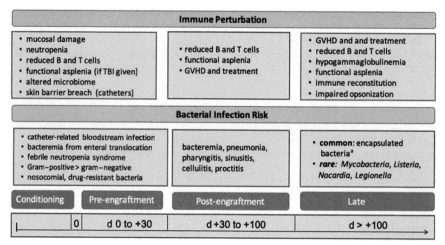

Fig. 1. Transplant phase, associated immune perturbation, and risk of specific infection syndromes. At the bottom of this figure, the transplant timeline is depicted, beginning with pretransplant conditioning. SCT occurs on day 0. After transplant, there is usually a 2-week to 4-week period during which the recipient has an entirely depleted bone marrow and low white blood cell and red blood cell counts, the pre-engraftment phase. By day 30, marrow recovery has usually occurred and some immune function is restored. Days 30 to 100 are known as the early postengraftment period or phase. The period after day 100 is referred to as late postengraftment. The occurrence of specific infection syndromes (bacterial infection risk) can be approximately assigned to one or more pretransplant or post-transplant periods (conditioning/pre-engraftment, early postengraftment, or late postengraftment). Similarly, there is a stereotypic set of immune defects (immune perturbations) that characterize each post-transplant period. For example, most bacterial BSIs occur during conditioning and pre-engraftment, as a result of the risk posed by intravascular devices, damage to the intestinal epithelium (leading to bacterial translocation to the blood) as a result of chemotherapy, conditioning or irradiation, and the absence of innate immune responses (neutrophils and monocytes) and T cells and B cells. [a] Most common: *Haemophilus influenzae* and *Streptococcus pneumoniae*; less common: *Neisseria meningitidis*. TBI, total body irradiation. (*Data from* Refs.[2–7])

organisms.[10] In US national surveillance data, SCT patients are the risk group with the highest incidence of CLABSI, with rates that exceed hospitalized patients who have acute leukemia or who are on general oncology units.[11] In the studies reviewed, CLABSI comprises between 16% and 41% of BSIs and affects 3% to 36% of SCT/HM patients.[12–14]

In comparison to past eras, bacterial infections remain common in the contemporary SCT and HM populations. A 1997 study of 66 German patients undergoing chemotherapy and autologous peripheral SCT found clinical or microbiologic evidence of infection in 48% of patients and bacteremia in 39%.[15] Other studies published in the 1990s reported a 10% to 30% incidence of bacteremia.[16–19] Published in 2014, a multicenter prospective study of 720 Spanish patients who underwent autologous SCT between 1998 and 2003 found bacterial infection had occurred in 25% and bacteremia in 20% of patients after transplant, respectively.[14] The contemporary studies reviewed in this article (from 2014 forward) demonstrate rates of bacteremia ranging from 7% to over 50% (**Table 1**).[12–14,20–38] In certain subgroups (allogeneic SCT) and geographic regions, the incidence of BSI has been reported to be as high as 75%.[20]

Pneumonia, skin and soft tissue infection, pharyngitis, sinusitis, gastrointestinal (GI) infections (including typhlitis, see Sunita Nathan and Celalettin Ustun's article, "Complications of Stem Cell Transplantation that affect Infections for the Stem Cell Transplant Recipient, with Analogies to the Hematologic Malignancy Patient," in this issue), perirectal abscess, proctitis, and urinary tract infections (UTIs) are also important infectious syndromes in this population. Several of these bacterial infection syndromes (pneumonia, pharyngitis, sinusitis, and GI infections) have clinical overlap with viral or fungal infection syndromes (pneumonia) or noninfectious processes (mucositis) or are polymicrobial in nature (perirectal abscess). As an example, data on the incidence and microbiologic etiology of pneumonia are scant in the SCT/HM literature. Available estimates of the frequency of bacterial pneumonia in the SCT population (see **Table 1**) range from 11% to 24%.[12,14,21–23] This lack of data reflects the difficulty in assigning a microbiologic etiology to pneumonia also seen in the general population. A large pneumonia etiology study in US inpatients found a definite cause of pneumonia in only 38% of cases, despite intensive investigation using both culture-based and non–culture-based tests.[39] An autopsy study in SCT has shown that diffuse alveolar hemorrhage or diffuse alveolar damage are common mimics of pneumonia in the SCT population.[40]

Similarly, UTIs are not well characterized in the SCT/HM population. Available data suggest rates may range from 4% to 20%.[12,21,22,24] Systematic surveys of bacterial skin and soft tissue infection in the SCT and HM population do not exist, to the authors' knowledge. Most of the available data consist of case reports of opportunistic pathogens with cutaneous presentations, such as nocardiosis, nontuberculous mycobacteria, and legionellosis.[41–44] In the studies reviewed in this article, skin and soft tissue infections make only small contributions (1% to 2%) to overall bacterial infection.[24,45]

Bacterial meningitis seems uncommon. One study suggests it may occur with a frequency 30-fold higher than among the non-SCT population.[46]

Atypical bacterial pathogens, such as *Legionella*, *Nocardia*, nontuberculous mycobacteria, and *Mycobacterium tuberculosis*, occur infrequently but are reported in outbreaks and in association with the hospital environment and vascular catheters.[22,25,44,47–52] Nocardia, with an estimated incidence of 0.3% to 1.7%, is most frequently seen in the late post-transplant period, almost always involves the lung, with frequent dissemination to the blood.[53] Infections due to these atypical organisms

Table 1
Frequency of bacterial infections in patients with hematologic malignancy or stem cell transplant

Reference	Location, Time Period, Study Design	Transplant Features	Population	Antibacterial Prophylaxis	Number and Percent of Bacterial Infections in Cohort	Bloodstream Infection Frequency, Etiology, and Resistance	Risk Factors[a] for Bacterial Infections or Bloodstream Infections	Mortality and Other Outcomes Associated with Bacterial Infections/ Bloodstream Infections

Wang et al,[23] 2018	Taiwan, single-center, 2005–2014, retrospective cohort study of BSIs and death within 45 d of SCT
	
	Comments
	• Stated all pts had Hickman catheters
	• Slight predominance of GN BSI
	• Early BSI only
	• BSI associated with higher mortality in autoSCT pts
		AlloSCT (55)
		• pSCT: 96%
		• MA: 69%
		• TBI: 33%
		• aGVHD: 55 (100%)
		• Grade 3–4 aGVHD: 7 (13%)
		• Median engraft: D17
		AutoSCT (50)
		• Median engraftment: D12
			105 adults
			AlloSCT (55)
			• Mean age: 30 y
			• Lymphoma: 3
			• AML: 20
			• ALL: 19
			• CML: 3
			• MDS: 3
			• Apl A: 7
			AutoSCT (50)
			• Mean age: 42 y
			• Lymphoma: 31
			• AML: 4
			• MM: 15
				• Universal
				• Levo 500 mg/d (2005–2010)
				• Levo 750 mg/d (2011–2014)
					• 117 episodes (4 non-BI)
					• 95/105 pts
					• FUO: 47/105 (45%)
					• BSI: 25/105 (24%)
					• PNA[f]: 25/105 24%
					• Septic shock[f]: 11/105 (10%)
					• Oral cavity[f]: 6/105 (6%)
					• Soft tissue[f]: 4/105 4%
					• GI infection[f]:
					• 1/105 (1%)
						• 28 total
						• 26 pre-engraft
						• 25 pts (24%)
						AlloSCT: 15/55 (27%)
						• 69 episodes
						AutoSCT: 10/50 (20%)
						• 48 episodes
						BSI overview
						• GP: 13/28 (46%)
						• GN: 14/28 (50%)
						• Ana: 1 (4%)
						GPB: 13
						  CoNS: 5 (38%)
						  • MR CoNS: 40%
						  Strep: 4 (30%)
						  • Pcn-R: 50%
						  • Clinda-R: 50%
						  • FQ-R: 50%
						  • Mac-R: 75%
						  SA: 1 (8%)
						  • Pcn-R
						  • MSSA
						  E faecium: 1
						  • Amp-R
						  • VRE
						GNB: 14
						  EC: 7 (54%)
						  • CFP-R: 14%
						  • FQ-R: 100%
						  • IMI-R: 0%
						  • MDR: 86%
							AlloSCT
							• Grade 3–4 aGVHD (2/55 (3.6%) had postengraft BSI coinciding with aGVHD)
							AutoSCT
							• Longer pre-engraft period
								AlloSCT mortality
								• Total: 7/55 (13%)
								• BSI: 5/55 (9%)
								• PNA: 1/55 (2%)
								• Higher mortality in pts with BSI than those without (33% vs 5%; P = .013)
								AutoSCT mortality
								• Total: 2/50 (4%)
								• BSI: 1/50 (2%)
								• PNA: 1/50 (2%)
								• No significant difference in mortality in BSI vs non-BSI pts (10% vs 2.5%; P = .36)
								AutoSCT other BSI outcomes
								• Engraft delayed in BSI pts (15 d vs 12 d; P = .002)
								• Longer hospital stay in BSI (25 d vs 21 d; P = .014)

Study	Description / Comments	Transplant characteristics	Patients	Prophylaxis	Onset	Resistance / Organisms	Outcomes	Mortality

Averbuch et al,[13] 2017	Large, international observational, prospective study of GNB and resistance, 2014–2015 (65 centers, 25 countries in Europe, Australia, and Asia). All BSIs from conditioning through 6 mo analyzed. Not an incidence study—all included pts had GN BSI
	
	Comments
	• High rates of abx R in Europe
	• Geographic pattern of more R in southeastern vs northwestern Europe
	• Mortality associated with FQ-R, carb-R, noncarb-R
	• Includes children, who had rates of
		Total: 591
		AutoSCT 231 (39%)
		AlloSCT 360 (61%)
		• Unrelated: 49%
		• MRD: 32%
		• MMRD: 19%
		stem cells
		• PBSCT: 76%
		• BMSCT: 17%
		• UCB: 5%
		Conditioning
		• MA: 68%
		• RIC: 32%
		aGVHD
		• Before BSI: 17%
		• At time of BSI: 17%
			591 pts
			Mean age: 51 y
			Children: 13%
			• Acute leukemia: 212 (36%)
			• Lymphoma: 25%
			• Plasma cell disorder: 18%
			• MDS/MP: 9%
				Adult alloSCT
				• FQ: 76%
				Adult autoSCT
				• FQ: 45%
				Pediatric alloSCT
				• FQ: 25%
				Pediatric autoSCT
				• FQ: 9%
					n/d	Kleb: 2 (15%)
						• CFP-R: 100%
						• IMI-R: 0%
						• FQ-R: 100%
						• MDR: 100%
						Acineto: 2
						• MDR: 100%
						• pan-R: 1
						Enterobacter: 1
						• MDR: 1
						Achromo: 1
						• MDR: 1
						Serratia: 1
						• MDR: 1
						
						655 GN BSI
						• BSI with 1 isolate: 84%
						• BSI with ≥2 isolates: 17%
						591 pts
						• Median onset: D8
						AlloSCT
						• FQ-R: 56%
						• Noncarb-R: 59%
						• Carb-R: 24%
						• MDR: 44%
						AutoSCT
						• FQ-R: 41%
						• Noncarb-R: 36%
						• Carb-R: 9%
						• MDR: 20%
						Total GN isolates: 704
						• EB: 73%
						• EC: 43%
						• KP: 18%
						• Other EB: 12%
						• NFRM GNR: 24%
						• PsA: 14%
						• Steno: 5%
						• Acineto: 2%
						• Other: 3%
							Overall GN BSI
							• Not a/w with
							  ○ Carb-R
							  ○ Non-carb[9]-R
							  ○ FQ-R
							Overall GN R
							• Rates higher in alloSCT unless community-acquired BSI
							• Rates higher in southeastern vs northwestern European countries
							  ○ Noncarb-R (55% vs 28%)
							  ○ Carb-R (21% vs 5%)
							  ○ FQ-R (54% vs 36%)
							  ○ MDR (39% vs 14%)
							R risk factors
							FQ-R
							• FQ ppx
							• Age
								7-d mortality
								• 38/589 (7%)
								• ↑ in noncarb-R vs noncarb-S (9% vs 2%; $P = .002$)
								• ↑ in carb-R vs carb-S (18% vs 4%; $P<.001$)
								• ↑ in MDR vs nonMDR (11% vs 4%; $P = .002$)
								Inappropriate therapy
								• 21% all GN BSI
								• 64% carb-R BSI
								• 46% MDR
								• 37% noncarb-R (all $P<.001$)

(continued on next page)

Table 1
(continued)

Reference	Location, Time Period, Study Design	Transplant Features	Population	Antibacterial Prophylaxis	Number and Percent of Bacterial Infections in Cohort	Bloodstream Infection Frequency, Etiology, and Resistance	Risk Factors[a] for Bacterial Infections or Bloodstream Infections	Mortality and Other Outcomes Associated with Bacterial Infections/ Bloodstream Infections
	resistance similar to adults • High CLABSI rates (36%)					CLABSI incid: 211/655 (36%) All GN • FQ-R: 50% • Carb-R: 19% • MDR: 35% • Noncarb-R: 50%[g] All EB • FQ-R: 57% • Noncarb-R[g]: 51% • Carb-R: 8% • MDR: 32% • AG-R: 33% • Colistin: 5% • Tigecycline: 6% EC • FQ-R: 65% • Noncarb-R[g]: 50% • Carb-R: 2% • MDR: 28% • AG-R: 32% • Colistin: 0% • Tigecycline: 2% P • FQ-R: 64% • Noncarb-R[g]: 67% • Carb-R: 25% • MDR: 52% • AG-R: 43% • Colistin: 7% • Tigecycline: 16% Enterobacter • FQ-R: 21% • Noncarb-R[g]: 49% • Carb-R: 7%	• Duration NP ↑ in EB BSI (57% in EB vs 31% in non-EB) Carb-R • On carb therapy • In ICU • Prior tx with other abx (excluding FQ, AG, βL/βLI)[h] • In-hospital days prior to BSI • ↑ in NFRM GNR MDR • On carb • On βL/βLI[h] • In-hospital days prior to BSI • ↑ in NFRM GNR Noncarb-R[g] • On ceph • Prior tx with other abx (excluding FQ, AG, βL/βLI)[h] • On βL/βLI[h] • In hospital • ↑ in adults vs children	

César-Arce et al,[12] 2017	210 SCT • Auto: 144 • Allo: 66 • MA: 93%	210 ps • Mean age: 38 y • Leukemia: 64 (31%) • HL: 32 (15%) • NHL: 52 (25%) • MDS/Apl A: 6 (3%) • MM: 56 (27%)	Allo • Ciprofloxacin (D0–35) • Metronidazole (D0–35) • T/S (D0–100) Auto • Ciprofloxacin (D 0–35)	Total infxns • Episodes: 184 (includes non-BI) • 109 pts • Incid: 22.4/1000 hospital days Presumed BI incid: • PNA[d]: 40 (19%) • BSI: 36 (33%) • UTI[e]: 30 (14%) • CLABSI: 28 (13%) • CDI: n/d	MDR: 23% • AG-R: 20% • Colistin: 0% • Tigecycline: 8% PsA • FQ-R: 30% • Noncarb-R[g]: 36% • Carb-R: 38% • MDR: 29% • AG-R: 27% • Colistin: 2% Steno • FQ-R: 27% • Noncarb-R[g]: 88% • Carb-R: 100% • MDR: 100% • AG-R: 100% • Colistin: 30% • Tigecycline: 0% • T/S-R: 19% Acineto • FQ-R: 70% • Noncarb-R[g]: 80% • Carb-R: 64% • MDR: 64% • AG-R: 46% • Colistin: 11% • Tigecycline: 67% BSI • Total: 69 (33% of pts) • CLABSI: 28 (13%) • Primary BSI: 36 (17%) • Secondary BSI: 5 (2%) • MDR: 25 (12%) • ESBL: 26 (13%) BSI overview • 110 isolates • MDR: 31/110 • ESBL: 27/110 • GNB: 71 (65%) • EC: 52 (47%)	• Allo vs auto: more MDR infxns (24% vs 6%; *P* = .0002) Overall 30-d mortality • 14/210 (7%), all due to neutropenia and infxn (not specified as BI) Overall 12-mo mortality • 59/210 (28%) • Allo: 44/66 (49%) • Auto: 27/144 (19%) • Any infxn vs no infxn: 75% vs 25%; *P*<.001
Mexico, single-center, 2009–2014. Retrospective, descriptive study of incid of all infxns within first year after SCT and outcomes at 30 d and 12 mo Comments • Includes all bacterial infxns within first year					

(continued on next page)

Table 1 (*continued*)

Reference	Location, Time Period, Study Design	Transplant Features	Population	Antibacterial Prophylaxis	Number and Percent of Bacterial Infections in Cohort	Bloodstream Infection Frequency, Etiology, and Resistance	Risk Factors[a] for Bacterial Infections or Bloodstream Infections	Mortality and Other Outcomes Associated with Bacterial Infections/Infections/Bloodstream Infections
						• ESBL EC: 26 (46%) • MDR PsA: 1 (1%) GPB: 39 (35%) • S epi: 13 (12%) ○ All CLABSI • VRE: 2 (2%) • MRSA: 1 (2%) All CLABSI as a % of BSI: 28/69 (41%)		• Does not distinguish between pre-engraft and postengraft BI/BSI • CLABSI contribution to BSI described (41%) • GN BSI predominate • High rates GN resistance • Infxns captured from D0–D365 post-transplant	Univariate analysis • Composite infxn and MDR BI associated with increase in 12-mo mortality Multivariate analysis • PNA a/w ↑ 12-mo mortality • BI or BSI not a/w 12-mo mortality
Girmenia et al,[38] 2017	Italy, 2014, prospective, multicenter (54 sites) descriptive study of pre-engraftment GN BSI and 4 m post-SCT mortality **Comments** • See text. • PsA comprised a larger fraction of GN BSI (14%) than most other studies. • Colonization with Carb-NS Kleb or ○ MDR PsA greatly increased risk of pre-engraft BSI with same isolate • Abx R a/w ↑ mortality • RFs of prior colonization/infxn	AlloSCT • 1118 pts • BMT: 43% • PBSCT: 55% • UCB: 3% • MRD: 27% • MMRD: 32% ○ 88% haplo • MUD: 26% • MMUD: 13% • MA: 74% • RIC: 22% • TCD: 40% AutoSCT • 1625 pts • PBSCT: 99.5% • BMT: 0.5% • RIC: 2% • MA: 91%	2743 pts AlloSCT • 1118 pts • Median age: 44 y • AML: 38% • ALL: 18% • MDS: 9% • NHL: 9% • HL: 6% • MM, plasma cell leukemia, amyloidosis: 5% • Apl A: 3% AutoSCT • 1625: pts • Median age: 56 y • AML: 3% • ALL: 1% • MDS: <0.1% • NHL: 27% • HL: 10%	AlloSCT • FQ in 860 (77%) AutoSCT • FQ in 1326 (82%)	Total MC BIs • 670 pts: 24% • 710 episodes AlloSCT • 341 pts (31%) • 366 MC BI episodes • GP BI: 193 pts (17%) • GN BI: 148 pts (13%) Clinical infxn episodes, alloSCT[†] • Total: 68 (6%) • PNA: 39 (4%) • Skin: 14 (1%) • GI tract: 6 (0.5%) AutoSCT • 344 pts (21%) • 329 MC BI episodes • GP BI: 172 pts (11%) • GN BI: 157 pts (10%) Clinical infxn episodes, autoSCT[†] • Total: 87 (5%)	AlloSCT D30 cum incid • GN BSI: 140 pts (17%) • 149 isolates ○ EC: 77 (52%) ○ Kp: 28 (19%) ○ All PsA: 21 (14%) ○ MDR PsA: 8 (5%) ○ Ceph-NS, carb-NS Kleb: 16 (11%) ○ GP BSI not reported AutoSCT D20 cum incidence GN BSI • GN BSI: 146 pts (9%) • 151 episodes ○ EC: 92 (61%) ○ Kp: 23 (15%) ○ All PsA: 13 (9%)	GN BSI in alloSCT • Ex vivo TCD lower risk (RR 0.13; P = .004) • Older age • Acute leukemia • Donor mismatch • Cord blood • Duration NP • Colonization with rGNB associated with pre-engraft BSI with same species, R pattern. Risk ratios for BSI of colonized/uncolonized were ○ Ceph-NS/carb-S EC (~RR: 7) ○ Carb-NS Kleb (~RR: 70) ○ nonMDR PsA (~RR: 48)	Death before engraft • Allo: 39% if GN BSI • Auto: 36% if GN BSI 4-mo survival, overall • Allo: 86% ○ No GN BSI: 88% • Auto: 97% ○ No GN BSI: 97.5% 4-mo survival in GN BSI • Allo ○ ceph-NS EC: 80% ○ nonMDR PsA: 62% ○ Carb-NS Kleb: 40% ○ MDR PsA: 25% • Auto ○ Ceph-S Kleb BSI: 86% ○ NonMDR PsA BSI: 83%

may justify targeted prophylaxis	• MM, plasma cell leukemia, amyloidosis: 52%
	• Solid tumors: 5%
		• PNA: 53 (3%)
		• GI tract: 20 (1%)
		• Skin: 12 (0.7%)
			○ Ceph-NS carb-NS Kleb 6 (4%)
			• GP BSI not reported
				• Pre-SCT BSI was RF for post-SCT BSI with same species, R pattern when pre-SCT BSI due to
				  ○ Ceph-NS/carb-S EC (~RR ≥6)
				  ○ Carb-NS Kleb (~RR ≥35)
				  ○ NonMDR PsA (~RR ≥13)
				• GN BSI in autoSCT
				• Lymphoma
				• Other diagnosis
				• Older age
				• No abx ppx
				• Colonization with
				  ○ Ceph-NS/carb-S Kp (~RR: 63)
				  ○ Carb-NS Kleb (~RR: 2714)
				  ○ MDR PsA (~RR: 7142) a/w with pre-engraft BSI with same species, R pattern
					○ Carb-NS Kleb BSI: 67%
					• 4-mo mortality in BSI
					• Allo: HR of death 2.1, with pre-engraft GN BSI (P<.001)
					• Auto: HR of death 2.4, with pre-engraft GN BSI (P = .01)

Schuster et al,[22] 2017	United States, 2006-2011, multicenter, prospective study of early and late post-transplant infxns occurring after SCT. Median follow-up: 413 d Comments • Moderate-sized study • Four US sites • Allows only estimates of % of bacterial PNA • No resistance data	AlloSCT • Total: 444 • MUD: 55% • MRD: 40% • MMURD: 5% • PBSCT: 87% • BMT: 12% • UCB: 1% • TCD: 2 (<1%) • MA: 72% • GVHD: 76%	431 adults (≥18 y) • Median age: 53 y • AML: 41% • NHL: 18% • Other: 13% • ALL: 9% • CML: 5% • HL: 2%	• Pts with BSI: 231/431(57%) • Episodes of BSI: 387 • Median onset: D48 Non-BSI infxn • CDI: 148/431 (33%) • >1 CDI episode: 38/148 (26%) • Median onset CDI: D27 • Bacterial PNA: ~67 pts (~15.5%) • UTI: 89 (20%) • Bacterial sinusitis: 2 (<1%)	• n/d Total BSIs: 387 • GP BSI: 244 (63%) • CoNS: 125 (32%) • VRE: 41 (11%) • Enterococcus: 39 (10%) • SA: 24 (6%) • MSSA: 17 (4%) • MRSA: 7 (2%) • GN BSI: 93 (24%) • PsA: 24 (6%) • EC: 20 (6%) • Steno: 6 (2%) • Polymicrobial: 50 (13%) • Anaerobic: 1 (<1%)	C difficile • MA conditioning regimen: OR 1.6; 95% CI 1.1-2.3 Crude mortality: 52% Mortality in BSI • GNB: 45% • GPB: 13% (P = .02) Mortality risk • CDI: OR 1.9; 95% CI, 1.3-2.9 • PNA: OR 1.8; 95% CI, 1.2-2.7

(continued on next page)

Table 1
(continued)

Reference	Location, Time Period, Study Design	Transplant Features	Population	Antibacterial Prophylaxis	Number and Percent of Bacterial Infections in Cohort	Bloodstream Infection Frequency, Etiology, and Resistance	Risk Factors[a] for Bacterial Infections or Bloodstream Infections	Mortality and Other Outcomes Associated with Bacterial Infections/ Bloodstream Infections
	• PsA most common GNB				• PNA: 30% (for MC PNA, 38/75 bacterial) • Nocardia: 0 • Mycobacteria: 0			
Slade et al,[35] 2017	United States, 2009–2015, single-center, retrospective cohort. Median follow-up: 218 d Comments • High incid of enterococcal infxn • VRE colonization a/w later BSI and ↑ mortality • CDI had no effect on survival and was not a/w GVHD • Few SA BIs	• Haploidnt pSCT with PTCy • No TCD • Median time to engraft: 17 d Conditioning • MA: 41% • RIC: 59% GVHD • Acute: 36% • Chronic: 43%	104 adults with HM • Median age: 50 y • AML: 67% • ALL: 11% • MDS: 11% • Other: 12%	• No routine ppx	• All BIs are MCIs Incid in pts • Total pts: 64/104 • GPC: 44/104 (42%) • GNR: 30/104 (29%) • Enterococcus 27/104 (26%) • VRE 23/104 (22%) • CoNS: 14/104 (13%) • Strep spp: 7/104 (7%) • PsA: 6/64 (9%) • CDI: 13/104 (13%) • rCDI: 3/13 (23%) Isolate freq • GPC: 63% • GNR: 57% • GPR (non-CDI): 5% • Enterococcus: 24% • VRE: 20% • CoNS: 10% • SP: 1% • non-SP Strep: 5% • CDI: 11% • PsA: 64% • EB: 27% • Steno: 6% • GN anaerobes: 1%	Total BIs: 146 Total pts: 64 Timing of BI due to enteric species • Pre-engraft: 26% • D31-100: 28% • >D100: 46% "Significant" BSI • Enterococcus: 18/64 (28%) • CoNS: 13/64 (20%) • SA 1/64 (2%) • GNR: 30/64 • PsA: 3/63 (5%)	BSI within 100 d • Mucositis • CVC VRE BSI • Prior colonization	• Overall mortality: 51/104 (49%) • BI a/w ↑ mortality • Enterococcal infxn a/w ↑ early mortality

| Weisser et al,[26] 2017 | Multicenter, prospective database of nosocomial BSI and PNA during hospital admission for SCT in setting of NP, 2002–2014. Survey data from 20 centers in Germany, Switzerland, Austria. During NP, weekly screening for BSI. Follow-up until discharge, transfer, or death. Data divided into 3 periods: 2002–2006, 2007–2010, and 2011–2014.

Comments
• GP BSIs predominates
• GN BSIs ↑ over study period
• No analysis of risk factors or associated mortality | • AutoSCT: 6537 (43%)
• AlloSCT: 8644 (60%)
• Stem cell source
  ○ PB: 97%
  ○ BM: 3%
  ○ UCB: <1% | 15,181 SCT
• Median age: 55 y
• AML: 27%
• MM: 26%
• NHL: 18%
• Other: 15%
• MDS: 5%
• CML: 3% | 2009–2014
AutoSCT: FQ 54%
AlloSCT: FQ 60% | All BSIs | Total pts with BSI 2388 (16%)
BSI incidence:
9%–32% (varied by center)
• GP BSI: 1529 (10%)
• GN BSI: 767 (5%)
• Anaerobic BSI:23 (0.2%)
• Monomicrobial BSI: 2219 (93%)

Isolated species
GP BSI
• CoNS: 933 (39%)
• Enterococci: 271 (11%)
  ○ VRE: 11%
• Strep: 190 (8%)
• SA: 50 (2%)
  ○ MRSA: 26%

GN BSI
• EC: 476 (20%)
• PsA: 93 (4%)
• Kleb: 69 (3%)
• Steno: 32 (1%)
• EB: ~582 (~24%)
  ○ ESBL: 11%

Trends 2002–2014
• GN BSI ↑, all (4% → 7%)
• GP BSI ↓, all (16% → 14%)
• EC ↑ (2.7% → 4.4% in all; 3.6% → 4.9% in auto; 1.1% → 3.8% in allo)
• Enterococci ↑ allo only (1.8% → 3.3%)
• No MRSA after 2010 | GP BSI
• AlloSCT vs autoSCT (RR 1.4; 95% CI 1.3–1.6) | Mortality rate during NP: 477 (3.1%) |

(continued on next page)

Table 1
(continued)

Reference	Location, Time Period, Study Design	Transplant Features	Population	Antibacterial Prophylaxis	Number and Percent of Bacterial Infections in Cohort	Bloodstream Infection Frequency, Etiology, and Resistance	Risk Factors[a] for Bacterial Infections or Bloodstream Infections	Mortality and Other Outcomes Associated with Bacterial Infections/Bloodstream Infections

						2002–2010
						• CoNS ↓
						  ○ 7% → 4%, all
						  ○ 8% → 6%, allo
						  ○ 8% → 2%, auto		

Zheng et al,[34] 2017	China, single-center, 2007–2014, retrospective study of pre-engraft BSI and outcomes; 5-y follow-up	• UCB
		• All unrelated
		• All MA
		  ○ Bu-CY
		  ○ TBI-Cy regimen
		  ○ No ATG
		  ○ No MTX
			226 pts considered high risk at diagnosis
			• ALL: 131
			• AML: 95
				• Cefdinir
				• T/S after engraft
				• IV IgG weekly D7–100, then monthly × 6 mo
					All BIs were pre-engraft BSI
					• Median onset after UCB: 4.5 d
						Total BSIs
						• 72/226 (32%) (69 episodes analyzed; 3 polymicrobial BSIs excluded)
						GN BSI: 44/69 (64%)
						• EC: 29 (42%)
						• Kleb: 8 (12%)
						• PsA: 4 (6%)
						GP BSI: 25/69 (36%)
						• VGS: 7 (10%)
						• E faecium: 6 (9%)
						• S epi: 4 (6%)
						• All Strep spp: 13 (19%)
						• All Staph spp: 5 (7%)
						• SA: 0
							• BSI ↑ in TBI-Cy regimen vs Bu-Cy ($P = .03$)	Mortality
								• BSI vs no BSI: no difference in D180 TRM, engraft, acute or chronic GVHD, or 5-y disease relapse
								• GN vs GP BSI: GN associated with increase in 180 d TRM (39% vs 8%; $P = .01$)
								Overall survival and disease-free survival at 5 y
								• BSI vs no BSI: no difference
								• GP vs GN BSI, OS: 79% vs 44% (HR 0.36; $P = .046$)
								• GP vs GN BSI, disease-free survival: 67% vs 43% ($P = .11$)

Ballen et al,[21] 2016	International registry study (CIBMTR), 2008–2011 Descriptive analysis of infxn incid (density)[b]	1781 SCTs • All first SCT • All alt donors • UCB: 568 pts • MUD: 930 ○ 82% pSCT	1781 adults • All >16 y old • All acute leukemia, in remission • AML: 1374 (77%) • ALL: 407 (23%)	n/d	1-y incid all BIs • UCB: 72% • MMUD: 65% • MUD: 59% • $P<.0001$	BSI episodes • 189 total • 100 pre-engraft • 80 postengraft	BI density • MMUD vs MUD: RR 1.2; $P = .03$ • UCB vs MUD: RR 1.6; $P<.001$	Univariate analysis of overall NRM • MMUD: 27% • UCB: 33% • MUD: 14% • $P<.0001$

Study	Population	Prophylaxis	BI epidemiology	Analysis / Outcomes
and mortality at 100 d and 1 y post-SCT in participating centers. Comments • 450 transplant centers in registry • BI, not BSI, outcomes analyzed • Excluded commensal bacteria from nonsterile body sites • Infxn density reported • Bacterial UTI confirmed • No resistance data • No CDI data • BI associated with worse outcome • UCB with sig higher rate of GN BI	• MMUD ○ 81% pSCT • MA: 71% • RIC: 29% • pts who received TCD, CD34 selection, and PTCy were excluded Median follow-up • MUD: 58 mo • MMUD: 56 mo • UCB: 46 mo • Median age ○ UCB: 43 y ○ MUD: 48 y ○ MMUD: 47 y		Types of BI • GP BSI: 70% of GP BI • GN BSI: 60% of GN BI • UTI: 16% of all BIs • PNA: n/d GNB • 60% BSI • UCB: 28% • MMUD: 23% • MUD: 21% • $P = .013$ GPB • 70% BSI • UCB: n/d • MMUD: n/d • MUD: n/d • GP BI density • MMUD, UCB (vs MUD) higher risk ($P<.001$) • GN BI density • UCB (vs MUD, MMUD): higher risk ($P = .003$) BI within 90 d • Lower with RIC vs MA: RR 0.59; $P<.0001$ BSI risk • Not analyzed separately	• aGVHD: RR 1.4; $P = .0001$ • cGVHD: RR 1.5; $P = .0024$ • SCT in 2010–2011 vs 2008-09: RR 0.94; $P = .02$ Multivariate analysis of overall mortality risk • BI vs no BI: RR 2.45; $P<.0001$ Multivariate analysis of NRM • BI vs no BI: RR 3.17; $P<.0001$
Styczynski et al,[24] 2016 Poland, 2012–2013, multicenter, retrospective cohort study Comments • Pediatric only • BI more common in allo vs auto, similar to published adult cohorts • BSI microbial epidemiology not described • Low mortality	308 SCT • 232 alloSCT • 76 autoSCT 2076 children • 308 SCT • 756 HM • 1012 solid tumors	Pcn, ceph, or cipro	Total incid: 26% (MCI)[o] Total episodes: 1,620[p] SCT incid: 34%[o] • BSI: 34% • GI: 12% • UTI: 4% • SSTI: 2% • CDI: 56/308 (18%) SCT episodes: 276[p] Non-SCT incid: 26%[o] • BSI: 26% • GI: 8% • UTI: 7% • SSTI: 2% Non-SCT episodes: 1344 BI cum incid SCT Overall BI incid (SCT and non-SCT): 26%[o] Overall BI episodes: 1,620[i] SCT incid: 34%[i] AutoSCT: 29% AlloSCT: 35% SCT episodes: 276[j] • GP: 145/276 (52.5%) • GN: 131/276 (47.5%) SCT pathogen freq[j] GP BI (145) • CoNS: 34/145 (23%) • SA: 7/145 (5%) • E faecium: 43/145 (30%) • E faecalis: 0/145 • Strep: 2/145 (1%)	• GP BI more common in SCT vs HM • Within SCT, BI more likely in alloSCT vs autoSCT • Crude SCT mortality: 4% • Crude HM mortality: 1.8% ($P = .03$)

(continued on next page)

Table 1
(continued)

Reference	Location, Time Period, Study Design	Transplant Features	Population	Antibacterial Prophylaxis	Number and Percent of Bacterial Infections in Cohort	Bloodstream Infection Frequency, Etiology, and Resistance	Risk Factors[a] for Bacterial Infections or Bloodstream Infections	Mortality and Other Outcomes Associated with Bacterial Infections/ Bloodstream Infections
					• 34% within 100 d • 40% within 180 d Non-SCT • 40% within 100 d • 60% within 180 d	• CDI: 56/145 (38%) • Other: <1% GN BI (131) • EC: 34/131 (26%) • Kleb: 30/131 (23%) • Enterobacter 38/131 (29%) • PsA: 9/131 (7%) • Steno: 9/131 (7%) Non-SCT incid: 26%[i] Non-SCT episodes: 1344[j] • GP: 488/1344 (36%) • GN: 856/1344 (64%) Non-SCT pathogen freq[j] GP BI (488)[j] • CoNS: 154/488 (32%) • SA: 48/488 (10%) • *E faecium*: 23/488 (5%) • *E faecalis*: 14/488 (3%) • Strep: 32/488 (7%) • CDI: 175/488 (36%) • Other: 21/488 (4%) • *E coli*: 270/856 (32%) • Kleb: 252/856 (29%) • Enterobacter: 143/856 (17%) • PsA: 77/856 (9%) • Steno: 13/856 (2%) • Other: 33/856 (4%)	• Advanced oncologic disease	
Young et al,[25] 2016	United States, multisite prospective, randomized trial	PBSCT or BMT from HLA-compatible	• 499 pts • 1347 infxn episodes BMT (249)	n/d	Total BIs • 810 episodes • 384 pts (77%)	Total BSIs • 413/1347 (30%) all infxns	BI risk	BI associated with lower survival (HR for death 1.49;

comparing survival and infxn episodes in BMT vs PBSCT, 2004–2009 Follow-up: 2 y

Comments
• Nice overview of all postSCT infxn
• Prolonged follow-up is strength
• No resistance data
• Late BI occurred, including late CDI

(matched) unrelated donors
• Majority received MA

• Median age: 44 y
• AML: 116
• ALL: 54
• CML: 27
• CMML: 4
• MDS: 46
• Graft failure: 9%
• cGVHD: 41%

PBSCT (250)
• Median age 44 y
• AML: 122
• ALL: 52
• CML: 32
• CMML: 3
• MDS: 37
• Graft failure: 3%
• cGVHD: 53%

CoNS
149 (39%) pts
224 (28%) BIs

Enterococci
82 (21%) pts
103 (13%) BIs

SA
29 (8%) pts
40 (5%) BIs

EC
34 (9%) pts
39 (5%) BIs

Kleb
29 (8%) pts
36 (4%) BIs

Pseud
25 (7%) pts
32 (4%) BIs

Enterobacter
12 (3%) pts
14 (2%) BIs

Steno
12 (3%) pts
13 (2%) BIs

CDI
123 (15%) BIs

Nocardia
5 (<1%) BIs

NTM
2 (<1%) BIs

BMT
• 431 (53%) total BI episodes

• 413/810 (51%) of BIs

BMT
• 219/431 (51%)
• 100-d cum incid: 45% ($P = .03$; BMT vs PBSCT)
• 2-y cum incid: 52% ($P = .092$; BMT vs PBSCT)

PBSCT
• 194/379 (51%)
• 100-d cum incid: 35%
• 2-y cum incid: 48% ($P = .092$; BMT vs PBSCT)

• Female gender
• aGVHD
• cGVHD
• CMV R$^+$

$P = .004$) in BMT/ PBSCT combined group

(continued on next page)

Table 1
(continued)

Reference	Location, Time Period, Study Design	Transplant Features	Population	Antibacterial Prophylaxis	Number and Percent of Bacterial Infections in Cohort	Bloodstream Infection Frequency, Etiology, and Resistance	Risk Factors[a] for Bacterial Infections or Bloodstream Infections	Mortality and Other Outcomes Associated with Bacterial Infections/Bloodstream Infections
Kikuchi et al,[31] 2015	Japan, single-center, 2006–2013, retrospective study of pre-engraft BSI and postengraft BSI and	• BMT: 122 (58%) • pSCT: 68 (33%) • UCB: 19 (9%) • MA: 122 (58%) • nonMA: 87 (42%) • MUD: 47%	209 adults • Median age: 45 y • 201/209 first transplant • All with CVC for receipt of	• FQ until engraft • T/S or inhaled pentamidine for PJP	• 201/249 (81%) • Cum incid pre-engraft: 48% (P = .002, BMT vs PBSCT) • 2-y cum incid: 72% (P = .003, BMT vs PBSCT) • CoNS: 123 (29%) • Enterococcus: 54 (13%) • CDI: 69 (16%) • EC: 16 (4%) PBSCT • 379 (47%) total BI episodes • 183/250 (73%) pts • Cum incid pre-engraft: 32% (P = .002; PBSCT vs BMT) • 2-y cum incid: 63% (P = .003; BMT vs PBSCT) • CoNS 101 (27%) • Enterococcus 49 (13%) • CDI 54 (14%) • EC 23 (6%)	All BSIs: 136 • GP BSI: 99 (73%) • GN BSI: 31 (23%) • Fungal BSI: 6 (4%) Pre-engraft • Total pts: 70/209 (34%) • Cum incid: 39% • Total episodes: 92 • Median onset: D9	Pre-engraft BSI • Longer time from diagnosis to transplant (>261 d)[r] (HR 2.2; P = .001)	Overall mortality • 45/209 (22%) Infxn-related mortality • 17/209

outcomes Follow-up: 180 d. Comments • GP/GN ratio (1.5 in 2007 vs 2.8 in 2013) • Most pts had mucositis (grade II–IV) • High rates of MR CoNS (96%) • GP: 57% FQ-R • GN: 24% FQ-R, 52% carb-R, 29% AG-R • No VRE • No ESBL GN	conditioning regimen • AML: 42% • ALL: 14% • MDS: 13% • lymphoma 10% • Apl A 7% • MRD: 24% • MMUD: 16% • Partial match, related: 12%		• All GP isolates: 62/92 (67%) • CoNS: 42/92 (46%) • E faecium: 8/92 (9%) • Coryneform: 3/92 (3%) • E faecalis: 3/92 (3%) • Other: 9 (10%) • All GN isolates: 26/92 (28%) • Steno: 8/92 (9%) • PsA: 6/92 (7%) • EC: 2/92 (2%) • Other: 9 (10%) • Fungal isolates: 4/92 (4%) Postengraft • Total pts: 33/209 (16%) • Cum incid: 17% • Total episodes: 44 • GP isolates: 37/44 (84%) • CoNS: 27/44 (61%) • E faecium: 3/44 (7%) • Coryneform: 2/44 (5%) • E faecalis: 1/44 (2%) • Other: 5/44 (11%) • GN isolates: 5/44 (11%) • Steno: 1/44 (2%) • PsA: 1/44 (2%) • EC: 1/44 (2%) • Other: 2/44 (5%)	• Failure to engraft (HR 2; P = .003) • High-risk disease at time of SCT (HR 1.9; P = .004) Postengraft BSI • None identified	○ 9 BSIs ○ 8 PNA BSI-attributable mortality • Pre-engraft: 5/70 (7%, all GN BSI) • Postengraft: 2/34 (6%, both GP BSI) Pre-engraft BSI vs no pre-engraft BSI • decreased OS at 180 d (70% vs 83%; P = .02)
Sanz et al,[28] 2015	Spain, single-center, 1997–2012, retrospective study of BSIs and outcomes at early (0–30 d), intermediate (31–100 d), late (101–365 d) • Single-unit UCBT • All MA with ATG	241 pts • Median age: 34 y • All had CVC • AML/MDS: 40% • ALL: 37% • CML: 12% • Other: 11%	• Cipro • T/S prior to UCBT and after neutrophil recovery • 100% BSIs	• 189 episodes • 134 pts Timing of BSI • 98/189 (52%) in early period (median D6) • 38/189 (20%) in intermediate period	• Reduced risk of BSI with more CD8+ cells in donor graft Crude D7 mortality rate • Overall: 12% • GN BSI: 18% • GP BSI: 7% • NRM greater for BSI within 7 d (RR 1.5; P = .04)

(continued on next page)

Table 1
(continued)

Reference	Location, Time Period, Study Design	Transplant Features	Population	Antibacterial Prophylaxis	Number and Percent of Bacterial Infections in Cohort	Bloodstream Infection Frequency, Etiology, and Resistance	Risk Factors[a] for Bacterial Infections or Bloodstream Infections	Mortality and Other Outcomes Associated with Bacterial Infections/Bloodstream Infections
	d), and very late (>365 d) periods after SCT. Median follow-up: 73 mo		• 95% HLA mismatched			• 41/189 (22%) in late period • 12/189 (6%) in very late period Cum incid BSI • D7: 21% • D14: 29% • D30: 34% • D100: 42% • D365: 52% • 4 y: 54% GN:GP BSI ratio • BSI < D30: GN/GP = .90 • BSI ≥D30: GN/GP = 1.6 GN pathogens EC: 31% PsA: 28%		Neutrophil recovery • BSI prior to D14 a/w lower likelihood of neutrophil recovery

Satlin et al,[36] 2015	Single-center, retrospective cohort study with 2 objectives
	1. Describe incid of BSI and NF within 30 d after SCT
	2. Describe BSI etiology, and MDR and CDI incid within 90 d post-SCT. Two periods were compared: January 2003–May 2006 and
		465 autoSCT
		• Conditioning: melphalan
		• Duration NP: median 7 d
		• Pts with CVC: 100%
			Total pts: 465
			• MM: 275
			  Period 1: 119
			  Period 2: 156
			Lymphoma: 190
			• Period 1: 88
			• Period 2: 102
				• Levo ppx initiated June 2006 in 95% MM pts	All BSI	Total BSIs, period 1 vs period 2
						• MM: 41% vs 15% (P<.001)
						• Lymphoma: 43% vs 47% (P = .5)
						NF in period 1 vs period 2
						• MM: 92% vs 61% (P<.001)
						• Lymphoma: 99% vs 97% (P = .6)
						BSI period 1
						MM
							• ↑ BSI in pts not on levo ppx (OR 3.7; P<.001)
							• ↑ NF in pts not on levo ppx (OR (5.55; P<.001)
							• Duration NP a/w ↑ BSI (RR 1.1; P = .001)
							• Levo ppx a/w trend toward ↑ levo-R EB BSI (P = .08)
							• Levo ppx a/w trend toward ↑ risk CDI (P = .12)
								Mortality in MM pts, both periods
								• At 30 d: 7/275 (2.5%)
								• At 90 d: 8/275 (4.3%)
								MM, period 1 (no ppx)
								• At 30 d: 4/127 (3.1%)
								• At 90 d: 8/127 (6.2%)[q]
								MM, period 2 (levo ppx)

June 2006–April 2010. Levo ppx was initiated during second period. Outcomes included sepsis, ICU admission, mortality at D30 and D90.

Comments
- Period with levo ppx a/w large drop in BSI incid among MM pts
- Among MM, decline in period 2 in incid for all BSI, BSI due to any GP, VGS, and CoNS
- Among MM, trend toward decline in GN BSI (P = .3) in period 2
- Among MM, trend toward ↑ risk of levo-R EB BSI and ↑ CDI in period 2

- 126 episodes
- 119 pts
- GP BSI: 31%[s]
- VGS: 10%[s]
- CoNS: 9%[s]
- Enterococci: 5%[s]
  - VRE: 67%[s]
- SA: 5%[s]
  - MRSA: 67%[s]
- GN BSI: 11%[s]
- EB: 9%[s]
- EC: 6%[s]
- Kp: 2%[s]
- Levo-R EB: 1%[s]
- CFTX-R EB: 0%[s]
- PsA: 0%[s]
- CDI: 3%[s]

Lymphoma[s]
- All BSIs: 43%
- GP BSI: 27%
- VGS: 6%
- CoNS: 8%
- Enterococci: 11%
  - VRE: 70%
- SA: 1%
  - MRSA: 0%
- GN BSI: 32%
- EB: 30%
- EC: 10%
- Kp: 15%
- Levo-R EB: 8%
- CFTX-R EB: 6%
- PsA: 0%
- CDI: 5%

BSI period 2
MM
- 116 episodes
- 156 pts
- All BSIs: 10%[s]
- GP BSI: 10%[s]
- VGS: 3%[s]
- CoNS: 0%[s]
- Enterococci: 5%[s]

- At 30 d: 4/148 (2.7%)
- At 90 d: 4/148 (2.7%)[q]

(continued on next page)

Table 1
(continued)

Reference	Location, Time Period, Study Design	Transplant Features	Population	Antibacterial Prophylaxis	Number and Percent of Bacterial Infections in Cohort	Bloodstream Infection Frequency, Etiology, and Resistance	Risk Factors[a] for Bacterial Infections or Bloodstream Infections	Mortality and Other Outcomes Associated with Bacterial Infections/ Bloodstream Infections

						○ VRE: 83%[s]
						• SA: 3%[s]
						  ○ MRSA: 100%[s]
						• GN BSI: 7%[s]
						• EB: 7%[s]
						• EC: 5%[s]
						• Kp: 0%[s]
						• Levo-R EB: 5%[s]
						• CFTX-R EB: 1%[s]
						• Carb-R EB: 1%[s]
						• PsA: 0%[s]
						• CDI: 7%[s]
						
						Lymphoma
						• No significant change from period 1
						• Trend toward
						  ○ ↓ CFTX-R EB (1%; *P* = .10)
						  ○ ↓ levo-R EB (2%; *P* = .08)		

Wang et al,[30] 2015	China, 2008–2014, single-center, retrospective cohort study of BSI during NF and 90-d survival Comment • Over entire study period, GN BSI more frequent than GPB BSI	SCT • Allo: 63 • Auto: 22	273 pts • Median age: 31 y • All with CVC • AML: 22 • ALL: 16 • NHL/HL: 13 • MM: 4 • Apl A: 2 • MDS: 2	• Levof	Only BSI reported	84/273 pts (31%) Episodes (84) • Median time to occurrence: D5 • GN BSI: 50 (60%) • GP BSI: 22 (26%) • Polymicrobial: 12 (14%) Isolates (108) GN • EC: 36 (33%) • Kleb: 24 (22%) • Steno: 3 (3%) • PsA: 3 (3%) GP • CoNS: 20 (19%) • Enterococcus: 3 (3%) • SA: 2 (2%)	n/d	• Overall mortality: 17/84 (20%) • BSI-related mortality: 11/84 (13%) Mortality risk factors • High-risk disease and alloSCT • Neutropenia for ≥15 d • GN BSI

| Blennow et al,[29] 2014 | • 521 alloSCT
Stem cell source
• BMT: 147 (28%)
• PBSCT: 331 (64%)
• UCB: 43 (8%)
Conditioning
• MA: 266 (51%)
• RIC: 255 (49%)
Matching
• HLA-ident: 194 (37%)
• MUD: 242 (46%)
• Mismatched: 85 (16%) | • 493 pts
• Median age: 37 y
• 156 y <18 y (30%)
• Acute leukemia: 220 (42%)
• lymphoma: 41 (8%)
• MDS: 65 (12%)
• Solid tumor: 38 (7%)
• Noncancer diagnosis: 82 (16%) | • Cipro from D1 until engraft | • Total BSIs: 126
• 3 Candida
• 1 M avium | All bacterial BSI
• Incid: 109/521 SCTs (21%)
• Bacterial episodes: 120
• Bacterial isolates: 122
• Median onset: D8
By era
• 2001–2004: 22% (55/247)
• 2004–2008: 54/247 (20%)
• 2001–2008: 32% (all CoNS, Corynebacterium included)
• 1975–1996: 27% (all CoNS, Corynebacterium included)
2001–2008
GP BSI
• 100/122 (82%)
• VGS: 43 (35%)
  ○ Median onset: D4
  ○ 21% pcn-R
• CoNS: 33/122 (27%)
• Enterococcus 18/122 (15%)
  ○ Median onset: D11
  ○ No VRE
• SA: 1 (<1%)
GN BSI
• 17/122 (14%)
• EC 9/122 (7%)
• Cipro-R EC: ~50%
• Acineto: 2/122 (2%)
• PsA: 1 (<1%)
• Fusobacterium: 4/122 (3%)
Polymicrobial
• 6/122 (5%) | All BSIs
• Unrelated donor
• UCBT
• pSCT protective
• VGS BSI protective
• RIC (vs MA)
• Higher number of nucleated cells in SCT product
CoNS BSI RF
• UCBT
Enterococcal BSI RF
• Prior SCT | D30 crude mortality
• BSI: 5.5%–8%
• No BSI: 1%
  ○ P = .01
D120 crude mortality
• All BSIs: 21%
• No BSI: 9%; P<.001
• VGS BSI: 27%
BSI-attributable mortality
• All: 4/120 (3.3%)
• CoNS: 0%
• VGS BSI: (3/43) 7%
• GN BSI: n/d
BSI a/w ↑ aGVHD before D100:
• RR 1.5 (95% CI, 1.04–21) |

Sweden, 2001–2008, single-center, retrospective study of pre-engraft[a] BSI. Comparison of 2 recent eras

• 2001–2004
• 2004–2008

to historic era

• 1975–1996

Follow-up: 120 d

Comments

• Overall BSI incid stable over 3 eras
• VGS ↓ over 3 eras
• Enterococcus ↑ over 3 eras
• GP/GN ratio fell from 9 to 4.2 between 2001–2004 and 2004–2008
• GN BSI rate ↑ over 3 eras (0.3%, 2.4%, 3.6%)
• FQ-R ↑ over eras
• BSI-attributable mortality low (3%), although 120 d crude mortality sig higher in BSI vs non-BSI (21% vs 9%) (investigators interpret as association of BSI with other risk factors for mortality)
• Investigators conclude cipro ppx remains appropriate

(continued on next page)

Table 1
(continued)

Reference	Location, Time Period, Study Design	Transplant Features	Population	Antibacterial Prophylaxis	Number and Percent of Bacterial Infections in Cohort	Bloodstream Infection Frequency, Etiology, and Resistance	Risk Factors[a] for Bacterial Infections or Bloodstream Infections	Mortality and Other Outcomes Associated with Bacterial Infections/Bloodstream Infections
Gudiol et al,[20] 2014	Spain, 2006–2013, single-center, retrospective study comparing pre-engraft and postengraft BSI **Comments** • MDR ↑ over 2 periods in study (2006–2009 and 2010–2013) • late BSI due to SP seen, a/w ↑ morbidity and mortality and GVHD • No analysis of overall BSI risk factors (no comparison to pts without BSI) • Only univariate analysis performed	400 SCT • Auto: 239 • Allo: 161	• Population characterized only for 189 episodes of BSI • Median age: 54 y • Acute leukemia 95 (50%) • MM: 47 (25%) • NHL: 18 (10%) • MDS: 12 (6%) • HL: 7 (4%) • CML: 5 (3%)	• Cipro through D60 (begun in 6/2011) • T/S (for PJP) after engraft	Bls that were not BSI-associated were not described Early BSI sources • CVC: 47% • Endogenous or unknown: 40% • Mucositis: 10% • Urinary: 1% • Respiratory: 1% Late BSI sources • CVC 37% • Endogenous or unknown: 30% • Respiratory: 14% • Urinary: 6% • GI: 5%	• 189 episodes in 172 pts ○ 100 early (pre-engraft) ○ 89 late (postengraft)[l] • Overall incid: 189/400 (47%) • BSI in alloSCT: 120/161 (75%) • BSI in autoSCT: 69/239 (29%) **GP BSI** • 115/189 (61%) • CoNS 66/189 (35%) • SP: 13/189 (7%, 12 as late BSIs) • Enterococcus: 12/189 (6%) • VGS: 11/189 (6%) • SA: 9/189 (5%) **GN BSI** • 62/189 (33%) • EC: 40/189 (21%) • PsA: 10/189 (5%) • Kleb: 9/189 (5%) • FQ-R GN: 33/62 (53%) • MDR GN: 13/62 (21%) **Other BSIs** • Polymicrobial: 11/189 (6%) • Anaerobes: 3/189 (2%)	Pre-engraftment BSI[m] • NP • Severe mucositis • CVC • MASCC score ≥21 • Unrelated donor • Prior chemo tx • Prior radiation • Antifungal ppx **Postengraft BSI** • AlloSCT • GVHD • RIC • Antibacterial ppx or prior abx tx • Parenteral nutrition • Concomitant infxn (CMV, CDI, other) • Urinary catheter • Steroid use • Prior/current CyA use • Prior hospital stay	48-h case fatality rate • All BSIs: 6% • Pre-engraft BSI: 2% • Postengraft BSI: 10% 30-d case fatality rate • All BSIs: 14% • Pre-engraft BSI: 4% • Postengraft BSI: 25% multivariate analysis, mortality risk • BSI due to VGS (OR 16; P = .03) • ICU admission

| Macesic et al,[33] 2014 | Australia, 2001–2010, single-center, retrospective study of all bacterial and candida infxns during admission for SCT and crude mortality at 7 d and 28 d after BSI.

Study period divided into 3 eras (2001–2004, 2004–2007, 2007–2010).

Comments
• Study led investigators to limit FQ use to pts receiving MA
• FQ-R bacteria more likely to be ESBL with R to fourth-gen ceph, carbs, AGs
• ESBL-R organisms more likely to have cross-resistance to FQs, fourth-gen ceph, carbs, AGs | 528 SCTs
• Allo: 244 (46%)
• Auto: 281 (53%)
• MA: 152 (29%)
• RIC: 92 (17%)
• aGVHD: 62%
• cGVHD: 65% | 528 SCT
508 pts
• MM: 152 (29%)
• AML: 132 (25%)
• NHL: 113 (21%)
• ALL: 40 (7%)
• HL: 37 (7%)
• CML: 15 (3%)
• CLL: 9 (2%)
• Other: 40 (6%) | • Cipro (beginning in 8/2005, cipro given during conditioning through engraft)
• TfS (allo) | • 380 BI episodes
• 605 total isolates
• 586 bacterial (97%)
• 19 Candida (3%)
• GPB predominated over GNB
• CDI n/d

Sources
• Blood: 380 (63%)
• Sputum: 79 (13%)
• Urine: 10 (10%)
• Wounds/surface sites: 45 (8%)
• Catheters: 14 (2%)
• BAL: 7 (1%)

GPB
• SA: 107 (34%)
• CoNS: 94 (30%)
• Enterococcus: 60 (19%)

GNB
• EC: 28%
• Kleb: 19%
• Pseud: 17%
• Enterobacter: 12%
• Acineto: 6%
• Steno: 6%

Trends across eras[n]
• SA ↓
• CoNS ↑, became most frequent
• Enterococcus ↑, mostly due to VRE
• VGS ↓
• GNB freq did not change
• FQ-R GNB ↑ (13% vs 36%)
• ESBL GNB ↑ (32% vs 51%)
• MDR ↑ (11% vs 22%) | • BSI incid: 212/508 (42%)
• 362 bacterial BSIs in 212 pts

GP BSI
• Total: 225/362 (62%)
• CoNS: 92/362 (25%)
  ○ 93% MR-CoNS
• Enterococcus: 45/362 (12%)
  ○ 38% VRE
• SA: 35/362 (10%),
  ○ 49% MRSA
• VGS: 33/362 (9%)

GP BSI trends across eras
• VRE BSI ↑: 7% vs 67%
• ↑ proportion of GP isolates: 55% vs 68%

GN BSI
• Total: 137/362 (38%)
• EC: 45/362 (12%)
• Kleb: 35/362 (10%)
• Enterobacter: 18/362 (5%)
• Pseud: 12/362 (3%)
• Acineto: 10/362 (3%)

GN BSI trends across eras[n]
• ↑ FQ-R: 12% vs 28% (P = .001)
• ↑ ESBL-R: 26% vs 36% (P = .04)
• No change in carb-R (8% vs 8%) | • RIC was RF for late BSI (>D100)
• AutoSCT was RF for early BSI (D7 to D29) | Overall mortality: 267/528 (51%)
7-d crude mortality after BSI
• 25/212 (12%)
• E faecium most frequent isolate (24%)

Factors a/w death 7 d after BSI
• Active disease at transplant
• MDR organism

28-d crude mortality
• 53/212 (25%)
• CoNS most frequent isolate in BSI death
• Enterococcus second most frequent in BSI death

Factors a/w death 28 d after BSI
• Active disease at transplant
• MDR organism
• Grade 4 aGVHD |

(continued on next page)

Table 1 (*continued*)

Reference	Location, Time Period, Study Design	Transplant Features	Population	Antibacterial Prophylaxis	Number and Percent of Bacterial Infections in Cohort	Bloodstream Infection Frequency, Etiology, and Resistance	Risk Factors[a] for Bacterial Infections or Bloodstream Infections	Mortality and Other Outcomes Associated with Bacterial Infections/Bloodstream Infections
Mikulska et al,[27] 2014	Large survey of BSI etiology and resistance, 39 centers (18 countries) in Europe and Near East, 2011 Comments • Contains qualitative data on resistance • Survey supports a trend of ↑ MDR over time and a relative ↑ in GN BSI • In comparison to published literature, supports a ↓ in PsA (10% vs 5%) and ↓ resistance rates for all bacteria, but an ↑ in enterococcal isolates	n/d	Large survey, children and adults	n/d	n/d	BSI composition (percentage) • GP BSI: 55% • CoNS: 24% • Enterococcus: 8% • VGS: 6% • SA: 5% • Other: 5% • GN BSI: 45% • EB: 30% • PsA: 5% • Acineto: 2% • Other: 3% Differences from prior published literature • ↓ ratio of GP:GN (1.2:1, not 1.5:1) • ↑ freq enterococcus (8% vs 5%) • ↑ freq EB (30% vs 24%) • ↓ freq PsA (5% vs 10%) • ↓ in MDR isolates • ↓ R rates, although still substantial, for ESBL-R GN, AG-R GNB, and carb-R PsA	n/d	n/d
Piñana et al,[14] 2014	Spain, 1998–2003, multicenter (24 sites), analysis of 2 historic cohorts for which BSI data were collected prospectively (pts registered in 2 prior	All autoSCT • PBSCT: 96% • BMT: 4%	720 adults • HM: 590 • Solid tumors: 70 • Other: 48 • TPN: 258 (8%) • CVC: ≥83%	• FQ: 45% • T/S: 14% • Both: 13% • Other: 1% • None: 27%	All BIs: 339/720 (47%) Total MC BIs: 195/720 (27%) BSI: 145/720 (20%) PNA: 60/145 (15%) CLABSI: 52/72 (7%)	All BSIs 145 pts (20%) 145 episodes GP BSI incid: 94/720 (13%) GN BSI incid: 62/720 (9%) GP pathogens	All BSIs • NP >9 d (RR 2.6; *P*<.001) GP BSI • PNP >5 d (RR 1.7; *P* = .03)	• TRM at D30: 13 (1.8%) • Total deaths with 30 d 5/145 (3%) • BSI not a/w mortality

prospective studies) Data captured: BSI during SCT admission, death by D30, CLABSI, PNA, other Follow-up: D60 after SCT Comments • Trend for more BSI in those who died (RR 1.9; P = .19) but not sig • At least 83% of pts with CVC (2% no CVC, 15% n/d) • Percent BSI due to CLABSI described (16%) • Not all PNA was MCI • No resistance data • No ↑ in mortality in pts with GN BSI • Conditioning regimen data missing for many					• Total: 94 (65%) • CoNS: 62 (43%) • Strep: 21 (15%) • SA: 5 (3%) GN pathogens • Total: 62 (43%) • E coli: 30 (21%) • PsA: 10 (7%) GP plus GN pathogens 11 (8%) CLABSI • In BSI: 23/145 (16%) • In total cohort: 23/720 (3%)		• TPN >5 d (RR 1.9; P = .008) GN BSI • NP >9 d (RR 5; P<.001) • FQ ppx (RR 0.5; P = .006)	
Srinivasan et al,[37] 2014	United States, 1990–2009, single-center, retrospective, cohort study of first infxn episode, death by D30 after SCT Mean follow-up duration: 8.73 y Comments • n/d on CVC BSI • Scant data on resistance • CDI more frequent in leukemia pts than solid tumor pts (14% vs 3%)	All autoSCT Comparison of 2 eras • 1990–1999: 128 pts • 2000–2009: 192 pts	Total pts: 385 • Infants • Children • Adolescents • Young adults (18–20) • Solid tumor: 241 (63%) • Lymphoma: 79 (21%) • Leukemia: 65 (17%)	• T/S	Note: spectrum of bacterial infxn not clearly defined Solid tumor/lymphoma • All: 33 (10%) • Median onset: 5 d • GP: 24 (8%) • GN: 11 (3%) • CDI: 11(3%) Leukemia: 65 • 32/65 (49%) • GP: 15 (23%) • GN: 3 (5%) • CDI: 9 (14%)	Solid tumor/lymphoma (320) • All BSIs: 23 (7%) • GPB: 12 (4%) • CoNS: 6 (2%) • Strep spp: 3 (1%) • Bacillus: 2 (1%) • SAB: 1 (0.3%) • GNB: 11 (3%) • Kleb: 5 (2%) • EC: 2 (1%) • Morganella: 1 (0.3%) • Proteus: 1 (0.3%) • Enterobacter: 1 (0.3%) Leukemia (65) All BSIs: 8 (12%)	• Leukemia • No association with transplant era	3 Deaths (0.7% total), all infxn-related • 2/3 (0.5%) due to BSI (all had leukemia and SCT before 2000)

(continued on next page)

Table 1
(continued)

Reference	Location, Time Period, Study Design	Transplant Features	Population	Antibacterial Prophylaxis	Number and Percent of Bacterial Infections in Cohort	Bloodstream Infection Frequency, Etiology, and Resistance	Risk Factors[a] for Bacterial Infections or Bloodstream Infections	Mortality and Other Outcomes Associated with Bacterial Infections/Bloodstream Infections
	• No noteworthy GN R • CD133-selected PBSCT and CD34+-selected BMT seem to be a/w a variety of different infxns							
Srinivasan et al,[32] 2013	United States, single-center, retrospective, 1990–2009. Follow-up for bacterial, viral, fungal, other infxns and outcomes for median of 2 y post-transplant. Follow-up for survival analysis: median of 8 y Comments • No adults	AlloSCT • MRD: 243 • MUD: 239 • Haplo: 176 • UCB: 0 Conditioning • MA: 597 (79%) • TBI: 497 (65%) • RIC: 162 (21%) • TCD: 365 (48%)	759 mostly children and adolescents • Mean age: 9.4 y • Excluded ages: >21 y • 15% infants • Leukemia: 502 (66%) • Lymphoma: 24 (3%) • MDS: 48 (6%) • Solid tumors: 27 (4%) • Hematologic/immune disorder: 17% • Other: 31 (4%) • aGVHD: 369 (49%) • cGVHD: 129 (17%)	• No FQs • T/S for 1 y • In cGVHD: pcn + T/S	1990–2009 (759) • Total: 426 (56%) • GP: 40% • GN: 16% 1990–1999 (329) • Total: 53% • GP: 39% • GN: 15% 2000–2009 (430) • Total: 58% • GP: 42% • GN: 17% CDI: 110/759 (14%)	By transplant era • 1990–2009: 225/759 (30%) • 1990–1999: 86/329 (26%) • 2000–2009: 139/430 (30%) By transplant phase • Median onset: 87 d • D0–D30: 59/759 (8%) • D31–D100: 73/735 (10%) • D101–D730: 93/622 (15%) By pathogen 225 total • S epi: 70 (31%) • VGS: 16 (7%) • Enterococci: 13 (6%) ◦ 7 VRE • Kleb: 18 (8%) • EC: 17 (8%) • Pseud: 14 (6%)	BI at 0–30 d • No BI RF identified BI at 31 d–100 d • Severe aGVHD • PBSCT BI at >100 d • cGVHD	Overall mortality due to infxn: 60 (8%) Overall mortality due to bacterial infxn: 12 (2%) • All BSIs • 9/12 GNB

Note: studies with fewer than 100 patients were not included.

Abbreviations: ↑, increased; ↓, decreased; ~, estimation by this investigator; βL/βLI, β-lactam/β-lactamase inhibitor (usually antipseudomonal βL/βLI); a/w, associated with; abx, antibiotic(s). Achromo-bacter; Acineto, acinetobacter; AG, aminoglycoside; aGVHD, acute graft-versus-host-disease; allo or alloSCT, allogeneic SCT; alt donor, alternative donor; mismatched unrelated donor, mismatched donor, un-related cord blood donor, or haploidentical cord blood donor); amp, ampicillin; ana, anaerobic; Apl A, aplastic anemia; ATG, antithymocyte globulin; auto or autoSCT, autologous SCT; BM/BMSCT, bone marrow stem cells or transplant using bone marrow stem cells; BI, bacterial infection; BSI, bloodstream infection; Bu, busulfan; carb, carbapenem; ceph, a member of the cephalosporin class; CFP, cefepime; CFTX, ceftriaxone; cGVHD, chronic GVHD; CI, confidence interval; CIBMTR, Center for International Blood and Marrow Transplant Research; cipro, ciprofloxacin; clinda, clindamycin; CMML, chronic myelomonocytic leukemia; CMV, cytomegalovirus; CRI, catheter-related infection; cum, cumulative; CVC, central venous catheterization; Cy, cyclophosphamide; CyA, cyclosporine; D/d, day; EB, enterobacteriaceae; EC, E coli; engraft, engraftment;

freq, frequency; FUO, fever of unknown origin; GENT, gentamicin; GNAB, gram-negative aerobic bacteria; GNR, gram-negative rods or bacilli; GPAB, GP aerobic bacteria; GPC, GP cocci; GPR, GP rods other than *C difficile;* haplo or haploSCT, haploidentically matched SCT; HL, Hodgkin Lymphoma; HR, Hazard Ratio; ident, identical; IMI, imipenem; incid, incidence; infxn, infection; Kleb, *Klebsiella* species (spp); KP, *Klebsiella pneumoniae*; levo, levofloxacin; mo, month; MA, myeloablative conditioning regimen; Mac, macrolide; MC/MCI, microbiologically confirmed/microbiologically confirmed infection; MDS, myleodysplastic syndrome; MMRD, mismatched related donor; MMUD, mismatched unrelated donor; MP, myeloproliferative disorder; MR, methicillin-resistant; MRD, matched related donor; MSSA, methicillin-susceptible Staphylococcus areus (SA); MTX, methotrexate; MUD, matched unrelated donor; OR, odds ratio; n/d, no data; NFRM GNR, nonfermentating gram-negative rods; NHL, Non-Hodgkin lymphoma; NP, neutropenia (defined as circulating neutrophils <1000/μL); NRM, nonrelapse mortality; NS, nonsusceptible; NTM, nontuberculous mycobacteria; OFX, ofloxacin; PB/PBSCT, peripheral blood SCT; pcn, penicillin; PNA, pneumonia; PNP, profound neutropenia (defined as circulating neutrophils <100/μL); ppx, antibiotic prophylaxis; PsA, *Pseudomonas aeruginosa*; Pseud, undifferentiated *Pseudomonal* species; PTCy, post-transplant cyclophosphamide; pt, patient; R/r, resistant or resistance; R+, recipient serologic status (eg, CMV R^+ indicates recipient has IgG antibody to CMV, indicating prior exposure); RF, risk factor; RIC, reduced intensity conditioning; RR, relative risk; S epi, *Staphylococcus epidermidis*; S, susceptible; sig, significant; SP, *Streptococcus pneumoniae*; Staph, undifferentiated *Staphylococcus* species, which may or may not include *Staphylococcus aureus*; Steno, *Stenotrophomonas* species; Strep, undifferentiated streptococci (excluding *Enterococcus* species and also often excluding SP); T/S, trimethoprim-sulfamethoxazole (Bactrim) antibiotic prophylaxis (generally targeting *Pneumocystis jirovecii*); TBI, total body irradiation; TCD, T-cell depletion; TPN, total parenteral nutrition; TRM, transplant-related mortality; tx, therapy; UCB/UCBT, umbilical cord blood as source of stem cells or transplantation using umbilical cord stem cells; y, year.

[a] Results of multivariate analysis presented.

[b] Infection density: infections per patient days of risk, a measure that accounts for the possibility of single or multiple infections occurring per patient over a defined risk period (often the first 100 days or the first year after transplant).

[c] Engraftment is usually defined as an absolute neutrophil count greater than 500/mL for greater than or equal to 3 consecutive days.

[d] No microbial etiology determined.

[e] Proportion due to bacteria versus fungal organisms not stated.

[f] Aside from BSI, unclear if culture-confirmed as bacterial.

[g] Noncarb-R: resistant to noncarbapenem, anti-PsA βL/βLIs (eg, piperacillin/tazobactam).

[h] βL/βLIs: anti-PsA βL/βLI.

[i] Pts with infxn.

[j] Infxn episodes.

[k] Sixteen patients that did not engraft were excluded from analysis.

[l] Includes 2 episodes of *Candidemia*.

[m] Pre-engraft versus postengraft, unadjusted comparison only.

[n] Frequency in 2001 to 2004 versus 2007 to 2010.

[o] % of patients with infection.

[p] Number or frequency of episodes or isolates.

[q] $P = .13$.

[r] Compared to transplant on or before 261 d after diagnosis.

[s] Frequency of pts with infxn.

[t] Unclear in study what percent represented bacterial, viral, fungal, or other infection.

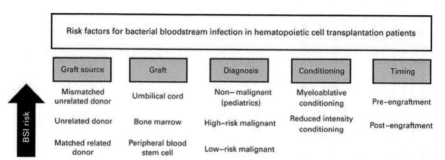

Fig. 2. Effect of various transplant factors on the risk of bacteremia in SCT. The risk of bacteremia depends on several transplant factors, including the degree of HLA compatibility between donor and recipient (risk rises for unrelated or mismatched donor-recipient pairs), the source of the stem cells (umbilical cord blood graft carries higher risk), the underlying hematologic or other disease, the conditioning regimen (myeloablative regimens are higher risk), and location in the transplant timeline (most bacteremias occur during preengraftment). (*From* Dandoy CE, Ardura MI, Papanicolaou GA, et al. Bacterial bloodstream infections in the allogeneic hematopoietic cell transplant patient: new considerations for a persistent nemesis. Bone Marrow Transplant 2017;52(8):1096; with permission.)

may be missed in the initial diagnostic workup and lead to high morbidity and mortality. With the possible exception of *Legionella*, antibiotic regimens recommended for first-line use in the prophylaxis and treatment of neutropenia and neutropenic fever (NF) are ineffective against these atypical pathogens.

Because of the limitations in the literature, this review focuses on BSIs, which, by definition, have microbiologic confirmation. We describe the available data on the incidence, microbial epidemiology, risk factors, resistance pattern, and outcomes of GP bacteria (GPB) and GN bacteria (GNB) found in the contemporary literature (2014 to present) (see **Table 1**).[a] Potential new diagnostic methods, emerging management strategies, and novel anti-infective agents also are reviewed.

GENERAL RISK FACTORS FOR BACTEREMIA (BLOODSTREAM INFECTION)

The risk of bacterial infection and BSI is not distributed evenly across the HM and SCT populations. Underlying disease, type of transplant (autologous, allogeneic, or cord blood), HLA-matching (matched, mismatched, and haploidentical), stem cell source, conditioning or chemotherapy agents, comorbidities, and age all modify risk (**Fig. 2**). Patients with AML, for example, have much greater risk of BSI than patients with Hodgkin or non-Hodgkin lymphoma, chronic lymphocytic leukemia (CLL), or multiple myeloma (MM).[54] Individuals with chronic graft-versus-host disease (GVHD), enduring T-cell and B-cell dysfunction caused by conditioning regimens, functional hyposplenism from total body irradiation, and hypogammaglobulinemia, continue to be at higher risk for bacterial infections during early and late postengraftment periods (see **Fig. 1**).

MICROBIAL EPIDEMIOLOGY OF BLOODSTREAM INFECTIONS

In the 1970s and 1980s, GNB were the predominant cause of bacteremia and were associated with significant mortality among neutropenic patients with cancer and

---

[a] See **Table 1**. Some studies reviewed contain a mixture of adults and children. One single large study investigating BSI in children and 2 studies surveying BSI in children and adolescents have been included for comparison.

the SCT population.[55–58] Beginning in the late 1980s, GPB increased in frequency and, in many studies, became the majority of BSI isolates,[59–64] although *P aeruginosa* (PsA) continued to comprise a large share of all bacteremia (14%–20% in some centers).[58,60] Among GP isolates, *Staphylococcus aureus* (SA), streptococci, coagulase-negative staphylococci (CoNS), and enterococci were the most frequently recovered, with SA accounting for 6% to 50% of all GPB infections.[63,65–67] Several factors likely contributed to this new pattern, including the adoption of fluoroquinolone (FQ) prophylaxis in cancer centers, evolving conditioning regimens, changing reliance on invasive devices (urinary catheters and venous catheters), and increasing outpatient management of cancer treatment.

In the current SCT literature, many studies report bacteremia rates of 20% to 30%, and a few centers have reported BSI rates as high as 50% to 75%.[20,22,25] Thus, it does not seem as if the incidence of BSI has declined much over the past 3 decades.[15–19] Infections due to GPB continue to be more frequent than those due to GNB in most studies, although the ratio of GP to gram-negative (GN) organisms may be slightly lower than before.[26,27] Most BSI events occur within the pre-engraftment period, with onset in the first 2 weeks to 4 weeks after SCT.[20,28–31,64,67] In studies where follow-up is extended to a year or more, most BSIs still occur within the first 90 days after SCT.[25,28,32] GPB still predominate over GNB in most centers. **Table 1** summarizes major studies of BSI in the HM and SCT population published since 2014.

Among GPB, CoNS, streptococci (including viridans group streptococci [VGS]), and enterococci are the most frequently isolated species. SA generally accounts for approximately 5% of GPB, and, overall, is probably less frequent than in the past.[28,29,33,62,63,65,68] In a few centers, however, SA BSI occurs at higher frequency and may comprise 13% to 18% of all isolates.[33,69] Enterococcal species, in particular *Enterococcus faecium*, are increasing or stable in frequency and represent 10% to 16% of all GP BSI isolates.[22,28–30,32,33,64,70] Enterococcal BSIs may occur later after SCT compared with BSI due to other organisms.[29,71] One study in Sweden found that the median onset for enterococcal BSI was 11 days post-transplant, compared with 4 days for VGS BSI.[29]

Streptococcus pneumoniae (SP) is an uncommon but important pathogen.[72] The incidence of invasive pneumococcal disease (IPD) among autologous and allogeneic SCT recipients is estimated at 696 per 100,000 patients and 812 to 956 per 100,000 patients, respectively.[73,74] By comparison, among the US population in 2016, the rate of IPD was 9.5/100,000.[75] Persons with HM also are at higher risk, in particular patients with MM, who have an estimated incidence of 674 cases/100,000 per year.[72] These recent estimates in the SCT and HM population are similar, if not a little higher, than those published previously.[76–78] The mortality associated with IPD in SCT patients is substantial, and ranges from 13% to 30% in recent studies.[74,76,78] Mortality rates in IPD, however, do not seem higher in SCT than in the general population.[77,79,80]

Traditionally, SP BSI has been described as a late post-SCT event, concentrated in patients with chronic GVHD.[3,78] In addition, in most centers, SP does not make a major contribution to BSI (see **Table 1**).[67] However, 1 center in Spain, remarkably, identified SP as the etiology of 7% of all BSIs and 13% of late-onset BSIs.[20] The median onset was 594 days after transplant. Only 3 of the 13 (23%) patients with SP BSIs had received the pneumococcal polysaccharide at the time of transplant. Youssef and colleagues[76] described 54 episodes of SP infections at a single institution between 1989 and 2005, with most patients, diagnosed in the late transplant period, as seen in prior eras.[77,78] Lymphoma and high doses of steroid (equivalent of $\geq$60 mg prednisone/day) were identified as risk factors. In this study, 69% of IPD occurred in patients without chronic GVHD, which was not found a risk factor.[76]

Among GNB, Enterobacteriaceae predominate, especially *Escherichia coli* and *Klebsiella pneumoniae* (Kp). *Pseudomonas* species, most often PsA, occur at a frequency of less than 1% to 14%.[20,28,29] A few cancer centers have reported a higher proportion of GNB than GPB as causes of BSI.[12,23,30,34,69,81,82] Most studies that provide a comparison observe a higher mortality rate in GN BSI than GP BSI (see **Table 1**).[13,30,67,83] Large surveys carried out in Europe have shown that the microbial composition of GN BSI as well as antibiotic resistance patterns vary across geographic regions, with southeastern Europe having high rates of resistance compared with northwestern Europe.[13] Kp carbapenemase (KPC)-Kp and highly resistant PsA species are frequently reported in some centers and throughout some countries, such as Italy,[38,45] and are associated with particularly high mortality.

TRENDS IN ANTIMICROBIAL RESISTANCE AND ASSOCIATED MORTALITY IN GRAM-POSITIVE BLOODSTREAM INFECTIONS
Coagulase-negative Staphylococci

Among GPBs commonly implicated in BSIs, CoNS species generally outpace all other GP organisms in frequency (see **Table 1**) and are often methicillin resistant. In 2014, a study of 548 patients who received SCT between 2001 and 2010 at a single center in Australia found that CoNS isolates were almost universally methicillin resistant (94%).[33] Similarly, a single center in Japan reported 96% of all CoNS isolates were methicillin resistant.[31] This extremely high rate of resistance among CoNS represents a change compared with prior eras.[15,67]

Enterococcus Species

Enterococci, including vancomycin-resistant enterococci (VRE), are now common BSI isolates. The Australian single-center investigators (discussed previously) detected a significant rise over a 10-year period in enterococcal infections from blood and non-blood sites. Most of the increase was attributable to *E faecium,* which comprised 12% of all BSI isolates over the period.[33] Vancomycin-resistance (VRE) rates consequently rose sharply: in 2001% to 2004%, 7% of isolates were VRE; in 2007% to 2010%, 64% of isolates were VRE. Similarly, Satlin and colleagues[84] reported that 80% of enterococcal BSI isolates were vancomycin-resistant and VRE accounted for 19% of all BSIs. Other studies report vancomycin-resistance rates of 22% to 85%.[32,35,64,85] A few centers have reported little or no VRE.[12,29,69]

Risk factors for VRE BSI in the SCT population include VRE colonization, previous use of vancomycin and other antibiotics (advanced β-lactams or higher-generation cephalosporins, anaerobic agents, and aminoglycosides), older age, comorbid conditions, reduced renal function, neutropenia, mucosal barrier injury from GVHD or *Clostridium difficile* infection (CDI), HLA-mismatch, and T-cell depletion.[71,84,86–90] Several studies have demonstrated increased mortality associated with VRE bacteremia in the SCT population.[35,91–93] It is unclear whether VRE is the direct cause of increased mortality or a marker for other causes of increased mortality.[94] For example, despite that VRE colonization is a risk factor for VRE BSI, 2 recent retrospective studies have shown that the addition of linezolid to empiric therapy for NF in colonized patients had no impact on mortality.[95,96]

Methicillin-resistant Staphylococcus aureus

Methicillin-resistant *Staphylococcus aureus* (MRSA) infections, including BSI, are a global issue. Several countries in Central America and South America and Asia have MRSA rates that exceed 50%.[97,98] In the United States, methicillin-resistant isolates account for up to 49% of SA BSIs.[99,100] There is a wide range in MRSA incidence across Europe. Northern European countries have rates between 1% and 10%. Southern Europe and eastern Europe have rates of 25% to 50%.[101] China, Australia, and Africa have similarly high rates.[98]

In the SCT and HM populations, the reported rate of MRSA BSI also varies widely.[12,27,69,102] An Australian center reported a stable 54% rate of methicillin resistance among *Staphylococcus aureus* (SA) isolates between 2001 and 2010.[33] Similarly, in a survey from Belarus, SA reported that 65% of SA strains were MRSA.[103] In contrast, a multicenter prospective European survey found very low rates of MRSA (0.1%).[26] Similarly, a recent survey of BSI during neutropenia in 20 transplant centers in Germany, Austria, and Switzerland noted that SA was the etiology of only 2% of BSI between 2002 and 2014. In this study, no MRSA BSIs occurred after 2010.[26]

Viridans Group Streptococci

VGS[b] are common BSI isolates in the SCT and HM population, where FQ prophylaxis is a recognized risk factor for VGS BSI.[104–107] Partial or complete resistance to penicillin and other β-lactams, such as ceftazidime and cefotaxime, has been widely observed among VGS since the 1990s.[108–111] Alcaide and colleagues[111] characterized 410 VGS strains consecutively isolated from blood cultures between 1986 and 1996 and found one-third of all isolates were penicillin resistant. *S mitis*, *S anginosus*, and *S sanguinis* (formerly known as *S sanguis*) represented 50%, 24%, and 18% of the isolates, respectively. A subsequent study from Spain analyzed the activity of various β-lactams against 89 clinical VGS strains and found 39% had some degree of penicillin resistance, 23% were highly penicillin-resistant, 54% were resistant to ceftazidime, 34% were resistant to cefepime, and 22% were resistant to ceftriaxone.[112]

Historically, VGS BSIs in the SCT/HM host has been associated with septic shock, acute respiratory distress syndrome, and a very high mortality rate.[109,113] Studies carried out when VGS comprised a large fraction of BSI suggested that a mortality benefit accrued to patients who received vancomycin for NF.[114–116] Data in support of this view largely derive from an era in which ceftazidime, an unreliable agent for VGS, was widely used for the empiric treatment of NF.[108,109,116] Gudiol and colleagues,[20] however, also recently reported a strong mortality association with VGS BSI (odds ratio [OR] 16; $P = .03$).

Shelburne and colleagues[117] examined the activity of penicillin and 3 advanced β-lactams widely used for initial treatment of NF (cefepime, meropenem, and piperacillin-tazobactam) against 48 VGS BSI clinical strains to determine which penicillin minimum inhibitory concentration (MIC) breakpoint[c] would best predict resistance to the advanced β-lactams. Ceftriaxone, cefepime, and piperacillin-tazobactam were effective for all VGS isolates with penicillin MICs of less than or equal to 2 μg/mL. In contrast, meropenem was effective for most, but not all, strains with penicillin MICs of less than or equal to 2 μg/mL. Thus, VGS isolates with a penicillin MIC greater than or equal to 2 μg/mL seemed to predict nonsusceptibility to advanced β-lactams.[117]

---

[b] VGS include *S anginosus* group (*S anginosus*, *S constellatus*, and *S intermedius*), *S mitis* group (*S mitis*, *S oralis*, and *S infantis*), *S sanguinis* group (*S sanguinis*, *S parasanguinis*, and *S gordonii*), *S bovis* group (*S gallolyticus* and *S lutetiensis*), *S mutans*, and *S salivarius*.

[c] The current breakpoint for penicillin resistance among VGS strains is an MIC of greater than or equal to 4 μg/mL. VGS strains with a penicillin MICs of 0.25 μg/mL to 2.0 μg/mL are considered intermediate; those with an MIC less than or equal to 0.12 μg/mL are considered susceptible.[118]

These investigators then identified and validated several factors associated with β-lactam–resistant VGS strains (defined as penicillin MIC of ≥ 2 μg/mL): β-lactam prophylaxis, receipt of a β-lactam within the preceding 30 days, and hospital-onset BSI.[117] Having any of the 3 risk factors predicted nonsusceptible VGS BSI with a sensitivity of 96%, specificity of 57%, positive predictive value of 34%, and negative predictive value of 98%. The investigators estimated that use of this prediction tool could reduce the unnecessary use of extra GP coverage by 42%. Interestingly, although 18% of all VGS isolates in this survey had a penicillin MIC greater than or equal to 2 μg/mL, these isolates were not associated with worse outcomes.

Kimura and colleagues[119] examined 28 episodes of breakthrough VGS BSI that occurred among 182 allogeneic SCT patients who had received levofloxacin prophylaxis for neutropenia. Five had VGS BSI-associated septic shock syndrome. None of strains was susceptible to levofloxacin and 21% were resistant to penicillin. All strains, however, were susceptible to piperacillin/tazobactam and meropenem and 95% were susceptible to cefepime. Mortality was similar in patients with or without VGS BSI.

Multiple other studies have noted similar rates of β-lactam resistance among VGS without a significant impact on mortality.[109,112,120] In summary, although penicillin resistance may now affect up to 60% of VGS strains, there is far less resistance among VGS to the antipseudomonal β-lactams in current use for empiric treatment of NF (piperacillin-tazobactam, cefepime, meropenem, and imipenem). Thus, the literature would suggest that for NF unaccompanied by septic shock or GP BSI, withholding additional GP coverage (with agents as vancomycin, glycopeptide derivatives, and daptomycin) remains appropriate. This management approach is supported by most guidelines.[121–126]

Streptococcus pneumoniae

For SP, both the frequency and the rate of resistance vary by country. In the United States, SP isolates causing IPD have the following resistance rates: 0.2% to levofloxacin, 0.4% to cefotaxime, 2.2% to penicillin, 12% to tetracycline, 31% to erythromycin.[75] In parts of Asia, SP resistance rates are much higher.[127,128]

Data as to whether outcomes are worse in patients with IPD who receive initial antibiotic therapy that is inadequate (misdirected or discordant) due to unappreciated strain resistance are conflicting.[129–131] In a non-SCT population in Spain, discordant therapy was associated with a very elevated risk of death (OR 10.6).[131] However, it is worth noting that in this study there were very high rates of resistance to antibiotics that may have been used for the entire course of treatment.

SP isolates obtained from 47 SCT patients diagnosed with IPD between 1989 and 2005 at the MD Anderson Cancer Center in Texas showed a striking amount of resistance; 41% were resistant to penicillin, 20% were resistant to imipenem, 21% were resistant to TMP-SMX, and 57% were resistant to azithromycin (only 3% were resistant to ceftriaxone). No deaths occurred in the 2 patients who initially received antibiotics to which their isolate was resistant.[76] In a separate study of IPD in patients with cancer (including SCT, HM, and solid tumors), initial misdirected therapy also did not result in increased risk of death, perhaps due to the small sample size.[132]

TRENDS IN ANTIMICROBIAL RESISTANCE AND ASSOCIATED MORTALITY IN GRAM-NEGATIVE BLOODSTREAM INFECTION

Most studies covered in this review observe increasing resistance of GNB causing BSI and other infections (see **Table 1**). Enterobacteriaceae (E coli, specifically) are the most common gram-negative species in most series. FQ prophylaxis has been associated with increased rates of extended-spectrum β-lactamase (ESBL)-mediated resistance and FQ resistance in *E coli* and other *Enterbacteriaceae*.[13,33] *E coli* and *Klebsiella* species with FQ resistance, ESBL-mediated resistance, carbapenem resistance, and/or multidrug resistance (MDR)[d] are now reported from diverse transplant centers (see **Table 1**). High rates of carbapenemase-producing *Enterobacteriaceae*, often Kp species, are reported in some regions and BSIs due to these pathogens are associated with increased mortality.[45,81,82] Highly resistant GNB represent a critical challenge to clinicians, transplant centers, and infection control programs.

Averbuch and colleagues[13] published a large, prospective analysis of antimicrobial resistance in GN BSIs, drawing data from 25 countries (65 centers) from eastern and western Europe, the Middle East, Australia, and China (see **Table 1**). All isolates from GN BSI occurring within 6 months of SCT were captured; 73% of the 704 GN isolates were Enterobacteriaceae. Among all GNB, *E coli* was the most frequently isolated (43%), followed by Kp (18%), PsA (14%), other Enterobacteriaceae (12%), and *Stenotrophomonas maltophilia* (5%). 50% of the GNB isolates in this study were resistant to FQs and noncarbapenems (ceftazidime, cefepime, and antipseudomonal β-lactam/β-lactamase inhibitor combinations). Close to 32% of total bacteria were aminoglycoside resistant and approximately 19% were carbapenem resistant. 35% of isolates were MDR, of which 50% also were carbapenem resistant. Although *A baumannii* comprised less than 2% of all GNB, 60% of strains were MDR.

Several interesting trends emerged from this large study. First, resistance rates in all categories considered (FQ, carbapenem, noncarbapenem, and MDR) were higher in countries in southeastern Europe (eg, Croatia, Greece, Israel, Italy, Portugal, Russia, Spain, and Turkey) than in northwestern Europe (eg, Austria, Belgium, Denmark, France, Germany, Sweden, Switzerland, and United Kingdom) (see **Table 1**).[13] Second, GN resistance across all antibiotic resistance categories was significantly higher in the allogeneic SCT group than the autologous group. For example, allogeneic SCT patients were twice as likely as autologous SCT patients to have a GN BSI with an MDR organism (44% vs 20%; *P*<.0001). Third, among centers that used FQs for antimicrobial prophylaxis during neutropenia, rates of FQ resistance were 3 times higher than centers that did not use FQ prophylaxis (74% vs 25%). Within the autologous SCT population, FQ prophylaxis was associated with acquisition of MDR pathogens and increased resistance to noncarbapenems. Risk factors for different categories of GN resistance analyzed in this study are listed in **Table 1**.

In contrast to the findings by Averbuch and colleagues,[13] another multicenter, prospective European survey of hospitalized neutropenic patients between 2002 and 2014 found much lower rates of resistance (see **Table 1**).[26] This study analyzed 2400 episodes of BSI from 36 sites. ESBL resistance was found in 10% of all Enterobacteriaceae and ESBL-resistant GN BSI occurred in only 64 of 2388 patients with BSI (2.7%). No increase in ESBL resistance was observed over 8 years of captured data and no carbapenem resistance was reported after surveillance was started in 2013.

In a study of GN BSI from 54 sites in Italy,[83] GNB resistance rates among allogeneic SCT patients were significantly higher than those seen in the autologous SCT group, similar to the findings of Averbuch and colleagues.[13] 38% of the PsA isolates in allogeneic SCT group were MDR strains compared with 7% in the autologous SCT group. In both groups, rectal colonization with carbapenem-resistant Kp and MDR PsA predicted BSI with those respective strains. In addition, having a BSI due to resistant GNB

---

[d] MDR is defined as nonsusceptibility to at least 1 agent in 3 or more antimicrobial categories.[133]

prior to transplant was associated with post-transplant BSI with the same isolate and resistance pattern (see **Table 1**).[83]

In several single-center studies, resistant GNB pose a particular problem.[12,20,23,30,31,33,34,81] Although it is possible that single-center studies introduce bias into the literature, results from larger studies (discussed previously)[13,26,83] support the view that GN resistance rates are high in many regions but also geographically variable.

Gram-negative BSI and GN BSI due to resistant organisms have been shown in multiple studies to be associated with increased mortality (see **Table 1**).[13,20,22,30,33,34,83,103] KPC-Kp BSI and MDR PsA, in particular, have been repeatedly associated with increased mortality(see **Table 1**).[45,81–83] In a large study in Italy, for example, KPC-Kp–colonized patients had a KPC-Kp BSI incidence of 39%, which was associated with 70% mortality.[45] In the study by Averbuch and colleagues,[13] early mortality was 3-fold to 4-fold higher in patients with any type of resistant GN BSI compared to BSI without resistant organisms. For example, mortality for BSI episodes due to carbapenem-resistant GNB was 18% versus 4% for carbapenem-susceptible GNB ($P<.001$). For MDR BSI episodes, mortality was 11% versus 4% for non-MDR BSI episodes ($P = .002$).

NEW APPROACHES TO MANAGEMENT OF BLOODSTREAM INFECTIONS
Molecular Diagnosis of Bloodstream Infections

In the best of circumstances, diagnosis of BSI prolongs hospital stay, adds expense, and may lead to additional procedures and morbidity. In other cases, the occurrence of BSI represents a greater likelihood of death. When the infecting organism also possesses MDR, the incorrect choice of empiric therapy may further elevate mortality. Novel diagnostic tools that are culture independent allow rapid and accurate pathogen identification. Use of these new molecular techniques has the potential to reduce the mortality that results from using incorrect empiric therapy for BSI.

Nucleic acid detection platforms can rapidly identify tens to hundreds of bacterial species, depending on the specific technology.[134] Positive blood cultures are not required. The molecular methods suitable for direct use on small volumes of blood include broad-range polymerase chain reaction (PCR) targeting 16S ribosomal RNA (rRNA) in bacterial species, followed by mass spectrometry or probe hybridization, PCR combined with in situ DNA hybridization and DNA melting analysis, and PCR followed by sequencing.[134,135] Platforms usually also detect *Candida* or other fungal species by simultaneously targeting 18S rRNA. Other techniques can be used to speed the identification of pathogens once blood cultures have turned positive. These methods include broad-range or multiplex PCR, sequencing, microarrays, and mass spectrometry.[135]

One example of a direct platform is SeptiFast (Roche Diagnostics GmbH, Mannheim, Germany), a technology that can identify 16 bacterial species as well as methicillin resistance in SA (*mecA* gene mutation). SeptiFast has variable sensitivity, specificity, and negative predictive value depending on the patient cohort to which it is applied. Sensitivity in hematology patients and patients with febrile neutropenia, for example, ranges from 26% to 95%, specificity from 78% to 88%, and negative predictive value from 66% to 99%.[134] Elges and colleagues[136] prospectively compared SeptiFast, blood culture, and a locally developed PCR method (for fungal pathogens only) in 205 BSI episodes in HM patients. They found a moderate correlation between BSI diagnosed by SeptiFast and blood culture, but SeptiFast identified more bacterial species (43 vs 38) and outperformed blood culture in diagnosing fungal

BSI. SeptiFast is commercially available in Europe but has not yet approved by the US Food and Drug Administration. Another platform, the IRIDICA PLEX-ID (Abbott Molecular, Des Plaines, Illinois), later known as the IRIDICA system, ID, can identify hundreds (up to 750) of bacterial species and 4 resistance markers (mecA, vanA, vanB, and KPC).[134] In patients with febrile neutropenia, IRIDICA PLEX-ID had a reported sensitivity of 45%, specificity of 93%, and negative predictive value of 80%.[134] Unfortunately, this product was discontinued by Abbott in 2017.[137]

Challenges faced by all molecular methods include false-positive results due to detection of DNA fragments from lysed bacteria, difficulty discriminating individual pathogens in polymicrobial bacteremia, and false-negative results in low-burden bacteremia. Further study of specific platforms in a variety of SCT and HM cohorts is needed.

Infection Control, Catheter Technology, and Antibiotic Stewardship

Infection control measures, including isolation, hand hygiene programs, cohorting, contact precautions, catheter care, and room and equipment disinfection, are critical to limiting health care transmission of drug resistant pathogens (**Box 1**).[138,139] Specific decontamination measures may include chlorhexidine-impregnated cleansing cloths, bleach applications to surfaces and equipment, and ultraviolet light. Catheter technology also is advancing rapidly. Antimicrobial peptides, antibiotics, or chlorhexidine-silver sulfadiazine coating can be applied to vascular catheters. CLABSI rates were lower with antibiotic-coated or chlorhexidine-silver sulfadiazine-coated catheters compared with standard catheters when used as part of a bundle.[140]

Antimicrobial stewardship programs are indispensable to reducing the rate of drug resistance and to designing care bundles for institutions with high rates of resistance.[139] Faced with increasing MDR, some centers and countries have begun to question or discontinue the standard practice of fluoroquinolone prophylaxis.[33,36,147,148] Other guideline groups, such as the Infectious Diseases Working Party (AGIHO) of the German Society of Hematology and Medical Oncology (DGHO) have placed more emphasis on discontinuing empiric antibiotics in stable, neutropenic patients after 7 days of defervescence.[122]

In 1 Italian center with a high rate of KPC-Kp infections, De Rosa and colleagues[149] devised a bundle of interventions to reduce BSI in patients with KPC-Kp rectal colonization. All hematology patients were screened with rectal swabs for MDR organisms at admission and weekly. Approximately 5% of SCT patients were found to have carbapenem-resistant Kp and received the Turin bundle: oral gentamicin for intestinal

Box 1		
Measures influencing risk of bacterial infection in patients undergoing hematopoietic stem cell transplant		
Benefit	**No Evidence of Benefit**	**Harm**
Hand washing	Oral hygiene	FQ use may increase prevalence
Oral FQs (GI	Low bacterial diet (cooked food)	of ESBL, MRSA, and VRE and
decontamination)	Contact isolation (gown, gloves)	increase risk of GVHD
Mask		
Vaccination		
Prophylactic penicillin or		
macrolide ($\downarrow$ risk SP)		
Immunoglobulin		
replacement		
Data from Refs.[125,141–146]		

decontamination prior to SCT, avoidance of levofloxacin prophylaxis (to prevent gut dysbiosis), and a regimen of tigecycline with piperacillin/tazobactam for NF (to avoid use of carbapenems). In cases of septic shock, a treatment regimen of colistin combined with tigecycline and high-dose meropenem was instituted. Two patients developed Kp bacteremia (no data were provided regarding antibiotic susceptibility of these isolates). None of the 5 colonized patients died or developed shock and 60% converted to negative rectal swabs. Prospective study of this bundle and its individual elements in an independent cohort is needed to confirm mortality benefits.

To date, the routine use of active screening cultures for MDR GNB remains controversial, although it is recommended in outbreak settings and in endemic sites.[138]

Bloodstream Infection Prediction Tools and Targeted Prophylaxis

Several groups have developed algorithms that predict bacteremia in SCT and HM patients using microbiome or clinical data. Taur and colleagues[150] characterized the intestinal diversity in patients undergoing allogeneic SCT by pyrosequencing variable regions in the bacterial 16S ribosomal RNA gene (16S rRNA) in fecal samples. Fecal samples were evaluated serially beginning prior to transplant and continuing until 35 days after transplant. Diversity was evaluated using the Shannon diversity index. Fecal biodiversity dropped significantly after transplant. Intestinal domination (representation of 30% of microbiome by a single bacterial taxon) by enterococcal species was associated with a 9-fold increased risk of VRE BSI ($P = .001$). Domination by Proteobacteria was associated with a 5-fold increased risk of GN BSI ($P = .047$); 22 of 94 patients (23%) developed bacteremia. In half of the BSI episodes, intestinal domination was apparent 1 week prior to BSI. Metronidazole was associated with enterococcal domination, whereas FQs were protective against Proteobacteria domination. A subsequent study by the same investigators found a correlation between reduced intestinal diversity and greater long-term mortality after transplant.[151]

In a small study of patients with non-Hodgkin lymphoma undergoing chemotherapy, Montassier and colleagues[152] found that clinical data did not predict BSI. Depletion of 13 taxonomic groups, however, predicted BSI and greater abundance of Erysipelotrichaceae and Veillonellaceae in fecal samples was associated with BSI.

In contrast, Webb and colleagues[71] were able to use clinical data to build a risk model that successfully predicted VRE BSI in leukemia and SCT patients. Predictive risk factors included VRE colonization, renal insufficiency, aminoglycoside use, receipt of antibiotics with antianaerobic activity, GI disturbance, severe neutropenia, and previous carbapenem or cephalosporin use. A score of 5 points or higher predicted BSI with a sensitivity of 77%, a specificity of 79%, and a negative predictive value of 99.9%. Validation of these microbiome-based and clinical prediction models in additional patient cohorts in different geographic regions is needed.

Novel Antimicrobials

Several new anti-infective agents have been approved by the US Food and Drug Administration or are in later stages of development (**Table 2**).[153,154] Many of these agents target high-priority, drug-resistant bacteria, such as carbapenem-resistant Enterobacteriaceae (CRE), ESBL-producing Enterobacteriaceae, MDR A baumannii, Pseudomonas, and other high-priority pathogens, such as MRSA and VRE. Among this group are new antibiotics in familiar classes (the aminoglycoside, plazomicin), founding members of new antibiotic classes (meropenem/vaborbactam, brilacidin, and murepavadin), and synthesized versions (mimetics) of antibacterial peptides and defensins (murepavadin and brilacidin). Collectively, these agents are chemically

Table 2
Selected novel anti-infective agents

Anti-infective (Brand Name)	Class/Mechanism	Targeted Pathogen	Development Phase
Meropenem/ vaborbactam (Vabomere)	Carbapenem + novel βLI	GN ESKAPE, CRE	FDA: August 2017
Plazomicin (Zemdri)	Aminoglycoside	GN ESKAPE, CRE	FDA: June 2018
Xerava (eravacycline)	Tetracycline	GN ESKAPE, CRE; ?CRAB	FDA: August 2018
Omadacycline	Tetracycline (oral)	GN ESKAPE, ?CRAB	FDA: October 2018
Cefepime + AAI101	Fourth-gen ceph + novel βLI	GN ESKAPE, ?CRE	Phase 3
Cefiderocol	Siderophore-βL comb	GN ESKAPE, CRE, CRAB, CR PsA	Phase 3
Ceftobiprole	Fifth-gen ceph with anti-MRSA activity		Phase 3
Imipenem/cilastatin + relebactam (MK-7655)	Carbapenem + novel βLI	GN ESKAPE; CRE, ?CR PsA	Phase 3
Murepavadin (POL7080)	Antimicrobial peptide mimetic	PsA, CR PsA	Phase 3
Sulopenem	Novel carbapenem	GN ESKAPE	Phase 3
Brilacidin	Defensin mimetic	Many susceptible and resistant GPB, GNB	Phase 2

Abbreviations: +, combined with; ?, indicates possible activity; βL/βLI, beta-lactam/beta-lactamase inhibitor; Ceph, cephalosporin; comb, combination; CRAB, carbapenem-resistant *A baumannii*; CR PsA, carbapenem-resistant PsA; FDA, date of approval by US Food and Drug Administration (month and year); gen, generation; GN ESKAPE, GN pathogens identified as public health priorities: Kp, *A baumannii*, PsA, and *Enterobacter* species; mimetic, synthesized version of antimicrobial peptide found in nature.

(*Data from* Pew Charitable Trusts. Antibiotics currently in global clinical development (updated Sept 2018). 2018. Available at: https://www.pewtrusts.org/-/media/assets/2018/09/antibiotics_currently_in_global_clinical_development_sept2018.pdf. Accessed December 25, 2019; and Mensa B, Howell GL, Scott R, et al. Comparative mechanistic studies of brilacidin, daptomycin, and the antimicrobial peptide LL16. Antimicrobial agents and chemotherapy 2014;58(9):5136–45.

and biologically ingenious, and have refreshed the toolbox needed to treat many of the highly resistant pathogens seen in SCT and HM patient populations.

SUMMARY

High rates of BSIs (20%–30%) are found in the SCT and HM populations, due to a unique and synergistic combination of profound immune suppression, mucosal barrier injury, and exposure to the health care environment. Most BSIs occur in the early post-transplant engraftment period, and up to one-third of BSIs are due to CLABSI.

In most studies, GPB occur at greater frequency than GNB, although some centers report that rates of GN BSI have recently increased.

The most frequently isolated species among GPB are CoNS, streptococci, and enterococci. A majority of CoNS are methicillin resistant. There is increasing resistance to penicillin and advanced β-lactams among VGS, but this trend has not affected mortality. The frequency of enterococci in BSI has increased along with the rate of VRE, which in some centers are the majority of enterococcal isolates. VRE

BSI has been associated in several studies with increased mortality. T-cell depletion, HLA-mismatch, mucositis, GVHD, CDI, older age, comorbidities (eg, renal failure and others), and receipt of vancomycin and other antibiotics are risk factors for VRE BSI. MRSA rates are low in many centers in Europe and some developing countries (eg, India and Egypt) but high in Latin America, Asia and the United States. SP, although infrequent, is an important cause of late transplant BSI. Some centers in Europe report low vaccination rates, which are a target for interventions.

Among GNB, *E coli* and *Klebsiella* species are the most frequent causes of BSI. In some centers, a large fraction of GNB are resistant to all agents in 1 or more antibiotic classes. Resistance rates are generally higher (often 2-fold) in allogeneic SCT compared with autologous SCT. FQ-mediated and ESBL-mediated resistance have been associated with FQ prophylaxis. BSI due to Kp, in particular KPC-Kp, is associated with very high mortality. Carbapenem resistance mediated by KPC is endemic in some regions (Italy and some other European centers). Risk factors for carbapenem resistance include length of hospitalization, ICU admission, prior use of antibiotics or carbapenem, and rectal colonization with KPC-Kp. Antibiotic treatment for suspected KPC-Kp should be guided by local epidemiology but may require 3 agents until susceptibility results are known. PsA isolates usually represent 5% or less of all BSIs but frequently have MDR, carbapenem resistance, and/or aminoglycoside resistance. *A baumannii* is also infrequent but usually highly drug resistant.

Infection control, new catheter technology, antibiotic stewardship, and the use of bundles for patients infected with highly resistant organisms all are important in management. Use of prediction tools, combined with an assessment of clinical features (septic shock and GPB), to select patients for whom additional GP coverage would be of benefit has not been extensively studied in SCT populations but should be. Such tools have great potential to improve antibiotic stewardship, without sacrificing safety, in this high-risk population. Several new anti-infectives have promise for the treatment of resistant pathogens, in particular GNB.

REFERENCES

1. Çelebi H, Akan H, Akçağlayan E, et al. Febrile neutropenia in allogeneic and autologous peripheral blood stem cell transplantation and conventional chemotherapy for malignancies. Bone Marrow Transplant 2000;26:211.

2. Sahin U, Toprak SK, Atilla PA, et al. An overview of infectious complications after allogeneic hematopoietic stem cell transplantation. J Infect Chemother 2016; 22(8):505–14.

3. Kulkarni S, Powles R, Treleaven J, et al. Chronic graft versus host disease is associated with long-term risk for pneumococcal infections in recipients of bone marrow transplants. Blood 2000;95(12):3683–6.

4. Wingard JR, Hsu J, Hiemenz JW. Hematopoietic stem cell transplantation: an overview of infection risks and epidemiology. Hematol Oncol Clin North Am 2011;25(1):101–16.

5. Demirer T, Gooley T, Buckner CD, et al. Influence of total nucleated cell dose from marrow harvests on outcome in patients with acute myelogenous leukemia undergoing autologous transplantation. Bone Marrow Transplant 1995;15(6): 907–13.

6. Tomblyn M, Chiller T, Einsele H, et al. Guidelines for preventing infectious complications among hematopoietic cell transplantation recipients: a global perspective. Biol Blood Marrow Transplant 2009;15(10):1143–238.

7. Rovira M, Mensa J, Carreras E. Infections after HSCT. In: Apperley J, Carreras E, Gluckman E, et al, editors. The EBMT handbook on haematopoietic stem cell transplantation. 6th edition. Paris (France): European School of Haematology and European Society for Bone Marrow Transplantation; 2012. p. 196–215.

8. Brown A. Neutropenia, fever, and infection. In: Brown AE, Armstrong D, editors. Infectious complications of neoplastic disease, controversies in management. New York: Yorke Medical Books; 1985. p. 19–34.

9. Dandoy CE, Ardura MI, Papanicolaou GA, et al. Bacterial bloodstream infections in the allogeneic hematopoietic cell transplant patient: new considerations for a persistent nemesis. Bone Marrow Transplant 2017;52(8):1091–106.

10. See I, Freifeld AG, Magill SS. Causative organisms and associated antimicrobial resistance in healthcare-associated, central line-associated bloodstream infections from oncology settings, 2009-2012. Clin Infect Dis 2016;62(10):1203–9.

11. Dudeck MA, Edwards JR, Allen-Bridson K, et al. National Healthcare Safety Network report, data summary for 2013, device-associated module. Am J Infect Control 2015;43(3):206–21.

12. César-Arce A, Volkow-Fernández P, Valero-Saldaña LM, et al. Complications and multidrug-resistant bacteria in patients with hematopoietic stem cell transplantation in the first 12 months after transplant. Transplant Proc 2017;49(6): 1444–8.

13. Averbuch D, Tridello G, Hoek J, et al. Antimicrobial resistance in gram-negative rods causing bacteremia in hematopoietic stem cell transplant recipients: intercontinental prospective study of the infectious diseases working party of the european bone marrow transplantation group. Clin Infect Dis 2017;65(11): 1819–28.

14. Piñana JL, Montesinos P, Martino R, et al. Incidence, risk factors, and outcome of bacteremia following autologous hematopoietic stem cell transplantation in 720 adult patients. Ann Hematol 2014;93(2):299–307.

15. Kolbe K, Domkin D, Derigs HG, et al. Infectious complications during neutropenia subsequent to peripheral blood stem cell transplantation. Bone Marrow Transplant 1997;19(2):143–7.

16. Wade J, Schimpf S. Epidemiology and prevention of infection in the compromised host. In: Rubin R, Young L, editors. Clinical approach to infection in the compromised host. New York: Plenum Press; 1988. p. 5–40.

17. Link H, Maschmeyer G, Meyer P, et al. Interventional antimicrobial therapy in febrile neutropenic patients. Study Group of the Paul Ehrlich Society for Chemotherapy. Ann Hematol 1994;69(5):231–43.

18. De Pauw BE, Deresinski SC, Feld R, et al. Ceftazidime compared with piperacillin and tobramycin for the empiric treatment of fever in neutropenic patients with cancer. A multicenter randomized trial. The Intercontinental Antimicrobial Study Group. Ann Intern Med 1994;120(10):834–44.

19. Freifeld AG, Walsh T, Marshall D, et al. Monotherapy for fever and neutropenia in cancer patients: a randomized comparison of ceftazidime versus imipenem. J Clin Oncol 1995;13(1):165–76.

20. Gudiol C, Garcia-Vidal C, Arnan M, et al. Etiology, clinical features and outcomes of pre-engraftment and post-engraftment bloodstream infection in hematopoietic SCT recipients. Bone Marrow Transplant 2014;49(6):824–30.

21. Ballen K, Woo Ahn K, Chen M, et al. Infection rates among acute leukemia patients receiving alternative donor hematopoietic cell transplantation. Biol Blood Marrow Transplant 2016;22(9):1636–45.

22. Schuster MG, Cleveland AA, Dubberke ER, et al. Infections in hematopoietic cell transplant recipients: results from the organ transplant infection project, a multicenter, prospective, cohort study. Open Forum Infect Dis 2017;4(2):ofx050.

23. Wang CH, Chang FY, Chao TY, et al. Characteristics comparisons of bacteremia in allogeneic and autologous hematopoietic stem cell-transplant recipients with levofloxacin prophylaxis and influence on resistant bacteria emergence. J Microbiol Immunol Infect 2018;51(1):123–31.

24. Styczynski J, Czyzewski K, Wysocki M, et al. Increased risk of infections and infection-related mortality in children undergoing haematopoietic stem cell transplantation compared to conventional anticancer therapy: a multicentre nationwide study. Clin Microbiol Infect 2016;22(2):179e1-10.

25. Young JH, Logan BR, Wu J, et al. Infections after transplantation of bone marrow or peripheral blood stem cells from unrelated donors. Biol Blood Marrow Transplant 2016;22(2):359–70.

26. Weisser M, Theilacker C, Tschudin Sutter S, et al. Secular trends of bloodstream infections during neutropenia in 15,181 haematopoietic stem cell transplants: 13-year results from a European multicentre surveillance study (ONKO-KISS). Clin Microbiol Infect 2017;23(11):854–9.

27. Mikulska M, Viscoli C, Orasch C, et al. Aetiology and resistance in bacteraemias among adult and paediatric haematology and cancer patients. J Infect 2014; 68(4):321–31.

28. Sanz J, Cano I, Gonzalez-Barbera EM, et al. Bloodstream infections in adult patients undergoing cord blood transplantation from unrelated donors after myeloablative conditioning regimen. Biol Blood Marrow Transplant 2015;21(4): 755–60.

29. Blennow O, Ljungman P, Sparrelid E, et al. Incidence, risk factors, and outcome of bloodstream infections during the pre-engraftment phase in 521 allogeneic hematopoietic stem cell transplantations. Transpl Infect Dis 2014;16(1):106–14.

30. Wang L, Wang Y, Fan X, et al. Prevalence of resistant gram-negative bacilli in bloodstream infection in febrile neutropenia patients undergoing hematopoietic stem cell transplantation: a single center retrospective cohort study. Medicine 2015;94(45):e1931.

31. Kikuchi M, Akahoshi Y, Nakano H, et al. Risk factors for pre- and post-engraftment bloodstream infections after allogeneic hematopoietic stem cell transplantation. Transpl Infect Dis 2015;17(1):56–65.

32. Srinivasan A, Wang C, Srivastava DK, et al. Timeline, epidemiology, and risk factors for bacterial, fungal, and viral infections in children and adolescents after allogeneic hematopoietic stem cell transplantation. Biol Blood Marrow Transplant 2013;19(1):94–101.

33. Macesic N, Morrissey CO, Cheng AC, et al. Changing microbial epidemiology in hematopoietic stem cell transplant recipients: increasing resistance over a 9-year period. Transpl Infect Dis 2014;16(6):887–96.

34. Zheng C, Tang B, Zhu X, et al. Pre-engraftment bloodstream infections in acute leukemia patients undergoing unrelated cord blood transplantation following intensified myeloablative conditioning without ATG. Ann Hematol 2017;96(1): 115–24.

35. Slade M, Goldsmith S, Romee R, et al. Epidemiology of infections following haploidentical peripheral blood hematopoietic cell transplantation. Transpl Infect Dis 2017;19(1):e12629.

36. Satlin MJ, Vardhana S, Soave R, et al. Impact of prophylactic levofloxacin on rates of bloodstream infection and fever in neutropenic patients with multiple

myeloma undergoing autologous hematopoietic stem cell transplantation. Biol Blood Marrow Transplant 2015;21(10):1808–14.

37. Srinivasan A, McLaughlin L, Wang C, et al. Early infections after autologous hematopoietic stem cell transplantation in children and adolescents: the St. Jude experience. Transpl Infect Dis 2014;16(1):90–7.

38. Girmenia C, Bertaina A, Piciocchi A, et al. Incidence, risk factors and outcome of pre-engraftment gram-negative bacteremia after allogeneic and autologous hematopoietic stem cell transplantation: an Italian Prospective Multicenter Survey. Clin Infect Dis 2017;65(11):1884–96.

39. Jain S, Self WH, Wunderink RG, et al. Community-acquired pneumonia requiring hospitalization among U.S. adults. N Engl J Med 2015;373(5):415–27.

40. Roychowdhury M, Pambuccian SE, Aslan DL, et al. Pulmonary complications after bone marrow transplantation: an autopsy study from a large transplantation center. Arch Pathol Lab Med 2005;129(3):366–71.

41. Baluch A, Pasikhova Y, Snyder M. Successful management of *Mycobacterium haemophilum* lower extremity cutaneous infection in a matched-unrelated donor stem cell transplant recipient. Transpl Infect Dis 2017;19(1):e12627.

42. Padrnos LJ, Blair JE, Kusne S, et al. Cutaneous legionellosis: case report and review of the medical literature. Transpl Infect Dis 2014;16(2):307–14.

43. Van Burik JA, Hackman RC, Nadeem SQ, et al. Nocardiosis after bone marrow transplantation: a retrospective study. Clin Infect Dis 1997;24(6):1154–60.

44. Shannon K, Pasikhova Y, Ibekweh Q, et al. Nocardiosis following hematopoietic stem cell transplantation. Transpl Infect Dis 2016;18(2):169–75.

45. Girmenia C, Rossolini GM, Piciocchi A, et al. Infections by carbapenem-resistant *Klebsiella pneumoniae* in SCT recipients: a nationwide retrospective survey from Italy. Bone Marrow Transplant 2015;50(2):282–8.

46. van Veen KE, Brouwer MC, van der Ende A, et al. Bacterial meningitis in hematopoietic stem cell transplant recipients: a population-based prospective study. Bone Marrow Transplant 2016;51(11):1490–5.

47. Sivagnanam S, Podczervinski S, Butler-Wu SM, et al. Legionnaires' disease in transplant recipients: a 15-year retrospective study in a tertiary referral center. Transpl Infect Dis 2017;19(5):e12745.

48. Mansi L, Daguindau E, Saas P, et al. Diagnosis and management of nocardiosis after bone marrow stem cell transplantation in adults: lack of lymphocyte recovery as a major contributing factor. Pathol Biol (Paris) 2014;62(3):156–61.

49. Wei MC, Banaei N, Yakrus MA, et al. Nontuberculous mycobacteria infections in immunocompromised patients: single institution experience. J Pediatr Hematol Oncol 2009;31(8):556–60.

50. Beswick J, Shin E, Michelis FV, et al. Incidence and risk factors for nontuberculous mycobacterial infection after allogeneic hematopoietic cell transplantation. Biol Blood Marrow Transplant 2018;24(2):366–72.

51. Zhao Z, Leow WQ. Concurrent hepatic tuberculosis and hepatic graft-versus-host disease in an allogeneic hematopoietic stem cell transplant recipient: a case report. Transplant Proc 2017;49(7):1659–62.

52. Fan WC, Liu CJ, Hong YC, et al. Long-term risk of tuberculosis in haematopoietic stem cell transplant recipients: a 10-year nationwide study. Int J Tuberc Lung Dis 2015;19(1):58–64.

53. Coussement J, Lebeaux D, Rouzaud C, et al. *Nocardia* infections in solid organ and hematopoietic stem cell transplant recipients. Curr Opin Infect Dis 2017;30(6):545–51.

54. Nørgaard M, Larsson H, Pedersen G, et al. Risk of bacteraemia and mortality in patients with haematological malignancies. Clin Microbiol Infect 2006;12(3): 217–23.

55. Funada H, Machi T, Matsuda T. Bacteremia complicating acute leukemia with special reference to its incidence and changing etiological patterns. Jpn J Clin Oncol 1988;18(3):239–48.

56. Funada H, Matsuda T. Changes in the incidence and etiological patterns of bacteremia associated with acute leukemia over a 25-year period. Intern Med 1998;37(12):1014–8.

57. Grigis A, Goglio A, Parea M, et al. Nosocomial outbreak of severe *Pseudomonas aeruginosa* infections in haematological patients. Eur J Epidemiol 1993;9(4): 390–5.

58. Rolston KV, Tarrand JJ. *Pseudomonas aeruginosa* - still a frequent pathogen in patients with cancer: 11-year experience at a comprehensive cancer center. Clin Infect Dis 1999;29(2):463–4.

59. Koll BS, Brown AE. The changing epidemiology of infections at cancer hospitals. Clin Infect Dis 1993;17(Suppl 2):S322–8.

60. Coullioud D, Van der Auwera P, Viot M, et al. Prospective multicentric study of the etiology of 1051 bacteremic episodes in 782 cancer patients. CEMIC (French-Belgian Study Club of Infectious Diseases in Cancer). Support Care Cancer 1993;1(1):34–46.

61. Safdar A, Rodriguez GH, Balakrishnan M, et al. Changing trends in etiology of bacteremia in patients with cancer. Eur J Clin Microbiol Infect Dis 2006;25(8): 522–6.

62. Worth LJ, Slavin MA. Bloodstream infections in haematology: risks and new challenges for prevention. Blood Rev 2009;23(3):113–22.

63. Gonzalez-Barca E, Fernandez-Sevilla A, Carratala J, et al. Prospective study of 288 episodes of bacteremia in neutropenic cancer patients in a single institution. Eur J Clin Microbiol Infect Dis 1996;15(4):291–6.

64. Wisplinghoff H, Seifert H, Wenzel RP, et al. Current trends in the epidemiology of nosocomial bloodstream infections in patients with hematological malignancies and solid neoplasms in hospitals in the United States. Clin Infect Dis 2003;36(9): 1103–10.

65. Del Favero A, Menichetti F, Bucaneve G, et al. Septicaemia due to gram-positive cocci in cancer patients. J Antimicrob Chemother 1988;21(Suppl C):157–65.

66. Whimbey E, Kiehn TE, Brannon P, et al. Bacteremia and fungemia in patients with neoplastic disease. Am J Med 1987;82(4):723–30.

67. Collin BA, Leather HL, Wingard JR, et al. Evolution, incidence, and susceptibility of bacterial bloodstream isolates from 519 bone marrow transplant patients. Clin Infect Dis 2001;33(7):947–53.

68. Balletto E, Mikulska M. Bacterial infections in hematopoietic stem cell transplant recipients. Mediterr J Hematol Infect Dis 2015;7(1):e2015045.

69. Batra U, Goyal P, Jain P, et al. Epidemiology and resistance pattern of bacterial isolates among cancer patients in a Tertiary Care Oncology Centre in North India. Indian J Cancer 2016;53(3):448–51.

70. Gudiol C, Royo-Cebrecos C, Laporte J, et al. Clinical features, aetiology and outcome of bacteraemic pneumonia in neutropenic cancer patients. Respirology 2016;21(8):1411–8.

71. Webb BJ, Healy R, Majers J, et al. Prediction of bloodstream infection due to vancomycin-resistant *Enterococcus* in patients undergoing leukemia induction or hematopoietic stem-cell transplantation. Clin Infect Dis 2017;64(12):1753–9.

72. Wong A, Marrie TJ, Garg S, et al. Increased risk of invasive pneumococcal disease in haematological and solid-organ malignancies. Epidemiol Infect 2010; 138(12):1804–10.

73. van Aalst M, Lotsch F, Spijker R, et al. Incidence of invasive pneumococcal disease in immunocompromised patients: a systematic review and meta-analysis. Travel Med Infect Dis 2018;24:89–100.

74. Torda A, Chong Q, Lee A, et al. Invasive pneumococcal disease following adult allogeneic hematopoietic stem cell transplantation. Transpl Infect Dis 2014; 16(5):751–9.

75. CDC. Active bacterial core surveillance report, emerging infections program network, Streptococcus pneumoniae. Atlanta (GA): Centers for Disease Control and Prevention; 2016.

76. Youssef S, Rodriguez G, Rolston KV, et al. *Streptococcus pneumoniae* infections in 47 hematopoietic stem cell transplantation recipients: clinical characteristics of infections and vaccine-breakthrough infections, 1989-2005. Medicine (Baltimore) 2007;86(2):69–77.

77. Kumar D, Humar A, Plevneshi A, et al. Invasive pneumococcal disease in adult hematopoietic stem cell transplant recipients: a decade of prospective population-based surveillance. Bone Marrow Transplant 2008;41(8):743–7.

78. Engelhard D, Cordonnier C, Shaw PJ, et al. Early and late invasive pneumococcal infection following stem cell transplantation: a European Bone Marrow Transplantation survey. Br J Haematol 2002;117(2):444–50.

79. van Lier A, McDonald SA, Bouwknegt M, et al. Disease burden of 32 infectious diseases in the Netherlands, 2007-2011. PLoS One 2016;11(4):e0153106.

80. Cohen C, Naidoo N, Meiring S, et al. *Streptococcus pneumoniae* serotypes and mortality in adults and adolescents in South Africa: analysis of National Surveillance Data, 2003 - 2008. PLoS One 2015;10(10):e0140185.

81. El-Mahallawy H, Samir I, Abdel Fattah R, et al. Source, pattern and antibiotic resistance of blood stream infections in hematopoietic stem cell transplant recipients. J Egypt Natl Canc Inst 2014;26(2):73–7.

82. Ghafur A, Devarajan V, Raj R, et al. Spectrum of bacteremia in posthematopoietic stem cell transplant patients from an Indian center. Indian J Cancer 2016;53(4):590–1.

83. Mikulska M, Del Bono V, Bruzzi P, et al. Mortality after bloodstream infections in allogeneic haematopoietic stem cell transplant recipients. Infection 2012;40(3):271–8.

84. Satlin MJ, Soave R, Racanelli AC, et al. The emergence of vancomycin-resistant enterococcal bacteremia in hematopoietic stem cell transplant recipients. Leuk Lymphoma 2014;55(12):2858–65.

85. Satwani P, Freedman JL, Chaudhury S, et al. A multicenter study of bacterial blood stream infections in pediatric allogeneic hematopoietic cell transplantation recipients: the role of acute gastrointestinal graft-versus-host disease. Biol Blood Marrow Transplant 2017;23(4):642–7.

86. Worth LJ, Thursky KA, Seymour JF, et al. Vancomycin-resistant *Enterococcus faecium* infection in patients with hematologic malignancy: patients with acute myeloid leukemia are at high-risk. Eur J Haematol 2007;79(3):226–33.

87. Mikulska M, Del Bono V, Prinapori R, et al. Risk factors for enterococcal bacteremia in allogeneic hematopoietic stem cell transplant recipients. Transpl Infect Dis 2010;12(6):505–12.

88. Zaas AK, Song X, Tucker P, et al. Risk factors for development of vancomycin-resistant enterococcal bloodstream infection in patients with cancer who are colonized with vancomycin-resistant enterococci. Clin Infect Dis 2002;35(10):1139–46.

89. Roghmann MC, McCarter RJ Jr, Brewrink J, et al. *Clostridium difficile* infection is a risk factor for bacteremia due to vancomycin-resistant enterococci (VRE) in VRE-colonized patients with acute leukemia. Clin Infect Dis 1997;25(5):1056–9.

90. Matar MJ, Safdar A, Rolston KV. Relationship of colonization with vancomycin-resistant enterococci and risk of systemic infection in patients with cancer. Clin Infect Dis 2006;42(10):1506–7.

91. Weinstock DM, Conlon M, Iovino C, et al. Colonization, bloodstream infection, and mortality caused by vancomycin-resistant *Enterococcus* early after allogeneic hematopoietic stem cell transplant. Biol Blood Marrow Transplant 2007; 13(5):615–21.

92. Vydra J, Shanley RM, George I, et al. Enterococcal bacteremia is associated with increased risk of mortality in recipients of allogeneic hematopoietic stem cell transplantation. Clin Infect Dis 2012;55(6):764–70.

93. Tavadze M, Rybicki L, Mossad S, et al. Risk factors for vancomycin-resistant *Enterococcus* bacteremia and its influence on survival after allogeneic hematopoietic cell transplantation. Bone Marrow Transplant 2014;49(10):1310–6.

94. Hefazi M, Damlaj M, Alkhateeb HB, et al. Vancomycin-resistant *Enterococcus* colonization and bloodstream infection: prevalence, risk factors, and the impact on early outcomes after allogeneic hematopoietic cell transplantation in patients with acute myeloid leukemia. Transpl Infect Dis 2016;18(6):913–20.

95. Kamboj M, Cohen N, Huang YT, et al. Impact of empiric treatment for vancomycin-resistant *Enterococcus* in colonized patients early after allogeneic hematopoietic stem cell transplantation. Biol Blood Marrow Transplant 2018. [Epub ahead of print].

96. Lisboa LF, Miranda BG, Vieira MB, et al. Empiric use of linezolid in febrile hematology and hematopoietic stem cell transplantation patients colonized with vancomycin-resistant *Enterococcus* spp. Int J Infect Dis 2015;33:171–6.

97. Seas C, Garcia C, Salles MJ, et al. *Staphylococcus aureus* bloodstream infections in Latin America: results of a multinational prospective cohort study. J Antimicrob Chemother 2018;73(1):212–22.

98. Stefani S, Chung DR, Lindsay JA, et al. Methicillin-resistant *Staphylococcus aureus* (MRSA): global epidemiology and harmonisation of typing methods. Int J Antimicrob Agents 2012;39(4):273–82.

99. Klein EY, Jiang W, Mojica N, et al. National costs associated with methicillin-susceptible and methicillin-resistant *Staphylococcus aureus* hospitalizations in the United States, 2010–2014. Clin Infect Dis 2019;68(1):22–8.

100. Kavanagh KT, Abusalem S, Calderon LE. The incidence of MRSA infections in the United States: is a more comprehensive tracking system needed? Antimicrob Resist Infect Control 2017;6:34.

101. Antimicrobial resistance surveillance in Europe 2017: annual report of the European antimicrobial resistance surveillance network (EARS-Net). Stockholm (Sweden): European Centre for Disease Prevention and Control; 2017. Available at: https://ecdc.europa.eu/en/publications-data/surveillance-antimicrobial-resistance-europe-2017.

102. Miles-Jay A, Podczervinski S, Stednick ZJ, et al. Evaluation of routine pretransplantation screening for methicillin-resistant *Staphylococcus aureus* in hematopoietic cell transplant recipients. Am J Infect Control 2015;43(1):89–91.

103. Stoma I, Karpov I, Milanovich N, et al. Risk factors for mortality in patients with bloodstream infections during the pre-engraftment period after hematopoietic stem cell transplantation. Blood Res 2016;51(2):102–6.

104. Choeyprasert W, Hongeng S, Anurathapan U, et al. Bacteremia during neutropenic episodes in children undergoing hematopoietic stem cell transplantation with ciprofloxacin and penicillin prophylaxis. Int J Hematol 2017;105(2):213–20.

105. Diekema DJ, Beach ML, Pfaller MA, et al. Antimicrobial resistance in viridans group streptococci among patients with and without the diagnosis of cancer in the USA, Canada and Latin America. Clin Microbiol Infect 2001;7(3):152–7.

106. Bochud P-Y, Calandra T, Francioli P. Bacteremia due to viridans streptococci in neutropenic patients: a review. Am J Med 1994;97(3):256–64.

107. Elting LS, Bodey GP, Keefe BH. Septicemia and shock syndrome due to viridans streptococci: a case-control study of predisposing factors. Clin Infect Dis 1992; 14(6):1201–7.

108. Freifeld AG, Razonable RR. Viridans group streptococci in febrile neutropenic cancer patients: what should we fear? Clin Infect Dis 2014;59(2):231–3.

109. Marron A, Carratalà J, González-Barca E, et al. Serious complications of bacteremia caused by viridans streptococci in neutropenic patients with cancer. Clin Infect Dis 2000;31(5):1126–30.

110. Carratala J, Alcaide F, Fernandez-Sevilla A, et al. Bacteremia due to viridans streptococci that are highly resistant to penicillin: increase among neutropenic patients with cancer. Clin Infect Dis 1995;20(5):1169–73.

111. Alcaide F, Liñares J, Pallares R, et al. In vitro activities of 22 beta-lactam antibiotics against penicillin-resistant and penicillin-susceptible viridans group streptococci isolated from blood. Antimicrob Agents Chemother 1995;39(10):2243–7.

112. Marron A, Carratalà J, Alcaide F, et al. High rates of resistance to cephalosporins among viridans-group streptococci causing bacteraemia in neutropenic cancer patients. J Antimicrob Chemother 2001;47(1):87–91.

113. Tunkel AR, Sepkowitz KA. Infections caused by viridans streptococci in patients with neutropenia. Clin Infect Dis 2002;34(11):1524–9.

114. Shenep JL, Hughes WT, Roberson PK, et al. Vancomycin, ticarcillin, and amikacin compared with ticarcillin-clavulanate and amikacin in the empirical treatment of febrile, neutropenic children with cancer. N Engl J Med 1988;319(16):1053–8.

115. Elting LS, Rubenstein EB, Rolston KV, et al. Outcomes of bacteremia in patients with cancer and neutropenia: observations from two decades of epidemiological and clinical trials. Clin Infect Dis 1997;25(2):247–59.

116. Feld R. Vancomycin as part of initial empirical antibiotic therapy for febrile neutropenia in patients with cancer: pros and cons. Clin Infect Dis 1999;29(3):503–7.

117. Shelburne SA, Lasky RE, Sahasrabhojane P, et al. Development and validation of a clinical model to predict the presence of β-lactam resistance in viridans group streptococci causing bacteremia in neutropenic cancer patients. Clin Infect Dis 2014;59(2):223–30.

118. Clinical and Laboratory Standards Institute. Performance standards for antimicrobial susceptibility testing: 24th informational supplement M100-S24. 26 edition. Wayne (PA): Clinical and Laboratory Standards Institute; 2016.

119. Kimura M, Araoka H, Yoshida A, et al. Breakthrough viridans streptococcal bacteremia in allogeneic hematopoietic stem cell transplant recipients receiving levofloxacin prophylaxis in a Japanese hospital. BMC Infect Dis 2016;16:372.

120. Han SB, Bae EY, Lee JW, et al. Clinical characteristics and antimicrobial susceptibilities of viridans streptococcal bacteremia during febrile neutropenia in patients with hematologic malignancies: a comparison between adults and children. BMC Infect Dis 2013;13:273.

121. Taplitz RA, Kennedy EB, Bow EJ, et al. Outpatient management of fever and neutropenia in adults treated for malignancy: American Society of Clinical

Oncology and Infectious Diseases Society of America Clinical Practice Guideline Update. J Clin Oncol 2018;36(14):1443–53.

122. Heinz WJ, Buchheidt D, Christopeit M, et al. Diagnosis and empirical treatment of fever of unknown origin (FUO) in adult neutropenic patients: guidelines of the Infectious Diseases Working Party (AGIHO) of the German Society of Hematology and Medical Oncology (DGHO). Ann Hematol 2017;96(11):1775–92.

123. Penack O, Becker C, Buchheidt D, et al. Management of sepsis in neutropenic patients: 2014 updated guidelines from the Infectious Diseases Working Party of the German Society of Hematology and Medical Oncology (AGIHO). Ann Hematol 2014;93(7):1083–95.

124. Averbuch D, Orasch C, Cordonnier C, et al. European guidelines for empirical antibacterial therapy for febrile neutropenic patients in the era of growing resistance: summary of the 2011 4th European Conference on Infections in Leukemia. Haematologica 2013;98(12):1826–35.

125. Freifeld AG, Bow EJ, Sepkowitz KA, et al. Clinical practice guideline for the use of antimicrobial agents in neutropenic patients with cancer: 2010 update by the infectious diseases society of america. Clin Infect Dis 2011;52(4):e56–93.

126. Lee D, Kim S, Kim S, et al. Evidence-based guidelines for empirical therapy of neutropenic fever in Korea. Korean J Intern Med 2011;26(2):220–52.

127. Song JH, Jung SI, Ko KS, et al. High prevalence of antimicrobial resistance among clinical Streptococcus pneumoniae isolates in Asia (an ANSORP study). Antimicrob Agents Chemother 2004;48(6):2101–7.

128. Kim SH, Song JH, Chung DR, et al. Changing trends in antimicrobial resistance and serotypes of Streptococcus pneumoniae isolates in Asian countries: an Asian Network for Surveillance of Resistant Pathogens (ANSORP) study. Antimicrob Agents Chemother 2012;56(3):1418–26.

129. Lujan M, Gallego M, Fontanals D, et al. Prospective observational study of bacteremic pneumococcal pneumonia: Effect of discordant therapy on mortality. Crit Care Med 2004;32(3):625–31.

130. Pallares R, Capdevila O, Linares J, et al. The effect of cephalosporin resistance on mortality in adult patients with nonmeningeal systemic pneumococcal infections. Am J Med 2002;113(2):120–6.

131. Bouza E, Pintado V, Rivera S, et al. Nosocomial bloodstream infections caused by Streptococcus pneumoniae. Clin Microbiol Infect 2005;11(11):919–24.

132. Kumashi P, Girgawy E, Tarrand JJ, et al. Streptococcus pneumoniae bacteremia in patients with cancer: disease characteristics and outcomes in the era of escalating drug resistance (1998-2002). Medicine (Baltimore) 2005;84(5):303–12.

133. Magiorakos AP, Srinivasan A, Carey RB, et al. Multidrug-resistant, extensively drug-resistant and pandrug-resistant bacteria: an international expert proposal for interim standard definitions for acquired resistance. Clin Microbiol Infect 2012;18(3):268–81.

134. Sinha M, Jupe J, Mack H, et al. Emerging technologies for molecular diagnosis of sepsis. Clin Microbiol Rev 2018;31(2) [pii:e00089-17].

135. Liesenfeld O, Lehman L, Hunfeld KP, et al. Molecular diagnosis of sepsis: New aspects and recent developments. Eur J Microbiol Immunol 2014;4(1):1–25.

136. Elges S, Arnold R, Liesenfeld O, et al. Prospective evaluation of the SeptiFast multiplex real-time PCR assay for surveillance and diagnosis of infections in haematological patients after allogeneic stem cell transplantation compared to routine microbiological assays and an in-house real-time PCR method. Mycoses 2017;60(12):781–8.

137. Özenci V, Patel R, Ullberg M, et al. Demise of polymerase chain reaction/electro-spray ionization-mass spectrometry as an infectious diseases diagnostic tool. Clin Infect Dis 2018;66(3):452–5.

138. Tacconelli E, Cataldo MA, Dancer SJ, et al. ESCMID guidelines for the management of the infection control measures to reduce transmission of multidrug-resistant Gram-negative bacteria in hospitalized patients. Clin Microbiol Infect 2014;20:1–55.

139. Trubiano JA, Worth LJ, Thursky KA, et al. The prevention and management of infections due to multidrug resistant organisms in haematology patients. Br J Clin Pharmacol 2015;79(2):195–207.

140. Pinese C, Jebors S, Echalier C, et al. Simple and specific grafting of antibacterial peptides on silicone catheters. Adv Healthc Mater 2016;5(23):3067–73.

141. Gardner A, Mattiuzzi G, Faderl S, et al. Randomized comparison of cooked and noncooked diets in patients undergoing remission induction therapy for acute myeloid leukemia. J Clin Oncol 2008;26(35):5684–8 (food).

142. Hayes-Lattin B, Leis JF, Maziarz RT. Isolation in the allogeneic transplant environment: how protective is it? Bone Marrow Transplant 2005;36:373 (isolation).

143. Imran H, Tleyjeh IM, Arndt CA, et al. Fluoroquinolone prophylaxis in patients with neutropenia: a meta-analysis of randomized placebo-controlled trials. Eur J Clin Microbiol Infect Dis 2008;27(1):53–63 (fluoroquinolones).

144. Cordonnier C, Calandra T, Meunier F. Guidelines from the first European conference on infections in leukaemia: ECIL1. Eur J Cancer Suppl 2007;5:1–60.

145. Cullen M, Baijal S. Prevention of febrile neutropenia: use of prophylactic antibiotics. Br J Cancer 2009;101(Suppl 1):S11–4.

146. Bow EJ. Fluoroquinolones, antimicrobial resistance and neutropenic cancer patients. Curr Opin Infect Dis 2011;24(6):545–53.

147. Slavin MA, Lingaratnam S, Mileshkin L, et al. Use of antibacterial prophylaxis for patients with neutropenia. Intern Med J 2011;41(1b):102–9.

148. Arnan M, Gudiol C, Calatayud L, et al. Risk factors for, and clinical relevance of, faecal extended-spectrum β-lactamase producing *Escherichia coli* (ESBL-EC) carriage in neutropenic patients with haematological malignancies. Eur J Clin Microbiol Infect Dis 2011;30(3):355–60.

149. De Rosa FG, Corcione S, Raviolo S, et al. Management of carbapenem-resistant K. pneumoniae in allogenic stem cell transplant recipients: the Turin bundle. New Microbiol 2017;40(2):143–5.

150. Taur Y, Xavier JB, Lipuma L, et al. Intestinal domination and the risk of bacteremia in patients undergoing allogeneic hematopoietic stem cell transplantation. Clin Infect Dis 2012;55(7):905–14.

151. Taur Y, Jenq RR, Perales M-A, et al. The effects of intestinal tract bacterial diversity on mortality following allogeneic hematopoietic stem cell transplantation. Blood 2014;124(7):1174–82.

152. Montassier E, Al-Ghalith GA, Ward T, et al. Pretreatment gut microbiome predicts chemotherapy-related bloodstream infection. Genome Med 2016;8(1):49.

153. Antibiotics currently in global clinical development (updated Sept 2018). Available at: https://www.pewtrusts.org/-/media/assets/2018/09/antibiotics_currently_in_global_clinical_development_sept2018.pdf?la=en&hash=BDE8590154A21A3167CB62A80D663534906C4308. Accessed February 2, 2019.

154. Mensa B, Howell GL, Scott R, et al. Comparative mechanistic studies of brilacidin, daptomycin, and the antimicrobial peptide LL16. Antimicrob Agents Chemother 2014;58(9):5136–45.

Clostridioides difficile Infection in the Stem Cell Transplant and Hematologic Malignancy Population

Elizabeth Ann Misch, MD[a,*], Nasia Safdar, MD, PhD[a,b]

KEYWORDS

- Stem cell transplant • Hematologic malignancy • *Clostridioides (Clostridium) difficile*
- Graft-versus-host disease

KEY POINTS

- *Clostridioides difficile* infection (CDI) in the stem cell transplant (SCT) population occurs at more than 9-fold the rate in the general population.
- Risk factors include allogeneic SCT, use of umbilical cord blood stem cells, neutropenia, myeloablative conditioning, chemotherapy, and possibly graft-versus-host disease (GVHD).
- CDI is associated with increased mortality, bacteremia, and GVHD in some studies.
- Current first-line therapies for primary or recurrent CDI are vancomycin and fidaxomicin for nonsevere and severe CDI. Intravenous metronidazole is recommended as adjunctive treatment of fulminant CDI, especially if ileus is present.
- Fecal microbiota transplant is highly effective for recurrent CDI and primary CDI. Pilot studies in SCT patients have shown safety and efficacy.

INTRODUCTION

Clostridioides difficile (CD) (previously known as *Clostridium difficile*) is an anaerobic, Gram-positive, spore-forming bacillus that is widespread in the natural environment (found in soils, puddle water, tap water, household surfaces, food, horses, and hay, among other sites), but whose main habitat is the gastrointestinal tract of young

Disclosure: The authors report no conflicts of interests. Nasia Safdar receives grant support from the National Institutes of Health (DP2AI44-244 and U01AI125053) and Agency for Health-care Research and Quality (R01HS026226 and R01HS025713).
[a] Department of Medicine, Division of Infectious Disease, University of Wisconsin School of Medicine & Public Health, 1685 Highland Drive, Centennial Building, 5th Floor, Madison, WI 53705, USA; [b] Department of Medicine, William S. Middleton Memorial Veterans Hospital, Madison, WI 53705, USA
* Corresponding author.
E-mail address: eamisch@medicine.wisc.edu

mammals.[1–3] CD colonizes the gut of up to 70% of neonates and infants and can form part of the commensal intestinal flora of asymptomatic adults.[4] However, since 1978, when it was first described as clindamycin colitis or antibiotic-associated pseudo-membranous colitis, CD has been recognized to cause a spectrum of human disease, ranging from mild diarrhea to severe illness and fulminant colitis, associated with ileus and bowel dilatation (megacolon), bowel perforation, and septic shock.[5–9] Between 2000 and 2005, a hypervirulent strain of CD, known as North American pulsed-field gel electrophoresis type 1, restriction endonuclease analysis group BI, and polymerase chain reaction (PCR) ribotype 027(NAP1/BI/027) spread globally.[10–12] The NAP1/027 strain is associated with increased toxin A and B production, produces binary toxin, and is fluoroquinolone-resistant. It harbors a deletion mutation in the TcdC gene (a negative regulator of toxin A and B transcription) that is thought to permit increased toxin production.[10,11] Coincident with the global emergence of NAP1/027, increasing reports of CD infection (CDI) in the stem cell transplant (SCT) and hematologic malignancy (HM) populations appeared in the literature.[13–22]

In the United States, CDI is the leading cause of health care–associated diarrhea, with an estimated incidence rate of 453,000 cases/y and 29,000 deaths, based on 2011 data.[23] The length of time spent in the hospital has been shown to have a linear relationship with the risk of CDI.[24] More than 90% of cases occur in association with prior or ongoing health care or hospitalization.[25] However, in contrast with the early 1980s, most CDI diagnoses are now made in the community or nursing home setting among individuals with recent health care exposure.[25]

Incidence, Risk Factors, and Outcomes in the Stem Cell Transplant Population

The usual risk factors for CDI in the general population (antecedent antibiotics, particularly fluoroquinolones, clindamycin, carbapenems, higher-generation cephalosporins; health care exposures; age >65 years; proton pump inhibitor use; or achlorhydria) also apply to the transplant population.[26,27] However, the incidence among SCT patients has been reported to be up to 9-fold higher among SCT patients and 6.5-fold higher among patients with undifferentiated cancer than for general inpatients.[19,28–30] In the contemporary literature, CDI occurs in adult SCT patients and patients with HM at a frequency of 3% to 33%.[31–37] Rates are higher in allogeneic compared with autologous transplant patients by approximately 2-fold.[27,29,38] CDI in the SCT population is often of mild to moderate severity[32,39,40] and in many studies does not significantly affect survival. CDI is most frequent in the first several weeks after SCT but may also occur in the late posttransplant phase.[33]

Well-known risk factors for CDI that are amplified in the SCT population include immune suppression, frequent antibiotic use, and health care exposure. Susceptibility to CDI in humans has been associated with lower levels of antibodies to CD toxins A and B.[41–43] SCT patients have low levels of protective antibodies because of myeloablative conditioning regimens and unreconstituted immunity following SCT. Several risk factors specific to the SCT and HM populations have been identified in the current literature and are highlighted in **Table 1**.

Lavallée and colleagues[39] performed a nested matched case-control study of 65 patients with CDI compared with 123 controls from the same allogeneic SCT cohort between 2002 and 2011. The study was performed at a single center in Quebec that had a high proportion of infection caused by the NAP1/027 strain. CDI was defined as diarrhea plus evidence of toxigenic CD (either Vero cell culture cytotoxicity assay or by an immunoassay to detect CD glutamate dehydrogenase and toxins A and B). The overall incidence of CDI in this cohort was 8.6% (65 out of 760), with approximately half the cases diagnosed in the early posttransplant period (by day 40). In a

Table 1
Predisposing and protective factors for *Clostridioides difficile* infection in the stem cell transplant and hematologic malignancy population

Predisposing Factors	
Male gender	Ref.[29]
Acute leukemia	Refs.[29,30]
Renal disease	Ref.[30]
Gastric ulcer	Ref.[30]
Prior hospitalization	Ref.[44]
Allogeneic (vs autologous) SCT	Refs.[19,21,29,38,45,46]
Umbilical cord blood SCT	Ref.[20]
Total body irradiation	Refs.[20,47]
Myeloablative conditioning	Refs.[32,36,46,48]
Chemotherapy	Refs.[21,44,49]
Neutropenia	Refs.[30,50]
Receipt of ≥1 high-risk antibiotic or recent antibiotic	Refs.[29,39,44,51,52]
Mucositis	Ref.[39]
Reciprocal association reported with GVHD	—
GVHD → CDI	Refs.[20,21,51,56]
CDI → GVHD	Refs.[18,21,45,47]
CMV reactivation	Ref.[39]
HSV or VZV reactivation	Ref.[39]
Precolonization with toxigenic strain	Refs.[32,49]
VRE colonization	Refs.[21,45]
Bacterial infection	Refs.[30,53]
Mechanical ventilation	Ref.[29]
Protective Factors	
TMP-SMX	Ref.[39]
Corticosteroids	Ref.[46]
Proton pump inhibitors	Ref.[46]
Colonization with nontoxigenic CD strains	Ref.[49]

Arrow (→) indicates direction of temporal relationship.
Abbreviations: CMV, cytomegalovirus; GVHD, graft-versus-host disease; HSV, herpes simplex virus; TMP-SMX, trimethoprim-sulfamethoxazole; VRE, vancomycin-resistant *Enterococcus*; VZV, varicella zoster virus.

multivariate analysis, use of trimethoprim-sulfamethoxazole was associated with a marked and significant reduction in the risk of CDI (odds ratio [OR], 0.07). CMV reactivation, HSV or VZV reactivation, and mucositis were all associated with significantly increased risk (OR, 6.2, 3.0, and 5.9, respectively). In a separate analysis of early versus late CDI, CMV reactivation and mucositis were associated with early CDI (OR, 22.1 and 13.2, respectively). Administration of CDI-promoting antibiotics (antipseudomonal penicillins, carbapenems, clindamycin, fluoroquinolones, and third-generation and fourth-generation cephalosporins) was associated with late CDI (OR, 4.5). In this study, acute GVHD was not associated with CDI in the multivariate analysis, in contrast with other reports.[18,21,45] Clinical manifestations of CDI were modest, with infrequent instances of severe disease (1 patient required colectomy, 2 died). Mortality in patients with CDI was similar to non-CDI controls.[39]

Alonso and colleagues[53] analyzed the incidence, severity, associated outcomes and risk factors for CDI occurring within the first year following umbilical cord blood transplant (UCBT) using a retrospective, case-cohort study design. Patients with CDI were identified from within a total cohort of 226 patients who underwent UCBT between 2003 and 2012. CDI was defined as diarrhea plus a positive stool assay for CD toxin (cell culture cytotoxicity assay, immunoassay for toxin A or toxin A and B combined, or PCR for the toxin gene) without another identified cause. Twenty-two patients (9.7%) in this cohort developed CDI within the first 100 days of transplant (incidence rate, 10.8 out of 10,000 person-days). Thirty patients had CDI within the first year (incidence rate, 5.6 out of 10,000 person-days), with a median onset of 38 days. A risk analysis was performed for total CDI and CDI within 100 days after transplant. In the multivariate analysis, only bacterial infection within 100 days of transplant was significant (hazard ratio [HR], 2.8; P = .03). Corticosteroid use, serum immunoglobulin (Ig) G levels, CD4 count, gut decontamination, transplant conditioning regimen, GVHD, mucositis, gastric acid suppression, and antibiotic exposure had no association with CDI risk. CDI was also not associated with increased mortality, although the investigators noted that markers of severe disease,[a] such as intensive care unit admission and increased serum creatinine (>1.5 mg/dL more than baseline), were seen in 9% and 32% of patients with CDI.[53] Recurrence rates were low (14%). A second, older study of a UCBT cohort from a single center in Japan found a similar rate of CDI (9%) and no association with increased mortality or GVHD.[54]

Dubberke and colleagues[51] prospectively evaluated risk factors for CDI in a cohort of 187 patients who underwent allogenic SCT at a single center (Barnes Jewish Hospital in St Louis, Missouri) between 2007 and 2010. CDI was defined as a positive toxin assay (enzyme immunoassay [EIA] for toxin A/B) and pertinent clinical symptoms occurring within the first year after transplant. Patients were followed for outcomes for a total of 30 months. Sixty-three (34%) patients were diagnosed with CDI, of whom 60% developed illness in the early posttransplant period (preengraftment phase, defined as within 30 days after transplant). Mild disease or moderate disease was seen in 73% of patients, whereas severe disease occurred in 27%. Risk factors for CDI in the preengraftment and postengraftment periods were analyzed separately. Absence of comorbid illness was significantly associated with protection from preengraftment CDI (OR, 0.3; 95% confidence interval [CI], 0.1 to 0.9). In the postengraftment period, relapse of primary disease, exposure to high-risk antibiotics, and GVHD (onset before CDI) were all significant risk factors for CDI (OR, 6.7, 11.8, and 7.8, respectively). No comparative analysis of mortality in patients versus controls was reported. However, death was not increased among those with severe CDI compared with patients with mild CDI.

---

[a] Severe CDI is variably defined in the literature: (1) leukocytosis with white cell count greater than or equal to 15,000 cells/mL and a serum creatinine level greater than 1.5 mg/dL[27]; (2) a score of 2 points or more in a scoring system including age more than 60 years (1 point), temperature greater than 38.3°C (1 point), albumin level less than 2.5 mg/dL (1 point), peripheral white blood cell count greater than 15,000 cells/mL (1 point), pseudomembranous colitis at endoscopy (2 points), or treatment in the intensive care (2 points)[67]; (3) grade 3 or higher diarrhea and/or colitis, with grade 3 diarrhea defined as 1 to 2 L of intestinal output per day[65]; (4) a score of 2 points or higher in a scoring system based on fever (1 point), ileus (1 point), systolic blood pressure (1 point), white blood cell count (0–2 points), and computed tomography findings (0–2 points).[66] Fulminant CDI, or severe CDI with complications, has been defined as CDI accompanied by hypotension (shock), ileus, or megacolon.[27]

Subsequently, the investigators augmented this study with a larger, prospective investigation of risk factors and outcomes associated with CDI among 385 SCT recipients.[35] The total cohort of SCT patients in this study included the 63 patients previously reported,[51] combined with 57 patients from 3 other transplant centers. All CDI episodes occurring within 1 year of SCT were counted, and patients were followed for 2.5 years after transplant. Diagnosis of CDI required a positive assay for CD (toxin immunoassay, PCR, or cellular cytotoxicity) and a clinical diagnosis of gastroenteritis. One-hundred and twenty patients developed CDI, with a median onset of 27 days posttransplant. Rates of CDI ranged from 12% to 38% among the centers. In a risk factor analysis, myeloablative conditioning, cardiovascular disease, GVHD during the past 30 days, and a comorbid condition were more common among patients with CDI. However, when the 63 patients from the previously published cohort were removed from the analysis, only myeloablative conditioning and GVHD in the past month remained significantly associated with CDI. Associations between antimicrobial exposure and CDI were not evaluated because of a lack of data on antibiotic administration.

Evaluated outcomes included subsequent bloodstream infection (BSI), GVHD, and death. Patients with CDI were more likely to experience BSI and GVHD with 30 days following the onset of CDI.[35] Mortality was similar between the two groups in the early posttransplant period. However, patients with CDI in the late posttransplant period (31 days after transplant) had increased mortality (HR, 1.8; $P = .007$) compared with controls.

Several other investigators have found myeloablative conditioning to be associated with increased risk of CDI.[32,36,46,48] Similarly, the association of CDI with mortality was found in a large study describing the incidence and associated outcomes of all infections occurring after transplant.[36] Schuster and colleagues[36] found that CDI was the most frequent bacterial infection caused by a single pathogen in their cohort, occurring in 148 of 444 (33%) enrolled subjects with a median onset at day 27 after SCT. Mortality was higher in patients with CDI (63%) compared with those without CDI (47%) (OR, 1.9; 95% CI, 1.3–2.9). CDI was also significantly more frequent in individuals who had received myeloablative conditioning compared with those who had not (OR, 1.6). Notably, this study relied on the same prospectively enrolled cohorts and transplant centers (University of Michigan, University of Alabama, University of Pennsylvania, and Washington University) as the 385-subject study described earlier[35] but spanned a longer period of enrollment (2006–2011).

Other investigators have also reported an association of CDI or recurrent CDI with mortality.[29,30,45,47,55,56] Guddati and colleagues[29] published an analysis of risk factors and outcomes for hospital-onset CDI in 344,407 SCT patients between 2000 and 2009 using a national administrative database of hospital discharges. A total of 6970 patients (4.7%) developed CDI, of whom 3678 had received autologous SCT (CDI rate of 5.5%) and 3292 had received allogeneic SCT (CDI rate of 8.4%). CDI was not associated with mortality during the so-called engraftment admission. However, during subsequent admissions, CDI was significantly associated with mortality in patients who also had GVHD. Mortality was 19% in patients with simultaneous CDI and GVHD, compared with 8% in patients with CDI without GVHD. Patients with GVHD but not CDI had a mortality of 12.5%.

Although the use of discharge International Classification of Diseases, Ninth Revision, codes to define CDI in this study was a limitation, the results suggest 2 divergent possibilities: (1) CDI is not always a mild illness in the SCT population and may be associated with greater risk of death; or (2) patients with GVHD and gastrointestinal symptoms are more likely to be diagnosed with CDI because of more frequent stool testing. It is unclear in the study by Guddati and colleagues whether the patients with GVHD and CDI died of fulminant CDI or died of severe GVHD with CD colonization. The investigators note that severe CDI was significantly less frequent in SCT compared with non-SCT patients in this database (see further discussion of severity in CDI below).

Diagnosis and Severity Assessment in the Stem Cell Transplant and Hematologic Malignancy Populations

Current methods for the diagnosis of CDI are imperfect and there is disagreement as to whether the best approach is to use a single, highly sensitive test or a combination of tests. Two older, gold standard reference methods, toxigenic culture (TC) and cell cytotoxicity neutralization assay (CNNA), are rarely used anymore. These reference assays involve cultivating the organism and then demonstrating the presence of toxin. The CNNA method requires 24 to 48 hours and has insufficient sensitivity (65%–85%).[27,57] In contrast, TC is very accurate but can take up to 5 days. It is thus impractical for patient care. The most frequently used laboratory tests have therefore become EIAs or nucleic acid amplification tests (usually PCR for toxin B). The EIAs target glutamate dehydrogenase (GDH), an enzyme present in toxigenic and nontoxigenic CD isolates, or, alternatively, toxins A and B. The EIA for GDH is highly sensitive but not specific. As a result, GDH is often combined with a PCR test or toxin EIA. As standalone tests, toxin EIAs are also not optimal, because of sensitivities that range from 67% to 92% when tested independently of the manufacturer.[58]

The NAAT (PCR) detects the gene for toxin B (tcdB) rather than its product. In contrast with the toxin EIAs, PCR for tcdB is highly sensitive and moderately specific.[58,59] However, this assay can detect strains that possess the toxin B gene but are not elaborating the toxin. Nonetheless, in the correct clinical context (ie, diarrheal stools in a hospitalized patient or person with recent antibiotic exposure), PCR for toxin B is the most sensitive test with the most acceptable specificity.[57,60] US guidelines recommend, for health care facilities with established standards for CD stool testing (liquid or unformed stools only), using PCR (NAAT) as a stand-alone test or using a multistep testing algorithm. The multistep algorithm might include, for example, GDH and toxin, PCR plus toxin, or GDH plus toxin, with discrepancies settled by PCR.[27] Standards for submitting fecal specimens to the laboratory for testing commonly specify liquid (unformed) stool consistency, new onset of at least 3 diarrheal episodes in 24 hours, and no receipt of laxatives in the preceding 48 hours.[27]

In the transplant population, the decision to use one or the other CD assay or testing algorithm has added complexity. First, the toxin EIA assays may perform poorly in immune-compromised patients,[61] raising the possibility of underdiagnosis of CDI in vulnerable patients. Second, SCT patients and patients with HM receiving chemotherapy are likely to have diarrhea for a variety of reasons other than CDI; for example, as a result of stem cell conditioning, exposure to antineoplastic agents, or supplemental feeding. In these patients, diarrheal symptoms may prompt more frequent testing for CDI, raising the possibility that an unknown subset of patients diagnosed with CDI by PCR may be merely colonized with a toxigenic CD strain. The conflation of CD colonization with CDI could explain the milder disease presentation among SCT patients that has been reported by some investigators, who have relied in whole or in part on PCR testing for CDI in their cohorts.[32,40,53,62,63] However, investigators who used EIA for GDH or toxin, followed by confirmation with culture-based methods (TC or CNNA) for CDI diagnosis, have also reported a mild spectrum of illness.[21,39,45,54] Some experts have suggested that lower estimates of severe disease in SCT patients and patients with HM stem from inappropriate criteria and have proposed other scoring systems.[27,64–67] Leukopenia, for example, is common after SCT and thus leukocytosis, one of the severity criteria in US guidelines, would be an insensitive measure of severe CDI. However, alternative severity scoring systems have not been prospectively validated or consistently applied in studies of CDI in the SCT population.[53,68]

Reported Association Between *Clostridioides difficile* Infection and Graft-versus-host Disease

Several studies have reported an association between preceding GVHD and CDI **(Table 1)**.[20,21,51,56] In contrast, others have found CDI to be a risk factor for subsequent GVHD.[18,21,45,47] A further set of studies uncovered no evidence of association in either direction.[22,32,39,52,62] These conflicting findings might be partially explained by differences in rates of GVHD, conditioning regimens, antibiotic prophylaxis, CDI strains, and donor-recipient compatibility across institutions. Other possible explanations include (1) the existence of a true association (either unidirectional or bidirectional) between CDI and GVHD that is inconsistently detected because of lack of power; (2) oversampling patients with GVHD for CDI and mistaking colonization for disease; (3) confounding because of an underlying cause common to both syndromes. The common cause that has been suggested is intestinal dysbiosis, described next.[69]

The Proposed Role of the Microbiome

Intestinal dysbiosis, or the loss of gastrointestinal microbial diversity and consequent alterations in intestinal metabolism, are features of both CDI and GVHD.[70–74] The healthy gut microbiome, which is dominated by anaerobic phyla such as Bacteroidetes and Firmicutes,[75] protects mammalian hosts from CD and other invasive bacteria through colonization resistance.[76,77] Colonization resistance is the summary of mechanisms by which commensal bacteria interact with host metabolic pathways to exclude pathogenic species.[78,79] For example, resistance to toxigenic strains of CD arises from the consumption of available nutrients by commensal species; elaboration of bacteriocins toxic to CD[79]; and the conversion of primary bile acids to secondary bile acids, which inhibit the germination of CD spores into replicating cells **(Fig. 1)**.[71,78] This host-bacteria mutualism is disrupted by antibiotics, which deplete resident microbial communities and result in outgrowth of toxin-producing CD and other pathogenic species (see **Fig. 1**).

Intestinal dysbiosis may similarly contribute to the immune pathogenesis of GVHD. Investigative work to support this hypothesis has largely been performed at Memorial Sloan Kettering Cancer Center (MSKCC). In one study, Taur and colleagues[80] determined that greater bacterial diversity in fecal samples collected before engraftment was associated with lower rates of transplant-related mortality after allogeneic SCT. Individuals with low microbial diversity had a hazard ratio of transplant-related mortality of 5.25 ($P = 0.014$). In a different study using stool samples prospectively collected 12 days after stem cell infusion, patients with higher fecal biodiversity had less GVHD-related mortality.[81] In addition, patients harboring a microbiome enriched with the bacterial genus *Blautia* experienced less mortality caused by GVHD and greater overall survival. Patients who did not receive anaerobic therapy had higher levels of *Blautia*. A shorter period on total parenteral nutrition was also associated with greater abundance of *Blautia*. Conditioning regimen had no impact. Interestingly, Commensal Clostridia are among the species contained within the *Blautia* genus.

More recently, researchers at MSKCC and an academic cancer center in Regensburg, Germany, investigated the impact of early administration of broad-spectrum antibiotics (used in 92% of Regensburg and 76% of MSKCC patients) on stool

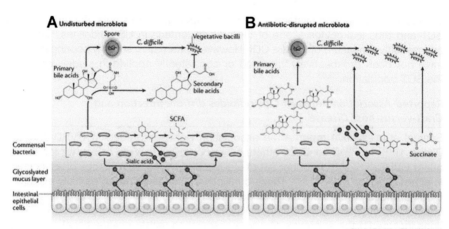

Fig. 1. Intestinal microbiota and colonization resistance. (*A*) In the healthy intestine, commensal bacteria convert primary bile acids into secondary bile acids, which inhibit the growth of CD. Commensal bacteria also convert carbohydrates into short-chain fatty acids (SCFAs), such as succinate, and produce sialidases that cleave sugars attached to gut epithelial cells and release sialic acid into the lumen. These molecules then serve as an energy source for the commensal bacteria. (*B*) Antibiotics deplete commensal bacterial populations, resulting in a buildup of primary bile acids that facilitate germination of CD spores. CD is then able to take advantage of the abundance of food sources (sialic acid and succinate) in the absence of competition from commensal bacterial communities. (*From* Abt MC, McKenney PT, Pamer EG. *Clostridium difficile* colitis: pathogenesis and host defense. Nat Rev Microbiol 2016;(14):615; with permission.)

biodiversity and outcomes.[82] Early administration was defined as receipt of additional antibiotics beyond the prophylactic regimen (to treat neutropenic fever or systemic infection) between day −7 and day 0. Late administration was defined as broad-spectrum antibiotics on day 0 or later. A small group received no additional antibiotics. Gut biodiversity was indirectly assessed through measuring the concentration of 3-indoxyl sulfate (3-IS), a metabolite of intestinal commensal bacteria, in the urine or by detection of commensal *Clostridiales* in fecal samples using reverse transcription PCR. Both groups received prophylactic antibiotics according to institutional protocols. No differences in intestinal biodiversity were seen between the three groups at baseline before SCT or before antibiotic administration. However, at both sites, the groups that received early antibiotic therapy had lower levels of the urinary marker 3-IS, measured between day 0 and day 28, and also less abundance of *Clostridiales* compared with the group receiving late or no antibiotic therapy. At both sites, there was an association between early antibiotic treatment and increased transplant-related mortality, including death from acute or chronic GVHD.[82] Taken together, the above studies suggest that maintaining the populations of commensal bacteria in the intestine may modulate the deleterious immune responses seen in GVHD and thus reduce transplant mortality.

At least 4 interventional studies of fecal microbiota transplant (FMT) and its impact on GVHD, colonization with antibiotic-resistant bacteria, and microbiome diversity have now been performed (reviewed in Ref.[83]). In a recent, open-label, uncontrolled pilot study, oral fecal microbiota capsules were given to 13 patients within 4 weeks of allogeneic stem cell transplant (median of 27 days after SCT).[84] Two patients developed GVHD, 1 of whom also had BSI. One patient developed severe abdominal pain, which was considered to be FMT-related, and 1 patient died of acute gastrointestinal GVHD. Overall survival was 85%. In this cohort, fecal microbial diversity increased, as measured by 3-IS concentrations in urine samples following FMT, compared with samples obtained before FMT. Unexpectedly, a significant contraction of microbiota diversity was not observed after SCT compared with pre-SCT baseline, when measured by 16S ribosomal RNA sequencing and no significant increase in microbiota diversity was seen after FMT when assessed by 16S ribosomal RNA sequencing on fecal samples. Thus, it is unclear whether performing 16S ribosomal RNA sequencing on stool specimens is not the optimal method of evaluating the gut microbiome or whether in this cohort the SCT procedure did not contract the intestinal microbiome as expected. The field will benefit from a randomized, prospective clinical trial of FMT to prevent GVHD that uses several different methodologies to assay intestinal biodiversity before and after SCT.

Management of Clostridioides difficile Infection in the Stem Cell Transplant and Hematologic Malignancy Population

Initial episode of Clostridioides difficile infection

Current standard care for the management of moderate to severe CDI in the United States involves withdrawal of the culpable antibiotic, when possible, and oral vancomycin (125 mg 4 times daily) or oral fidaxomicin (200 mg twice daily) given for 10 days.[27] Metronidazole (500 mg orally 3 times daily) is a less-effective, second-line agent, most often used for mild cases of CDI. Zar and colleagues[67] showed the superiority of vancomycin compared with metronidazole for patients with severe CDI. Among the patients with severe disease in this study, 28% had underlying malignancy. A later, retrospective study of CDI in patients with HM[85] showed no difference in outcomes between individuals treated with vancomycin compared with those treated with metronidazole. Thirty-seven percent of patients had severe disease, and treatment efficacy averaged only 50% (vancomycin) to 54% (metronidazole) for the initial episode. This study, apart from being retrospective, was likely underpowered to detect a difference between the two agents.[85] Subsequent studies, not focused on the SCT population, have clearly established that vancomycin is superior to metronidazole and reduces mortality in severe CDI.[86,87] In a large trial by Johnson and colleagues,[86] oral vancomycin had an efficacy of 81%, compared with 73% for metronidazole.

For fulminant CDI, high-dose oral vancomycin (500 mg 4 times daily) and intravenous metronidazole (same dose as oral administration) are recommended.[27] Vancomycin by the rectal route (instillation) should be considered for patients with ileus. For patients with fulminant CDI, surgical intervention may be required for cases involving megacolon, refractory septic shock, or colon perforation. Surgical options include total or subtotal colectomy or, alternatively, diverting loop ileostomy with colonic lavage followed by antegrade vancomycin flushes.[27,88] Fluid and electrolyte support are other important aspects of management. Gastric acid inhibitors and antimotility drugs should be avoided.[89] Institution-wide infection control measures, including accommodation in private rooms or cohorting, contact precautions, appropriate hand washing (soap and water), and room and equipment disinfection, are key to limiting health care transmission of infection.[27]

Recurrent Clostridioides difficile infection: vancomycin, fidaxomicin, bezlotoxumab, and fecal microbiota transplant

Recurrent CDI is seen in 15% to 35% of patients after a first episode.[90–92] Within the SCT population, recurrence rates are similar.[21,53] Risk factors for CDI relapse include older age, proton pump inhibitors, exposure to antibiotics during or after CDI treatment, strain type, inadequate anti-CD antibodies, severity of CDI, immune compromise, underlying disease, and prior episodes of CDI.[27] According to current US guidelines, second or higher episodes of CDI may be treated with vancomycin at standard doses (125 mg 4 times a day) for 10 days followed by a tapering dose over several weeks. However, the success rate after a second course of vancomycin for recurrent CDI was only 64% in one large trial.[93] Other options for treating recurrent CDI include vancomycin followed by rifaximin, fidaxomicin for 10 days, bezlotoxumab, or FMT.

Fidaxomicin is a macrocyclic antibiotic with potent activity against CD and CD spores but no activity against Gram-negative aerobes or anaerobes.[94,95] Consequently, stool microbial diversity is relatively preserved in fidaxomicin-treated patients.[96]

In 2 unrelated, randomized, double-blind, controlled trials (NCT00468728 and NCT00314951), fidaxomicin was equivalent to vancomycin in the initial response to treatment and was associated with lower levels of recurrent disease compared with vancomycin.[90,91] CDI recurrence rates of 13% to 15% and 25% to 27% were seen for fidaxomicin and vancomycin, respectively, in these 2 trials.[90,91] A subsequent post hoc analysis compared responses to fidaxomicin and vancomycin in patients with (183) and without cancer (922).[97] One-third of those with cancer had a diagnosis of HM. Overall treatment responses were lower among patients with cancer than those without cancer (79% vs 87%), and the duration of diarrhea was nearly twice as long in patients with cancer. In patients without cancer, cure rates for fidaxomicin and vancomycin were not different (89% and 89%, respectively). However, in patients with cancer, treatment with fidaxomicin resulted in a trend toward a higher rate of initial cure (85%) compared with vancomycin (74%) ($P = .065$). The odds of sustained response, defined as initial cure plus the absence of recurrence at 28 days posttreatment, were 2.6-fold higher in patients with cancer treated with fidaxomicin compared to vancomycin ($P = .003$).[97]

The US Food and Drug Administration approved bezlotoxumab, a monoclonal antibody against CD toxin B, in 2016 for secondary prophylaxis of CDI in patients at high risk of recurrence. In 2 large, double-blind, randomized, placebo-controlled trials, MODIFY I and MODIFY II,[98] a single infusion of bezlotoxumab, in addition to standard care for CDI (mostly vancomycin or metronidazole), was associated with a significantly lower CDI recurrence rate compared with placebo (16%–17% vs 26%–28%).[98] Approximately 20% of patients in these two trials were immune-compromised. A post hoc analysis in the immunocompromised subgroup showed a 36% recurrence rate in patients who received placebo compared with 19% in patients treated with bezlotoxumab.[99] No trials of bezlotoxumab in the SCT population have been performed, to our knowledge. Cost limits the use of bezlotoxumab. The average wholesale cost of a vial is estimated to be $3800 to $4560.[100,101] In addition, higher rates of heart failure and increased mortality in patients with a history of heart failure have been observed after bezlotoxumab treatment.[102]

FMT was first used in 4 cases of pseudomembranous colitis in 1958. Subsequently, it was successful in a case of documented CDI in 1983 (see excellent historical review in Ref.[103]). Between 1958 and 2008, approximately 100 case reports of FMT used for recurrent CDI were published, with a success rate of 89%.[104] Van Nood and colleagues[105] compared the efficacy of FMT via duodenal infusion with vancomycin for treatment of recurrent CDI in a small, open-label, randomized controlled trial. Immune-suppressed patients were not included in this trial, nor were patients who were critically ill. Enrolled patients had experienced a median of 3 CDI episodes.

Most of the group that received FMT were cured after a single infusion (13 out of 16, or 81%), and 15 out of 16 (94%) were cured with either 1 or 2 infusions. In comparison, only 4 out of 13 patients (31%) treated with vancomycin achieved cure. In a more recent study, Hvas and colleagues[106] showed that FMT given after 4 to 10 days of vancomycin in patients with recurrent CDI was superior to 10 days of fidaxomicin or 10 days of vancomycin. Clinical resolution was seen in 92% of patients treated with FMT, compared with 42% of those who received fidaxomicin and 19% of those who were treated with vancomycin.

Modes of delivery of FMT include oral capsules, colonoscopy, nasogastric or naso-duodenal tube, or retention enema.[104] There is little difference in the rates of success across these different modes of fecal preparation and delivery.[107] The presumed mechanism by which FMT works is by replenishing depleted populations of intestinal commensal bacteria and restoring colonization resistance against CD. Several studies have shown that FMT is associated with an increase in short-chain fatty acids and secondary bile acids, a more diverse intestinal microbiome (enriched for *Bacteroides*, *Lachnospiraceae*, and *Clostridiales*), and a reduction in *Proteobacteria*.[105,108,109]

Restoration of metabolic products associated with commensal flora after FMT has been shown in SCT patients.[84] However, FMT has not been widely used in the SCT population because of concerns that donor stool may introduce as-yet uncharacterized pathogenic viruses, bacteria, or other organisms into intensely immune-suppressed hosts. Several case reports of successful FMT after SCT or in patients with HM have been published[110–112] and at least 3 small, retrospective studies of FMT for recurrent CDI have been performed in allogeneic SCT patients (reviewed in Ref.[83]). No serious side effects or infections have been reported.

Hefazi and colleagues[113] published a case series of FMT used in 23 patients with cancer, including 13 with HM, for recurrent CDI. They reported an 87% success rate and no adverse events or infections. Most patients had completed chemotherapy at least 12 weeks before the FMT. A systemic review of the use of FMT for CDI in immune-compromised patients, which included 44 studies and 303 patients, reported an 87% success rate, a mortality of less than 1%, and a treatment-related infection rate of 1.6%.[114] A randomized controlled trial of autologous FMT for prophylaxis of CDI in allogeneic SCT patients (NCT02269150) is ongoing. Enrolled subjects will be followed for 1 year after SCT for CDI events.

Clostridioides difficile Infection Prophylaxis: Vancomycin and Fidaxomicin

Ganetsky and colleagues[115] examined the efficacy of vancomycin for primary prophylaxis of CDI in a retrospective study of 105 consecutive SCT patients at a single center. In this study, 0 out of 50 (0%) patients who received vancomycin during their SCT admission developed CDI, compared with 11 out of 50 (20%) patients not on prophylaxis. A second, retrospective study of CDI in allogeneic SCT patients found no difference in the incidence of CDI among patients with a history of CDI who received vancomycin prophylaxis (17% CDI), patients with a history of CDI who received no prophylaxis (14%), and patients without a history of CDI who received no prophylaxis (11%). Details of the timing and duration of vancomycin administration as well as the length of follow-up for CDI detection are not available.[116] A further clinical trial is underway to examine the effect of oral vancomycin prophylaxis on CD stool bacterial loads in patients with stool samples that are positive for CD by PCR but negative for CD toxin by EIA (NCT03030248).

Mullane and colleagues[117] recently published the results of a randomized controlled trial comparing oral fidaxomicin with placebo for primary prevention of CDI in SCT patients on fluoroquinolone prophylaxis (DEFLECT-1). The primary end point, prophylaxis failure, included all confirmed CDI, any use of CDI antibiotics, as well as missing assessment for CDI as failures. No difference in prophylaxis failure between fidaxomicin and placebo was seen. However, most failures were imputed from missing data. A sensitivity analysis that compared fidaxomicin with placebo, in which prophylaxis failure was more narrowly defined as confirmed CDI or use of anti-CDI agents, found a significantly lower rate of failure for fidaxomicin versus placebo (4% vs 11%; $P = .001$). Thus, it seems that fidaxomicin may be effective in reducing rates of CDI in SCT patients on fluoroquinolones and other antibiotics often given during engraftment.

Novel Agents for Clostridioides difficile infection

Multiple agents are currently under study for the treatment or prevention of CDI. This armamentarium includes new antimicrobials or repurposed drugs, such as ridinilazole,[118,119] cadazolid,[120] and niclosamide[121]; small molecules, such as bacteriocins directly toxic to CD[122]; spores from nontoxigenic CD strains[123,124]; probiotics[125]; and commensal bacteria bioengineered to overexpress the CD surface adhesin (and thereby competitively outbind CD at the epithelial cell-intestinal lumen interface).[126] A full discussion of the many anti-CD agents in development is beyond the scope of this article but may be found in 2 excellent reviews.[120,127]

SUMMARY

CDI is the leading cause of infectious diarrhea in hospitalized patients in the United States. The incidence of CDI is greater in the SCT and HM population, where rates are up to 9-fold higher than for the general population. Although most reports describe mild to moderate disease, CDI in immune-suppressed hosts may be severe, and several studies have found associations with unfavorable outcomes, including mortality, subsequent BSI, and GVHD. Unique risk factors for CDI in SCT patients and patients with HM include receipt of allogeneic (as opposed to autologous) transplant, use of cord blood stem cells, total body irradiation, myeloablative conditioning, chemotherapy, neutropenia, mucositis, herpes virus reactivation, and GVHD. CDI usually occurs within the first month following transplant, although late onset has also been described. The underlying pathophysiology of CDI involves a disruption of commensal microbial communities in the gut, leaving underoccupied niches that are exploited by toxin-producing strains of CD and other pathogens. Intestinal injury, from conditioning regimens, chemotherapy, or infection, is also a precursor to GVHD and may explain the bidirectional association between GVHD and CDI found in the literature.

Diagnostic tests for CDI are imperfect in that PCR testing for toxin B cannot distinguish between colonization and infection, and toxin immunoassays are insufficiently sensitive to rule out disease. Currently recommended antibiotic therapies for primary and recurrent CDI in SCT are identical to those for the general population. Of all the management approaches in use today for recurrent CDI, FMT has shown the greatest efficacy. However, many cancer centers have not adopted routine use of FMT for recurrent CDI in SCT and HM patients because of concerns about safety. Several case reports, small series, and retrospective studies have shown that FMT is effective and safe in SCT patients and patients with HM, and a randomized controlled trial of autologous FMT for prophylaxis of CDI in allogeneic SCT patients (NCT02269150) is underway.

New treatment approaches for CDI are urgently needed, given the frequency of this infection in SCT patients and its association in several studies with nontrivial outcomes, such as GVHD and transplant-related mortality. An abundance of novel therapeutics for CDI is currently in development. In addition, FMT, which is highly effective, may soon become an acceptable option for CDI prophylaxis and treatment and is being explored as a potential preventive measure for GVHD.

REFERENCES

1. Janezic S, Potocnik M, Zidaric V, et al. Highly divergent *Clostridium difficile* strains isolated from the environment. PLoS One 2016;11(11):e0167101.

2. Rodriguez C, Taminiau B, Van Broeck J, et al. *Clostridium difficile* in food and animals: a comprehensive review. In: Donelli G, editor. Advances in Microbiology, infectious diseases and public health, vol. 4. Cham (Switzerland): Springer International Publishing; 2016. p. 65–92.

3. Allen SD, Emery CL, Lyerly DM. Clostridium. In: Murrray PR, Baron EJ, Jorgensen JH, et al, editors. Manual of clinical microbiology, vol. 1, 8th edition. Washington, DC: American Society for Microbiology; 2003. p. 835–56.

4. Lees EA, Miyajima F, Pirmohamed M, et al. The role of *Clostridium difficile* in the paediatric and neonatal gut - a narrative review. Eur J Clin Microbiol Infect Dis 2016;35(7):1047–57.

5. Bartlett JG, Moon N, Chang TW, et al. Role of *Clostridium difficile* in antibiotic-associated pseudomembranous colitis. Gastroenterology 1978;75(5):778–82.

6. Lyerly DM, Krivan HC, Wilkins TD. *Clostridium difficile*: its disease and toxins. Clin Microbiol Rev 1988;1(1):1–18.

7. Johnson S, Gerding DN. *Clostridium difficile*-associated diarrhea. Clin Infect Dis 1998;26(5):1027–34 [quiz: 1035–6].

8. Efron PA, Mazuski JE. *Clostridium difficile* colitis. Surg Clin North Am 2009;89(2): 483–500.

9. Hurley BW, Nguyen CC. The spectrum of pseudomembranous enterocolitis and antibiotic-associated diarrhea. Arch Intern Med 2002;162(19):2177–84.

10. McDonald LC, Killgore GE, Thompson A, et al. An epidemic, toxin gene-variant strain of *Clostridium difficile*. N Engl J Med 2005;353(23):2433–41.

11. Warny M, Pepin J, Fang A, et al. Toxin production by an emerging strain of *Clostridium difficile* associated with outbreaks of severe disease in North America and Europe. Lancet 2005;366(9491):1079–84.

12. Loo VG, Poirier L, Miller MA, et al. A predominantly clonal multi-institutional outbreak of *Clostridium difficile*-associated diarrhea with high morbidity and mortality. N Engl J Med 2005;353(23):2442–9.

13. Gorschluter M, Glasmacher A, Hahn C, et al. *Clostridium difficile* infection in patients with neutropenia. Clin Infect Dis 2001;33(6):786–91.

14. Glasmacher A, Ziske C, Hahn C, et al. *Clostridium difficile* infection in patients with neutropenia. Clin Infect Dis 2001;33(6):786–91.

15. Arango JI, Restrepo A, Schneider DL, et al. Incidence of *Clostridium difficile*-associated diarrhea before and after autologous peripheral blood stem cell transplantation for lymphoma and multiple myeloma. Bone Marrow Transplant 2006;37(5):517–21.

16. Fortin É, Dionne M, Hubert B, et al. A portrait of the geographic dissemination of the *Clostridium difficile* North American Pulsed-Field Type 1 Strain and the Epidemiology of *C. difficile*-Associated Disease in Québec. Clin Infect Dis 2007;44(2):238–44.

17. Schalk E, Bohr UR, König B, et al. *Clostridium difficile*-associated diarrhoea, a frequent complication in patients with acute myeloid leukaemia. Ann Hematol 2009;89(1):9.

18. Dubberke ER, Reske KA, Srivastava A, et al. *Clostridium difficile*-associated disease in allogeneic hematopoietic stem-cell transplant recipients: risk associations, protective associations, and outcomes. Clin Transplant 2010;24(2):192–8.

19. Chopra T, Chandrasekar P, Salimnia H, et al. Recent epidemiology of *Clostridium difficile* infection during hematopoietic stem cell transplantation. Clin Transplant 2011;25(1):E82–7.

20. Willems L, Porcher R, Lafaurie M, et al. *Clostridium difficile* infection after allogeneic hematopoietic stem cell transplantation: incidence, risk factors, and outcome. Biol Blood Marrow Transplant 2012;18(8):1295–301.

21. Alonso CD, Treadway SB, Hanna DB, et al. Epidemiology and outcomes of *Clostridium difficile* infections in hematopoietic stem cell transplant recipients. Clin Infect Dis 2012;54(8):1053–63.

22. Kamboj M, Xiao K, Kaltsas A, et al. *Clostridium difficile* infection after allogeneic hematopoietic stem cell transplant: strain diversity and outcomes associated with NAP1/027. Biol Blood Marrow Transplant 2014;20(10):1626–33.

23. Lessa FC, Mu Y, Bamberg WM, et al. Burden of *Clostridium difficile* infection in the United States. N Engl J Med 2015;372(9):825–34.

24. Gerding DN, Johnson S. *Clostridium difficile*-associated diarrhea. Clin Infect Dis 1998;26(5):1027–34.

25. Gerding DN, Lessa FC. The epidemiology of *Clostridium difficile* infection inside and outside health care institutions. Infect Dis Clin North Am 2015;29(1):37–50.

26. Bartlett JG. *Clostridium difficile*: progress and challenges. Ann N Y Acad Sci 2010;1213(1):62–9.

27. McDonald LC, Gerding DN, Johnson S, et al. Clinical practice guidelines for *Clostridium difficile* infection in adults and children: 2017 update by the Infectious Diseases Society of America (IDSA) and Society for Healthcare Epidemiology of America (SHEA). Clin Infect Dis 2018;66(7):e1–48.

28. Kamboj M, Son C, Cantu S, et al. Hospital-onset *Clostridium difficile* infection rates in persons with cancer or hematopoietic stem cell transplant: a C3IC network report. Infect Control Hosp Epidemiol 2012;33(11):1162–5.

29. Guddati AK, Kumar G, Ahmed S, et al. Incidence and outcomes of *Clostridium difficile*-associated disease in hematopoietic cell transplant recipients. Int J Hematol 2014;99(6):758–65.

30. Selvey LA, Slimings C, Joske DJL, et al. *Clostridium difficile* infections amongst patients with haematological malignancies: a data linkage study. PLoS One 2016;11(6):e0157839.

31. Satlin MJ, Vardhana S, Soave R, et al. Impact of prophylactic levofloxacin on rates of bloodstream infection and fever in neutropenic patients with multiple myeloma undergoing autologous hematopoietic stem cell transplantation. Biol Blood Marrow Transplant 2015;21(10):1808–14.

32. Kinnebrew MA, Lee YJ, Jenq RR, et al. Early *Clostridium difficile* infection during allogeneic hematopoietic stem cell transplantation. PLoS One 2014;9(3):e90158.

33. Young JH, Logan BR, Wu J, et al. Infections after transplantation of bone marrow or peripheral blood stem cells from unrelated donors. Biol Blood Marrow Transplant 2016;22(2):359–70.

34. Slade M, Goldsmith S, Romee R, et al. Epidemiology of infections following haploidentical peripheral blood hematopoietic cell transplantation. Transpl Infect Dis 2017;19(1):1–10.

35. Dubberke ER, Reske KA, Olsen MA, et al. Epidemiology and outcomes of *Clostridium difficile* infection in allogeneic hematopoietic cell and lung transplant recipients. Transpl Infect Dis 2018;20(2):e12855.

36. Schuster MG, Cleveland AA, Dubberke ER, et al. Infections in hematopoietic cell transplant recipients: results from the organ transplant infection project, a multicenter, prospective, cohort study. Open Forum Infect Dis 2017;4(2):ofx050.

37. Styczynski J, Czyzewski K, Wysocki M, et al. Increased risk of infections and infection-related mortality in children undergoing haematopoietic stem cell transplantation compared to conventional anticancer therapy: a multicentre nationwide study. Clin Microbiol Infect 2016;22(2):179.e1-10.

38. Zacharioudakis IM, Ziakas PD, Mylonakis E. *Clostridium difficile* infection in the hematopoietic unit: a meta-analysis of published studies. Biol Blood Marrow Transplant 2014;20(10):1650–4.

39. Lavallée C, Labbé AC, Talbot JD, et al. Risk factors for the development of *Clostridium difficile* infection in adult allogeneic hematopoietic stem cell transplant recipients: a single-center study in Québec, Canada. Transpl Infect Dis 2017; 19(1):e12648.

40. Salamonowicz M, Ociepa T, Frączkiewicz J, et al. Incidence, course, and outcome of *Clostridium difficile* infection in children with hematological malignancies or undergoing hematopoietic stem cell transplantation. Eur J Clin Microbiol Infect Dis 2018;37(9):1805–12.

41. Johnson S, Gerding DN, Janoff EN. Systemic and mucosal antibody responses to toxin A in patients infected with *Clostridium difficile*. J Infect Dis 1992;166(6): 1287–94.

42. Kyne L, Warny M, Qamar A, et al. Asymptomatic carriage of *Clostridium difficile* and serum levels of IgG antibody against toxin A. N Engl J Med 2000;342(6): 390–7.

43. Leav BA, Blair B, Leney M, et al. Serum anti-toxin B antibody correlates with protection from recurrent *Clostridium difficile* infection. Vaccine 2010;28(4):965–9.

44. Aldrete S, Kraft CS, Magee MJ, et al. Risk factors and epidemiology of *Clostridium difficile* infection in hematopoietic stem cell transplant recipients during the peri-transplant period. Open Forum Infect Dis 2015;2(Suppl 1) [abstract: S235].

45. Trifilio SM, Pi J, Mehta J. Changing epidemiology of *Clostridium difficile*-associated disease during stem cell transplantation. Biol Blood Marrow Transplant 2013;19(3):405–9.

46. Scardina TL, Martinez EK, Balasubramanian N, et al. Evaluation of risk factors for *Clostridium difficile* infection in hematopoietic stem cell transplant recipients. Pharmacotherapy 2017;37(4):420–8.

47. Chakrabarti S, Lees A, Jones SG, et al. *Clostridium difficile* infection in allogeneic stem cell transplant recipients is associated with severe graft-versus-host disease and non-relapse mortality. Bone Marrow Transplant 2000;26(8):871–6.

48. Boyle NM, Magaret A, Stednick Z, et al. Evaluating risk factors for *Clostridium difficile* infection in adult and pediatric hematopoietic cell transplant recipients. Antimicrob Resist Infect Control 2015;4:41.

49. Cannon CM, Musuuza JS, Barker AK, et al. Risk of *Clostridium difficile* infection in hematology-oncology patients colonized with toxigenic *C. difficile*. Infect Control Hosp Epidemiol 2017;38(6):718–20.

50. Yoon YK, Kim MJ, Sohn JW, et al. Predictors of mortality attributable to *Clostridium difficile* infection in patients with underlying malignancy. Support Care Cancer 2014;22(8):2039–48.

51. Dubberke ER, Reske KA, Olsen MA, et al. Risk for *Clostridium difficile* infection after allogeneic hematopoietic cell transplant remains elevated in the postengraftment period. Transplant Direct 2017;3(4):e145.

52. Vehreschild MJ, Weitershagen D, Biehl LM, et al. *Clostridium difficile* infection in patients with acute myelogenous leukemia and in patients undergoing allogeneic stem cell transplantation: epidemiology and risk factor analysis. Biol Blood Marrow Transplant 2014;20(6):823–8.

53. Alonso CD, Braun DA, Patel I, et al. A multicenter, retrospective, case-cohort study of the epidemiology and risk factors for *Clostridium difficile* infection among cord blood transplant recipients. Transpl Infect Dis 2017;19(4):e12728.

54. Hosokawa K, Takami A, Tsuji M, et al. Relative incidences and outcomes of *Clostridium difficile* infection following transplantation of unrelated cord blood, unrelated bone marrow, and related peripheral blood in adult patients: a single institute study. Transpl Infect Dis 2014;16(3):412–20.

55. Mani S, Rybicki L, Jagadeesh D, et al. Risk factors for recurrent *Clostridium difficile* infection in allogeneic hematopoietic cell transplant recipients. Bone Marrow Transplant 2016;51:713.

56. Chang K, Kreuziger LMB, Angell K, et al. Recurrence of *Clostridium difficile* infection after total colectomy in an allogeneic stem cell transplant patient. Bone Marrow Transplant 2012;47:610–1.

57. Wilcox M, Planche T, Fang F, et al. Point-counterpoint: what is the current role of algorithmic approaches for diagnosis of *Clostridium difficile* infection? J Clin Microbiol 2010;48(12):4347–53.

58. Wilcox MH. Evaluation report: Clostridium difficile toxin detection assays (CEP08054). London: Centre for Evidence-Based Purchasing, National Health Service (UK); 2009.

59. Tenover FC, Novak-Weekley S, Woods CW, et al. Impact of strain type on detection of toxigenic *Clostridium difficile*: comparison of molecular diagnostic and enzyme immunoassay approaches. J Clin Microbiol 2010;48(10):3719–24.

60. Tenover FC, Baron EJ, Peterson LR, et al. Laboratory diagnosis of *Clostridium difficile* infection can molecular amplification methods move us out of uncertainty? J Mol Diagn 2011;13(6):573–82.

61. Erb S, Frei R, Strandén AM, et al. Low sensitivity of fecal toxin A/B enzyme immunoassay for diagnosis of *Clostridium difficile* infection in immunocompromised patients. Clin Microbiol Infect 2015;21(11):998.e9-15.

62. Bruminhent J, Wang Z-X, Hu C, et al. *Clostridium difficile* colonization and disease in patients undergoing hematopoietic stem cell transplantation. Biol Blood Marrow Transplant 2014;20(9):1329–34.

63. Crobach MJT, Vernon JJ, Loo VG, et al. Understanding *Clostridium difficile* colonization. Clin Microbiol Rev 2018;31(2). e00021-17.

64. Wang MS, Evans CT, Rodriguez T, et al. *Clostridium difficile* infection and limitations of markers for severity in patients with hematologic malignancy. Infect Control Hosp Epidemiol 2013;34(2):127–32.

65. Dubberke E, Sadhu J, Gatti R, et al. Severity of *Clostridium difficile*-associated disease (CDAD) in allogeneic stem cell transplant recipients: evaluation of a CDAD severity grading system. Infect Control Hosp Epidemiol 2007;28(2):208–11.

66. Belmares J, Gerding DN, Parada JP, et al. Outcome of metronidazole therapy for *Clostridium difficile* disease and correlation with a scoring system. J Infect 2007; 55(6):495–501.

67. Zar FA, Bakkanagari SR, Moorthi KMLST, et al. A comparison of vancomycin and metronidazole for the treatment of *Clostridium difficile*–associated diarrhea, stratified by disease severity. Clin Infect Dis 2007;45(3):302–7.

68. Alonso CD, Marr KA. *Clostridium difficile* infection among hematopoietic stem cell transplant recipients: beyond colitis. Curr Opin Infect Dis 2013;26(4): 326–31.

69. Shallis RM, Terry CM, Lim SH. Changes in intestinal microbiota and their effects on allogeneic stem cell transplantation. Am J Hematol 2018;93(1):122–8.

70. Schaffler H, Breitruck A. *Clostridium difficile* - from colonization to infection. Front Microbiol 2018;9:646.

71. Abt MC, McKenney PT, Pamer EG. *Clostridium difficile* colitis: pathogenesis and host defence. Nat Rev Microbiol 2016;14(10):609–20.

72. Khoruts A, Hippen KL, Lemire AM, et al. Toward revision of antimicrobial therapies in hematopoietic stem cell transplantation: target the pathogens, but protect the indigenous microbiota. Transl Res 2017;179:116–25.

73. Peled JU, Hanash AM, Jenq RR. Role of the intestinal mucosa in acute gastrointestinal GVHD. Blood 2016;2016(1):119–27.

74. Staffas A, Burgos da Silva M, van den Brink MR. The intestinal microbiota in allogeneic hematopoietic cell transplant and graft-versus-host disease. Blood 2017; 129(8):927–33.

75. Turnbaugh PJ, Hamady M, Yatsunenko T, et al. A core gut microbiome in obese and lean twins. Nature 2008;457:480.

76. Ballen K, Woo Ahn K, Chen M, et al. Infection rates among acute leukemia patients receiving alternative donor hematopoietic cell transplantation. Biol Blood Marrow Transplant 2016;22(9):1636–45.

77. Ng KM, Ferreyra JA, Higginbottom SK, et al. Microbiota-liberated host sugars facilitate post-antibiotic expansion of enteric pathogens. Nature 2013; 502(7469):96–9.

78. Sorbara MT, Pamer EG. Interbacterial mechanisms of colonization resistance and the strategies pathogens use to overcome them. Mucosal Immunol 2019; 12(1):1–9.

79. Rea MC, Dobson A, O'Sullivan O, et al. Effect of broad- and narrow-spectrum antimicrobials on *Clostridium difficile* and microbial diversity in a model of the distal colon. Proc Natl Acad Sci U S A 2011;108(Supplement 1):4639–44.

80. Taur Y, Jenq RR, Perales M-A, et al. The effects of intestinal tract bacterial diversity on mortality following allogeneic hematopoietic stem cell transplantation. Blood 2014;124(7):1174–82.

81. Jenq RR, Taur Y, Devlin SM, et al. Intestinal Blautia is associated with reduced death from graft-versus-host disease. Biol Blood Marrow Transplant 2015;21(8): 1373–83.

82. Weber D, Jenq RR, Peled JU, et al. Microbiota disruption induced by early use of broad-spectrum antibiotics is an independent risk factor of outcome after allogeneic stem cell transplantation. Biol Blood Marrow Transplant 2017;23(5): 845–52.

83. DeFilipp Z, Hohmann E, Jenq RR, et al. Fecal microbiota transplantation: restoring the injured microbiome after allogeneic hematopoietic cell transplantation. Biol Blood Marrow Transplant 2019;25(1):e17–22.

84. DeFilipp Z, Peled JU, Li S, et al. Third-party fecal microbiota transplantation following allo-HCT reconstitutes microbiome diversity. Blood Adv 2018;2(7): 745–53.

85. Parmar SR, Bhatt V, Yang J, et al. A retrospective review of metronidazole and vancomycin in the management of Clostridium difficile infection in patients with hematologic malignancies. J Oncol Pharm Pract 2013;20(3):172–82.

86. Johnson S, Louie TJ, Gerding DN, et al. Vancomycin, metronidazole, or tolevamer for Clostridium difficile infection: results from two multinational, randomized, controlled trials. Clin Infect Dis 2014;59(3):345–54.

87. Stevens VW, Nelson RE, Schwab-Daugherty EM, et al. Comparative effectiveness of vancomycin and metronidazole for the prevention of recurrence and death in patients with Clostridium difficile infection. JAMA Intern Med 2017; 177(4):546–53.

88. Neal MD, Alverdy JC, Hall DE, et al. Diverting loop ileostomy and colonic lavage: an alternative to total abdominal colectomy for the treatment of severe, complicated Clostridium difficile associated disease. Ann Surg 2011;254(3):423–7 [discussion: 427–9].

89. Debast SB, Bauer MP, Kuijper EJ. European Society of Clinical Microbiology and Infectious Diseases: update of the treatment guidance document for Clostridium difficile infection. Clin Microbiol Infect 2014;20:1–26.

90. Cornely OA, Crook DW, Esposito R, et al. Fidaxomicin versus vancomycin for infection with Clostridium difficile in Europe, Canada, and the USA: a doubleblind, non-inferiority, randomised controlled trial. Lancet Infect Dis 2012;12(4): 281–9.

91. Louie TJ, Miller MA, Mullane KM, et al. Fidaxomicin versus vancomycin for Clostridium difficile infection. N Engl J Med 2011;364(5):422–31.

92. Huebner ES, Surawicz CM. Treatment of recurrent Clostridium difficile diarrhea. Gastroenterol Hepatol 2006;2(3):203–8.

93. Cornely OA, Miller MA, Louie TJ, et al. Treatment of first recurrence of Clostridium difficile infection: fidaxomicin versus vancomycin. Clin Infect Dis 2012; 55(Suppl 2):S154–61.

94. Babakhani F, Bouillaut L, Gomez A, et al. Fidaxomicin inhibits spore production in Clostridium difficile. Clin Infect Dis 2012;55(Suppl 2):S162–9.

95. Goldstein EJC, Babakhani F, Citron DM. Antimicrobial activities of fidaxomicin. Clin Infect Dis 2012;55(suppl_2):S143–8.

96. Tannock GW, Munro K, Taylor C, et al. A new macrocyclic antibiotic, fidaxomicin (OPT-80), causes less alteration to the bowel microbiota of Clostridium difficileinfected patients than does vancomycin. Microbiology 2010;156(11):3354–9.

97. Cornely OA, Miller MA, Fantin B, et al. Resolution of clostridium difficile–associated diarrhea in patients with cancer treated with fidaxomicin or vancomycin. J Clin Oncol 2013;31(19):2493–9.

98. Wilcox MH, Gerding DN, Poxton IR, et al. Bezlotoxumab for prevention of recurrent clostridium difficile infection. N Engl J Med 2017;376(4):305–17.

99. Gerding DN, Kelly CP, Rahav G, et al. Bezlotoxumab for prevention of recurrent Clostridium difficile infection in patients at increased risk for recurrence. Clin Infect Dis 2018;67(5):649–56.

100. Lee Y, Lim W, Bloom C, et al. Bezlotoxumab (Zinplava) for Clostridium difficile infection. P T 2017;42:735–8.

101. Bezlotoxumab (Zinplava) for prevention of recurrent Clostridium difficile infection. Med Lett Drugs Ther 2017;59(1517):49–50.

102. Gerding DN, Johnson S. Bezlotoxumab. Clin Infect Dis 2018;68(4):699–704.

103. Bakken JS, Borody T, Brandt LJ, et al. Treating *Clostridium difficile* infection with fecal microbiota transplantation. Clin Gastroenterol Hepatol 2011;9(12):1044–9.

104. Bakken JS. Fecal bacteriotherapy for recurrent *Clostridium difficile* infection. Anaerobe 2009;15(6):285–9.

105. van Nood E, Vrieze A, Nieuwdorp M, et al. Duodenal infusion of donor feces for recurrent *Clostridium difficile*. N Engl J Med 2013;368(5):407–15.

106. Hvas CL, Jorgensen SMD, Jorgensen SP, et al. Fecal microbiota transplantation is superior to fidaxomicin for treatment of recurrent *clostridium difficile* infection. Gastroenterology 2019. [Epub ahead of print].

107. Khan MY, Dirweesh A, Khurshid T, et al. Comparing fecal microbiota transplantation to standard-of-care treatment for recurrent *Clostridium difficile* infection: a systematic review and meta-analysis. Eur J Gastroenterol Hepatol 2018;30(11):1309–17.

108. Seekatz AM, Theriot CM, Rao K, et al. Restoration of short chain fatty acid and bile acid metabolism following fecal microbiota transplantation in patients with recurrent *Clostridium difficile* infection. Anaerobe 2018;53:64–73.

109. Jalanka J, Mattila E, Jouhten H, et al. Long-term effects on luminal and mucosal microbiota and commonly acquired taxa in faecal microbiota transplantation for recurrent *Clostridium difficile* infection. BMC Med 2016;14(1):155.

110. de Castro CG, Ganc AJ, Ganc RL, et al. Fecal microbiota transplant after hematopoietic SCT: report of a successful case. Bone Marrow Transplant 2015;50(1):145.

111. Trubiano JA, George A, Barnett J, et al. A different kind of 'allogeneic transplant': successful fecal microbiota transplant for recurrent and refractory *Clostridium difficile* infection in a patient with relapsed aggressive B-cell lymphoma. Leuk Lymphoma 2015;56(2):512–4.

112. Mittal C, Miller N, Meighani A, et al. Fecal microbiota transplant for recurrent *Clostridium difficile* infection after peripheral autologous stem cell transplant for diffuse large B-cell lymphoma. Bone Marrow Transplant 2015;50(7):1010.

113. Hefazi M, Patnaik MM, Hogan WJ, et al. Safety and efficacy of fecal microbiota transplant for recurrent *Clostridium difficile* infection in patients with cancer treated with cytotoxic chemotherapy: a single-institution retrospective case series. Mayo Clin Proc 2017;92(11):1617–24.

114. Shogbesan O, Poudel DR, Victor S, et al. A systematic review of the efficacy and safety of fecal microbiota transplant for *Clostridium difficile* infection in immunocompromised patients. Can J Gastroenterol Hepatol 2018;2018:1394379.

115. Ganetsky A, Han JH, Hughes ME, et al. Oral vancomycin is highly effective in preventing *Clostridium difficile* infection in allogeneic hematopoietic stem cell transplant recipients. Blood 2016;128(22):2225.

116. Pereiras MA, Urnoski E, Wynd M, et al. Does oral vancomycin prophylaxis for clostridium difficile infection improve allogeneic hematopoietic stem cell transplant outcomes? Biol Blood Marrow Transplant 2017;23(3):S395.

117. Mullane KM, Winston DJ, Nooka A, et al. A randomized, placebo-controlled trial of fidaxomicin for prophylaxis of *Clostridium difficile*-associated diarrhea in adults undergoing hematopoietic stem cell transplantation. Clin Infect Dis 2019;68(2):196–203.

118. Goldstein EJC, Citron DM, Tyrrell KL, et al. Comparative *in vitro* activities of SMT19969, a new antimicrobial agent, against *Clostridium difficile* and 350 gram-positive and gram-negative aerobic and anaerobic intestinal flora isolates. Antimicrob Agents Chemother 2013;57(10):4872–6.

119. Vickers RJ, Tillotson GS, Nathan R, et al. Efficacy and safety of ridinilazole compared with vancomycin for the treatment of *Clostridium difficile* infection: a phase 2, randomised, double-blind, active-controlled, non-inferiority study. Lancet Infect Dis 2017;17(7):735–44.

120. Petrosillo N, Granata G, Cataldo MA. Novel antimicrobials for the treatment of *Clostridium difficile* infection. Front Med 2018;5:96.

121. Tam J, Hamza T, Ma B, et al. Host-targeted niclosamide inhibits C. difficile virulence and prevents disease in mice without disrupting the gut microbiota. Nat Commun 2018;9(1):5233.

122. Gebhart D, Lok S, Clare S, et al. A modified R-type bacteriocin specifically targeting *Clostridium difficile* prevents colonization of mice without affecting gut microbiota diversity. MBio 2015;6(2) [pii:e02368-14].

123. Gerding DN, Meyer T, Lee C, et al. Administration of spores of nontoxigenic *Clostridium difficile* strain M3 for prevention of recurrent C difficile infection: a randomized clinical trial. JAMA 2015;313(17):1719–27.

124. Gerding DN, Sambol SP, Johnson S. Non-toxigenic *Clostridioides* (formerly *Clostridium) difficile* for Prevention of *C. difficile* infection: from bench to bedside back to bench and back to bedside. Front Microbiol 2018;9:1700.

125. Barker AK, Duster M, Valentine S, et al. A randomized controlled trial of probiotics for *Clostridium difficile* infection in adults (PICO). J Antimicrob Chemother 2017;72(11):3177–80.

126. Vedantam G, Kochanowsky J, Lindsey J, et al. An engineered synthetic biologic protects against *Clostridium difficile* infection. Front Microbiol 2018;9:2080.

127. Darkoh C, Deaton M, DuPont HL. Nonantimicrobial drug targets for *Clostridium difficile* infections. Future Microbiol 2017;12(11):975–85.

Herpes Virus Infections Other than Cytomegalovirus in the Recipients of Hematopoietic Stem Cell Transplantation

Sanjeet Singh Dadwal, MD

KEYWORDS

- Herpes simplex virus (HSV) • Varicella zoster virus (VZV)
- Human herpes virus 6 (HHV6) • Human herpes virus 7 (HHV7)
- Epstein-Barr virus (EBV) • Human herpes virus 8 (HHV8)
- Hematopoietic stem cell transplantation (HSCT) • Acyclovir (ACV)

KEY POINTS

- Herpesviruses other than cytomegalovirus (CMV) lead to significant morbidity in hematopoietic stem cell transplantation (HSCT) recipients.
- Herpes simplex virus (HSV) and varicella zoster virus (VZV) reactivation has decreased with antiviral prophylaxis. Breakthrough infection with acyclovir-resistant HSV is an emerging problem, whereas VZV infection is mostly encountered after the discontinuation of prophylaxis.
- Asymptomatic HHV6 viremia after allogeneic HSCT is common, and the role for prophylaxis or preemptive therapy is not well defined.
- Varying clinical syndromes are seen with Epstein-Barr virus infection; posttransplant lymphoproliferative disorder is the most serious.
- Human herpes virus 7 (HHV7) and HHV8 are uncommon after HSCT, and clinical description of disease is limited to case reports or small case series.

INTRODUCTION

Herpes Virus Infections Hematopoietic Stem Cell Transplantation Recipients

All herpes viruses have similar morphologic appearance and are composed of 4 structural components: electron dense core containing double-stranded viral DNA, icosahedral capsid, tegument, and lipid envelope. Herpes simplex viruses (HSV) 1 and 2

Disclosures: Consultant/speaker bureau: Merck; Advisory Board: Merck, Clinigen, Janssen; Investigator: Merck, Gilead, Ansun, AiCuris, Chimerix, Shire, Oxford Immunotec.
City of Hope National Medical Center, 1500 East Duarte Road, Duarte, CA 91010, USA
E-mail address: sdadwal@coh.org

Infect Dis Clin N Am 33 (2019) 467–484
https://doi.org/10.1016/j.idc.2019.02.012
0891-5520/19/© 2019 Elsevier Inc. All rights reserved.

id.theclinics.com

belong to subfamily Alphaherpesvirinae; human herpes virus 6 (HHV6) and HHV7 belong to Betaherpesvirinae, whereas Epstein-Barr virus (EBV) and HHV8 belong to Gammaherpesvirinae.[1] Latency is the hallmark of herpes viruses, and reactivation in the setting of various stressors or immunosuppression leads to clinical disease.

Early on with the advent of HCT, herpes viruses were identified as a frequent cause of morbidity. In the absence of antiviral prophylaxis, HSV and varicella zoster virus (VZV) were frequently encountered in the early post–hematopoietic stem cell transplantation (HSCT) period.[2,3] These infections have become relatively uncommon in the setting of antiviral prophylaxis with acyclovir,[4,5] although late-onset disease remains a problem.[6] Acyclovir-resistant (ACVr) HSV infection has emerged in the setting of prophylaxis and can be severe,[7] and cases with multidrug-resistant HSV have been described.[8,9] It is a challenge to treat resistant HSV due to the toxicities of the second- and third-line agents, foscarnet and cidofovir. VZV infection following HSCT tends to occur upon discontinuation of or noncompliance with antiviral prophylaxis. There are 2 Food and Drug Administration (FDA) -approved vaccines for prevention of herpes zoster: a live-attenuated vaccine (Zostavax) and a nonlive subunit VZV vaccine (Shingrix)[10,11]; the latter is also effective in preventing herpes zoster in autologous HSCT.[12]

HHV6 infection occurs mostly after allogeneic HSCT, and its management remains challenging from the standpoint of surveillance and treatment in the context of reactivation. However, there is no doubt in its role in causing encephalitis.[13,14] HHV7 infection has been infrequently reported in HSCT,[15,16] and disease association has been suggested on the basis of case reports.[17–19] EBV and HHV8 (Kaposi sarcoma herpes virus) infections can lead to posttransplant lymphoproliferative disorder (PTLD) and Kaposi sarcoma (KS), respectively, mostly in the setting of allogeneic HSCT.[20,21] Management of EBV-related PTLD is challenging, although strategies using EBV-specific CD8 lymphocytes are promising.[20]

EPIDEMIOLOGY AND CLINICAL FEATURES OF ALPHAHERPESVIRNINAE (HERPES SIMPLEX VIRUS AND VARICELLA ZOSTER VIRUS) IN HEMATOPOIETIC STEM CELL TRANSPLANTATION
General Considerations

Latency is the hallmark of these viral infections. Disease following HSCT is related to reactivation of the virus, whereas primary infection is uncommon.[2,3,22] These viruses are neurotropic with HSV establishing latency in the trigeminal or sacral ganglia and upon reactivation results in eruptions in the labial or anogenital areas, whereas VZV establishes latency in the dorsal root ganglia and reactivation resulting in dermatomal zoster. Both viruses can lead to disseminated disease, which is largely dependent on the net state of immunosuppression, primarily cell-mediated immunity. Innate immunity, including natural killer cells, plays an important role in controlling these viral infections.[23–25]

Herpes Simplex Virus: Epidemiology

HSV 1 and 2 belong to the genus *Simplexvirus* of the subfamily Alphaherpesvirinae.[1] In the absence of antiviral prophylaxis, 70% to 80% of seropositive HSCT recipients developed HSV disease during preengraftment period with median time to onset of 3 weeks after HSCT.[2] In the current era of antiviral prophylaxis in seropositive recipients, the rate of infection has decreased significantly.[5,26] Moreover, acyclovir prophylaxis in the allogeneic HSCT is associated with significant reduction in mortality (relative risk of 0.79 and number needed to treat of 12).[5] HSV breakthrough infections occur with isolates that are susceptible or resistant to acyclovir. In a study by Kakiuchi and colleagues,[27] oral swabs were collected before HCT and then weekly after HCT through day 100. Testing for HSV revealed that 15% (39/268 HCT) had HSV shedding, and testing for susceptibility to acyclovir found that 11 had ACVr virus (11/39, 28%). One hundred-day mortality was significantly higher in the ACVr group compared with groups with no infection or acyclovir-sensitive HSV. Relapsed malignancy was a significant risk factor for ACVr HSV in this study. Another situation of HSV break-through infection is treatment with intermittent or weekly dosing of cidofovir.[28] Regarding ACVr, HSV epidemiology, in a retrospective study over a 10-year period (2002–2011) from France, did not show increased ACVr in immunocompetent persons. In the allogeneic HSCT cohort, ACVr increased from 14.3% in the 2002 to 2006 period to 46.5% in the 2007 to 2011 period (P = .005).[29] In other studies, an increase in ACVr has been observed with a lower dose of acyclovir prophylaxis and prolonged periods of immunocompromised state.[9,30] Apart from acyclovir preventing HSV disease, Erard and colleagues[31] demonstrated that longer duration of prophylaxis after HSCT correlated with HSV disease and ACVr HSV disease. There was 0% probability of HSV and ACVr HSV disease in those treated for greater than 1 year versus 3.9% and 0.2% probability of HSV and ACVr HSV disease, respectively, in those treated for 1 year. Percentages of 31.6% and 1.3% HSV and ACVr HSV disease were noted, respectively, in those treated until only 30 days after HCT. This study supports the prolonged duration of acyclovir prophylaxis as a protection against development of acyclovir resistance.

Herpes Simplex Virus: Clinical Presentation

Oropharyngeal/orofacial infection (nasolabial fold, vermilion border of lips, buccal mucosa, tongue, throat, cheeks), presents with localized pain and vesicle formation. Vesicles tend to evolve into ulcerative lesions that are often painful and can be quite destructive (**Fig. 1**). Oropharyngeal disease can be masked by or confused with mucositis related to the chemotherapy.[32] In the setting of unchecked oropharyngeal infection, it can spread to the esophagus by contiguous spread often facilitated by the presence of the nasogastric tube. HSV esophagitis presents with nausea, odynophagia, and chest pain.[33] Endoscopy with esophageal biopsy is necessary to confirm the diagnosis and to document resolution upon completion of therapy. Graft-versus-host disease (GVHD) and other viral infections, such as cytomegalovirus (CMV) and VZV, need to be excluded. Intestinal HSV infection is uncommon; literature is limited to case reports that suggest diagnosis is often delayed and associated with high mortality.[34–36] Hepatitis due to HSV is associated with marked elevation of transaminases, abdominal pain, and fever, and often there is no rash.[37] The respiratory disease manifests with tracheobronchitis and necrotizing pneumonia in the setting of contiguous

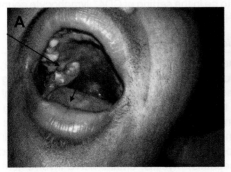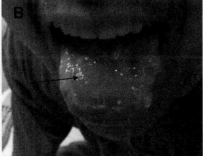

Fig. 1. (*A, B*) Severe ACVr HSV ulcerations. Ulcerations of palate and tongue (*Arrows*).

spread from oropharynx, whereas interstitial pneumonitis is encountered in disseminated disease[38]; the latter is associated with high mortality.[7,39] Clinically, patients may have fever, chest pain, cough, and hypoxemia. The central nervous system (CNS) is less frequently involved in HSCT. HSV 1 is more likely to be associated with encephalitis, whereas HSV 2 is more likely to be associated with meningitis. HSV infection needs to be ruled out in an HSCT patient presenting with CNS symptoms suggestive of infection.[40] Other uncommon syndromes that are associated with HSV include erythema multiforme,[41,42] herpetic whitlow, and involvement of the eye. Genital HSV is less frequent than oropharyngeal HSV and commonly involves the genital area, perianal skin, buttocks, and hips, and a severe outbreak can be associated with urinary retention.[43,44]

Diagnostic evaluation is based on clinical suspicion and the body site involved. Clues to the diagnosis include the presence of a vesicular rash, ulcerations that are often shallow, and scraping of the vesicle base/ulcer for viral inclusion (Tzanck smear), and direct fluorescent assay (DFA) can provide rapid diagnosis. Polymerase chain reaction (PCR) should be obtained from the vesicle fluid or from the ulcer base, along with viral culture. HSV PCR from plasma and deep tissue biopsy may be required in the context of visceral disease or disseminated disease with organ involvement. Cerebrospinal fluid (CSF) HSV PCR in suspected CNS disease should be obtained. Antiviral susceptibility should be requested in the instance of breakthrough infection. Because ACVr has been noted even in the absence of prior acyclovir use, perhaps obtaining antiviral susceptibility on all HSV isolates could be justified in this patient population. Often the diagnosis of ACVr HSV is clinical because the phenotypic assay is time consuming.[45] With the progress in molecular diagnostics, next-generation sequencing may help identify ACVr HSV rapidly and the mutations conferring resistance.[46] Radiographic evaluation should be based on the organ system affected.

Varicella Zoster Virus: Epidemiology

Primary varicella infection is uncommon after HSCT, and the burden is primarily from reactivation with herpes zoster. Locksley and colleagues[47] observed that 80% of HSCT recipients who developed varicella or herpes zoster were not on antiviral prophylaxis and most cases occurred within the first 9 months of HSCT. Visceral dissemination and mortality were comparable among those with herpes zoster or primary varicella infection. Mortality of 9.7% was observed, and a significant number suffered from postherpetic neuralgia (25%), although higher rates have been reported.[48] Antiviral prophylaxis has been very effective in reducing the rates of herpes zoster, especially with prolonged course following HSCT.[49]

The primary risk factor for development of herpes zoster is the lack of VZV-specific cell-mediated immunity, and these tend to be in the setting of CD4$^+$ lymphocyte count less than 200/μL, allogeneic HSCT, GVHD, and cord HSCT.[50–52]

Varicella Zoster Virus: Clinical Presentation

The most common presentation is dermatomal distribution of a vesicular rash. It may or may not present with the classic prodromal symptoms of burning pain or itching. The most common dermatomes affected are thoracic followed by lumbar, cervical, cranial, and sacral.[47] In some situations, the presentation can be highly atypical. Diagnosis is established by microbiologic confirmation by maintaining a high index of suspicion (Fig. 2). Cutaneous dissemination occurs in a third of patients (Fig. 3), and in such patients, there is a high risk for visceral dissemination and deep-seated infections: encephalitis, pneumonitis, hepatitis, myelitis, cranial nerve involvement, and retinitis (progressive outer retinal necrosis). Primary visceral disease is

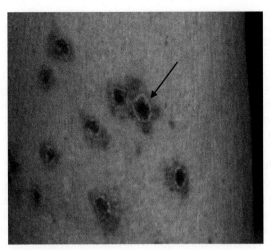

Fig. 2. Atypical disseminated herpes zoster in a cord HSCT patient. Atypical lesion (*arrow*).

uncommon; in a series of 10 cases, the majority presented with abdominal pain, fever, abnormally elevated transaminases, and pancreatic enzymes, and none had rash at initial presentation. Rash developed 6 days after abdominal pain (range, 4–10 days), and diagnosis was established 7 days after onset of symptoms (range, 4–14 days). This condition is a diagnostic challenge with an associated mortality up to 50%.[53]

Diagnosis relies heavily on clinical suspicion and history. Serology is not helpful in establishing the diagnosis; identification of the virus is the key, by PCR or DFA because culture is not a sensitive test. The scraping of the vesicle base for DFA and Tzanck smear provides rapid diagnosis; however, PCR is suggested because it is more sensitive than culture.[54] In the situation of atypical skin lesion, a biopsy is recommended, with immunostains/PCR for VZV. For suspected visceral disease plasma for VZV, PCR is suggested,[55] and appropriate imaging studies and diagnostic procedures, such as endoscopic examination of the gastrointestinal tract with biopsy (gut, liver) for confirmation of diagnosis, PCR on CSF evaluation for CNS infection, and vitreal aspirate for ophthalmic involvement, are recommended.

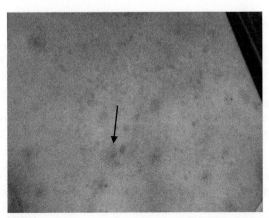

Fig. 3. Disseminated herpes zoster, which appears as primary varicella. Vesicle with erythematous base (*arrow*).

EPIDEMIOLOGY AND CLINICAL FEATURES OF BETAHERPESVIRINEA (HUMAN HERPES VIRUS 6 AND HUMAN HERPES VIRUS 7) IN HEMATOPOIETIC STEM CELL TRANSPLANTATION
General Considerations

In contrast to Alphaviruses, Betaherpesviruses infect and establish latency in a much wider reservoir. Latent HHV6 is found in peripheral blood mononuclear cells, bone marrow progenitor cells, natural killer cells, salivary glands, bronchial glands, oligo-dendrocytes, and astrocytes. HHV7 primarily infects CD4$^+$ T cells. Both viruses are acquired early in life, during childhood.[56]

Epidemiology: Human Herpes Virus 6

HHV6A and HHV6B are distinct viruses with HHV6B mostly causing disease after HSCT (accounts for 98% of HHV6 infections) and is the topic of this discussion. The mode of transmission is via saliva, and infection occurs in childhood years.[57] The primary illness during childhood is "roseola infantum," a febrile illness that is self-limited. In allogeneic HSCT, the infection is due to the reactivation of recipient HHV6; however, donor-derived infection is possible.[58,59] The risk factors of HHV6 reactivation include cord HSCT, HLA mismatched donor, unrelated donor, acute GVHD, and steroid use.[13,60,61] Reactivation is observed in 40% to 50% of HSCT recipients at a median of 3 weeks following transplantation.[62] Most patients are asymptomatic, and viremia resolves spontaneously. An important aspect noted with HHV6 virus is its integration to the germ-line cells leading to "chromosomally" integrated HHV6 (ci-HHV6), and it occurs in approximately 1% of the population. The ci-HHV6 can be donor derived and is associated with very high viral loads especially from the whole blood (>5.5 million copies/mL of whole blood) that do not change with antiviral therapy.[63] Most HSCT recipients with this entity are asymptomatic, and its role in causing illness is not well defined.[64–66]

CNS involvement is the main concern with HHV6B; it is the most common cause of seizure in HSCT patients, especially with a higher incidence in cord HSCT.[67,68] HHV6B reactivation with high viral load has been noted to be a risk factor for development of encephalitis[61,62]; however, preemptive therapy has not been effective in preventing CNS disease.[69,70] In fact, some cases of encephalitis have occurred in the absence of systemic viremia that argues against value of preemptive therapy in the context of treatment-related toxicities.

Clinical Presentation: Human Herpes Virus 6

HHV6B has been implicated in CNS disease, manifesting with encephalitis complicated by seizures, delirium, and memory deficits.[67,71] Patients often present with sudden deterioration, fever, confusion, and antegrade amnesia. Imaging with MRI may show medial temporal lobe encephalitis (often bilateral-hippocampal area)[72] (**Fig. 4**), CSF pleocytosis with lymphomononuclear predominance, and elevated protein level.[73] The clinical presentation coupled with imaging findings and demonstration of HHV6B in the CSF by PCR is considered confirmatory of the diagnosis of encephalitis.

Febrile illness with rash, bone marrow suppression/graft loss, delayed platelet engraftment, risk for CMV reactivation, and development of acute GVHD, hepatitis, and potential role in idiopathic pneumonia syndrome has been reported with HHV6.[74–76] Graft failure association has been strongest in cord HSCT.[77] Meanwhile, clinical significance of ci-HHV6 in causing disease among HSCT recipients is not well defined, with instances of antiviral treatment in asymptomatic patients.[65,78]

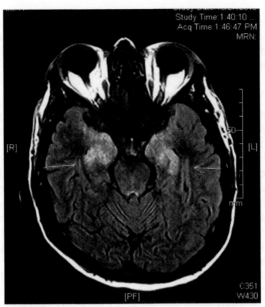

Fig. 4. MRI of HHV6 encephalitis with temporal lobe involvement. Temporal lobe enhancement (*arrows*).

Diagnosis of HHV6 infection relies on a careful assessment of the clinical presentation, risk factors, time to onset of symptoms after HSCT, and organ involvement. HHV6 reactivation in an asymptomatic patient does not establish disease.[66] There are no established guidelines for HHV6B surveillance, and variability exists across transplant centers in monitoring approaches. Appropriate samples need to be tested for viral load: plasma in the setting of systemic illness (febrile rash with no other explanation), delayed engraftment, or graft failure; bronchoalveolar lavage fluid in patients with idiopathic pneumonia; and CSF fluid in patients with CNS symptoms. Whole blood PCR does not correlate well with active replication.[79] High viral loads are noted with ci-HHV6, especially from whole blood samples, and could be a clue for this condition. Imaging with MRI of the brain is important to evaluate CNS infection. Electro-encephalogram should be performed in patients with seizures.

Human Herpes Virus 7: Epidemiology and Clinical Features in Hematopoietic Stem Cell Transplantation

HHV7 is tropic to the CD4+ cells; infection is typically acquired early in childhood, and transmission is via saliva.[56] In a recent prospective study of 105 patients monitored with a multiplex PCR assay starting pre-HSCT and then weekly until day 42, post-HCT had a reactivation rate of 8.6%.[15] Others have reported rates of up to 60%.[80] Weak association has been noted between HHV7 and encephalitis, with one report each of brain stem encephalitis,[19] meningitis with optic neuritis in another,[18] and a case of myelitis.[17]

EPIDEMIOLOGY AND CLINICAL FEATURES OF GAMMAHERPESVIRINAE (EPSTEIN-BARR VIRUS AND HUMAN HERPES VIRUS 8) IN HEMATOPOIETIC STEM CELL TRANSPLANTATION
General Considerations

Both EBV and HHV8 infect B cells and establish lifelong latency. The presence of significant immunosuppression, especially the blunted T-cell response, is the major risk factor for EBV reactivation. Selective T-cell depletion, both ex vivo and in vivo, is associated with development of EBV viremia and development of PTLD.[81] HHV8 infects CD19$^+$ B cells but is also found in endothelial cells, salivary glands, and monocyte-macrophage cells.[82]

Epidemiology of Epstein-Barr Virus

EBV infection following HSCT is either a reactivation or a result of a primary infection in a seronegative recipient from the seropositive donor cells or from an EBV-infected person. The incidence of EBV viremia after HSCT ranges from 0.1% to 63% and varies by the type of HSCT, defined level of viremia, screening methodology, and assay sensitivity.[83] In cord HSCT, EBV reactivation in the absence of EBV-specific T-cell response can evolve rapidly and lead to PTLD.[84,85] PTLD is a major complication of EBV infection, and incidence ranges from 1.2% to 12.9% with a median time to onset of 2 to 4 months[83] after HSCT. The highest risk occurs in recipients of cord HSCT, whereas very low rates occur among recipients of haploidentical HSCT who have received cyclophosphamide after transplant.[86] PTLD is a devastating illness, and the ability to predict its development helps intervene early. Uhlin and colleagues[87] identified the following 6 risk factors; HLA mismatch, EBV mismatch, splenectomy, use of reduced intensity conditioning, mesenchymal stromal cell treatment, and acute GVHD grades II-IV. Cumulative incidence of EBV-PTLD increases dramatically with increasing number of risk factors from 0.4% in patients with 1 risk factor (inclusive of antithymocyte globulin) to 40% with the presence of 5 risk factors. Others have reported a similar approach to predict EBV-PTLD that would enable targeted surveillance and preemptive treatment.[86]

Clinical Features of Epstein-Barr Virus

The clinical presentation of PTLD can be highly variable, from a localized involvement to a disseminated disease with infiltration of multiple organ systems, fever (B symptoms), and sepsis with organ failure. Mortality related to PTLD is high.[88]

Other syndromes that have been noted with EBV include infectious mononucleosis, hepatitis, hairy leukoplakia, gastrointestinal involvement, meningoencephalitis, and pneumonitis.[89] EBV can lead to hemophagocytic lymphohistiocytosis.[90] It can also lead to mucocutaneous ulcerations of the oral and gut mucosa and the skin.[91]

Diagnostic recommendations have been recently reviewed[83] and relies heavily on tissue biopsy confirmation of PTLD (excisional biopsy is preferred), and routine ancillary pathology techniques, such as EBV-encoded RNA in situ hybridization, should be performed. EBV viremia alone does not confirm PTLD. EBV viral load surveillance from whole blood is suggested in the context of preemptive monitoring.[83,92] In the setting of CNS PTLD, PCR should be performed on the CSF. Biopsy may be required to confirm diagnosis. Imaging is required to localize the extent of the disease, and PET scan may assist in diagnosis and staging.[93]

Epidemiology of Human Herpes Virus 8 and Clinical Features

HHV8 transmission is via saliva in children and young adults, whereas sexual transmission has been shown in men who have sex with men.[82,94] There is varied geographic prevalence with high seroprevalence in sub-Saharan Africa (>30%–40%) followed by Mediterranean (10%–20%) and Asia/United States (<10%).[82] In the HSCT, reactivation is uncommon (0%–1% detection of HHV8 DNA in blood), and natural history is not well described.[95] In HSCT patients, it has been associated with bone marrow failure,[96] fever with rash and hepatitis,[97] and KS.[21,98] Most of the KS have occurred in the immunosuppressed allogeneic HSCT, and the presence of diffuse disease is associated with high mortality.[21]

MANAGEMENT
Management of Herpes Simplex Virus and Varicella Zoster Virus in Hematopoietic Stem Cell Transplantation

The mainstay of therapy for HSV and VZV is prevention in the post-HSCT phase. Acyclovir (or Valtrex) prophylaxis in the HSV-seropositive recipient starting with the conditioning regimen for the HSCT is standard. The duration of prophylaxis for HSV is suggested for a period of 1 month after HSCT (both autologous and allogeneic); however, prolonged prophylaxis to 1 year after allogeneic HCT is recommended for VZV prevention (or longer based on immune status).[49,99] Prolonged prophylaxis is also protective against development of ACVr HSV infection.[31] Intravenous formulation of acyclovir should be used in the setting of mucositis or GVHD of the gut where absorption is a concern. Mucocutaneous HSV infection is treated with acyclovir 5 mg/kg every 8 hours (renal dose adjusted), with 10 to 12 mg/kg every 8 hours for tissue invasive disease. In suspected ACVr HSV, viral culture and test for phenotypic resistance assay should be obtained. Genotypic methods are not readily available for clinical care. Next-generation sequencing is promising not only for rapid diagnosis but also for providing novel resistance mechanisms.[46] The commonest mechanism of antiviral resistance against acyclovir in HSV is a thymidine kinase deficiency, whereas mutations in the DNA polymerase result in foscarnet and cidofovir resistance.[100,101] Foscarnet is the drug of choice for ACVr HSV,[101] although high-dose continuous infusion of acyclovir in a small series was shown to be effective.[102] The use of foscarnet is limited by toxicities that range from electrolyte abnormalities, to nephrotoxicity, and ulcerations (genital and oral; **Fig. 5**) with foscarnet.[103] Cidofovir is notorious for nephrotoxicity and uveitis as well as loss of intraocular pressure. For ACVr HSV mucocutaneous disease, topical application of cidofovir and imiquimod (local immune modulator that acts by upregulating TLR) has been used with success.[104,105] Pritelivir, a helicase-primase inhibitor currently being evaluated in clinical trials, has excellent activity against HSV, including ACVr HSV.[106] CMX001 (Brincidofovir) has been used for ACVr HSV.[107] A vaccine is not yet available for HSV.

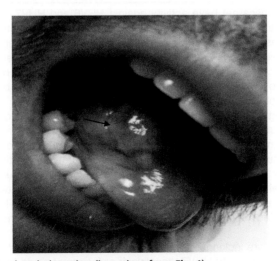

Fig. 5. Foscarnet-related ulceration (in patient from **Fig. 1**).

In patients with localized herpes zoster, oral antiviral therapy with valacyclovir or acyclovir until crusting of the lesions is suggested. However, the intravenous route should be used in when absorption from the gastrointestinal tract is questionable. Patients with herpes zoster with cutaneous dissemination, disseminated with visceral involvement or with ophthalmic involvement, should be hospitalized and treated with 10 mg/kg of acyclovir intravenously every 8 hours.[108] The organs involved should be taken into account when deciding duration of therapy and therapy should be continued until resolution of all lesions (with crusting) is achieved. Airborne precautions should be used in hospitalized patients to prevent nosocomial transmission. The helicase primase inhibitor Amenamevir is effective against VZV and is approved in Japan for treatment of herpes zoster among immunocompetent patients.[109]

Vaccines for the prevention of herpesvirus infections are discussed in (See Mini Kamboj and Monika K. Shah's article, "Vaccination of the Stem Cell Transplant Recipient and the Hematologic Malignancy Patient," in this issue). Varicella vaccine (Varivax) is a live-attenuated vaccine recommended for the prevention of varicella in VZV-seronegative HSCT recipients. It is recommended at or 2 years after autologous HSCT, and similarly in allogeneic HSCT patients who are no longer immunosuppressed (absence of GVHD, off all immunosuppressive therapy, and in some cases documentation of CD4 count >200).

Two vaccines for the prevention of herpes zoster are FDA approved: Zostavax (live-attenuated vaccine) and Shingrix (glycoprotein E/ASO1B adjuvant subunit vaccine).[10,11] Zostavax has not been studied in the setting of HSCT, with the exception of a single-center case series in multiple myeloma patients.[110] It is currently not recommended in HSCT patients due to of lack of safety data. In autologous HSCT recipients, Shingrix used in a 2-dose series, the first at 50 to 70 days after HSCT and the second at 2 months thereafter, was efficacious and safe in preventing herpes zoster.[12] It has not been studied in the allogeneic HSCT, thus the lack of data on its safety and efficacy in this population. Another inactivated herpes zoster vaccine was efficacious and safe in autologous HSCT, although it had a decline in efficacy beyond the first year of HCT.[111]

Management of Human Herpes Virus 6 and Human Herpes Virus 7

Ganciclovir and foscarnet have activity against HHV6 and HHV7. Prophylactic and preemptive therapy with antiviral agents has been mostly ineffective in preventing end-organ disease with HHV6.[69,70] Some centers use a risk-adapted surveillance approach, following HHV6 viral load cutoffs to use antiviral agents, with a resulting suggested reduction in disease. However, because of spontaneous resolution of viremia in most patients without treatment, and most reactivations being asymptomatic, routine prophylaxis or preemptive therapy is not suggested.

In the context of HHV6 encephalitis, treatment with ganciclovir or foscarnet should be instituted immediately. Ganciclovir dose is 5 mg/kg every 12 hours, and foscarnet is 90 mg/kg every 12 hours; both medications need to be renally dose adjusted. Minimum duration of therapy is 21 days or until a negative HHV6 PCR in CSF, whichever is later, based on the expert opinion by this author. Supportive care involving rehabilitative efforts among those patients with sequelae of CNS disease should be undertaken early on.[112] Last, in patients with ci-HHV6, treatment should be avoided unless there is a very high suspicion for end-organ disease from ci-HHV6.

Treatment data are lacking in patients with HHV7 infection. In situations with high likelihood of disease due to HHV7, ganciclovir or foscarnet could be used.

Management of Epstein-Barr Virus in Hematopoietic Stem Cell Transplantation

Antiviral agents may have activity in the setting of a lytic infection but are ineffective in the context of PTLD. Monitoring of EBV viral load by PCR from whole blood in high-risk patients is recommended. This monitoring allows preemptive treatment of EBV viremia with rituximab among those at high risk for development of PTLD,[83,113] and has been effective in reducing the development of PTLD. Other interventions include a reduction in immunosuppression if feasible. Because T-cell depletion is a major reason for PTLD development, adoptive transfer of EBV-specific CD8 T cells has been used (review by Rouce and colleagues[81]). However, this approach is limited by concomitant treatment with corticosteroids, which is commonplace in the management of GVHD. The manufacturing process is also tedious, and efforts are underway to counter that by developing "off-the-shelf" EBV-specific or polyvirus-targeted T-cell products. Vaccine development for EBV is an active area of research but not close to clinical application.[114,115]

Management of Human Herpes Virus 8

Antivirals (acyclovir, ganciclovir, and cidofovir) have in vitro activity against HHV8 but are not effective with KS. KS related to HHV8 requires reduction of immunosuppression or use of an mammalian target of rapamycin–based regimen following the observation of sirolimus leading to regression of KS, suggesting antineoplastic activity. Chemotherapy with agents, such as taxanes and anthracyclines, with or without radiation treatment, is suggested for diffuse KS. No new therapies appear to be on the horizon.[116]

SUMMARY

The burden of illness related to herpes viruses in HSCT patients is not insignificant. Although HSV infection is effectively controlled with prophylaxis, ACVr and multi-drug-resistant HSV infections are significant and difficult problems. The helicase primase inhibitor Pritelivir has excellent activity against ACVr HSV and would be an important development if found to be successful in ongoing clinical trial in immunocompromised patients. VZV management will undergo modification with the availability of nonlive vaccines, and helicase primase inhibitor Amenamevir is a new development (not yet available in the United States). Management of HHV6 is challenging and will continue to evolve, whereas models to predict development of HHV6 encephalitis could be useful. EBV-related PTLD remains a challenge, and future management is likely to use more of the "EBV-specific or polyvirus" T-cell immunotherapy either prophylactically or therapeutically with technological improvements. HHV7 and HHV8 are very uncommon after HSCT, and their management will largely be expert opinion until more data are available.

REFERENCES

1. Davison AJ. Introduction: definition and classification of human herpesviruses. 1st edition. Cambridge (England): Cambridge University Press; 2007.
2. Meyers JD, Flournoy N, Thomas ED. Infection with herpes simplex virus and cell-mediated immunity after marrow transplant. J Infect Dis 1980;142(3):338–46.
3. Meyers JD, Sullivan KM, Flournoy N, et al. Infection with Varicella-zoster virus after marrow transplantation. J Infect Dis 1985;152(6):1172–81.
4. Wade JC, Newton B, Flournoy N, et al. Oral acyclovir for prevention of herpes simplex virus reactivation after marrow transplantation. Ann Intern Med 1984; 100(6):823–8.

5. Yahav D, Gafter-Gvili A, Muchtar E, et al. Antiviral prophylaxis in haematological patients: systematic review and meta-analysis. Eur J Cancer 2009;45(18): 3131–48.

6. Sahoo F, Hill JA, Xie H, et al. Herpes zoster in autologous hematopoietic cell transplant recipients in the era of acyclovir or valacyclovir prophylaxis and novel treatment and maintenance therapies. Biol Blood Marrow Transplant 2017;23(3): 505–11.

7. Ljungman P, Ellis MN, Hackman RC, et al. Acyclovir-resistant herpes simplex virus causing pneumonia after marrow transplantation. J Infect Dis 1990; 162(1):244–8.

8. Chen Y, Scieux C, Garrait V, et al. Resistant herpes simplex virus type 1 infection: an emerging concern after allogeneic stem cell transplantation. Clin Infect Dis 2000;31(4):927–35.

9. Chakrabarti S, Pillay D, Ratcliffe D, et al. Resistance to antiviral drugs in herpes simplex virus infections among allogeneic stem cell transplant recipients: risk factors and prognostic significance. J Infect Dis 2000;181(6):2055–8.

10. Available at: https://www.fda.gov/BiologicsBloodVaccines/Vaccines/Approved Products/ucm136941.htm. Accessed February 19, 2019.

11. Available at: https://www.fda.gov/biologicsbloodvaccines/vaccines/approved products/ucm581491.htm. Accessed February 19, 2019.

12. Javier de la Serna LC, Campora L, Pranatharthi C, et al. Efficacy and safety of an adjuvanted herpes zoster subunit vaccine in autologous hematopoietic stem cell transplant recipients 18 years of age or older: first results of the phase 3 randomized, placebo-controlled ZOE-HSCT clinical trial. Paper presented at: Tandem. Salt Lake City (UT), 2018.

13. Ogata M, Fukuda T, Teshima T. Human herpesvirus-6 encephalitis after allogeneic hematopoietic cell transplantation: what we do and do not know. Bone Marrow Transplant 2015;50(8):1030–6.

14. Scheurer ME, Pritchett JC, Amirian ES, et al. HHV-6 encephalitis in umbilical cord blood transplantation: a systematic review and meta-analysis. Bone Marrow Transplant 2013;48(4):574–80.

15. Inazawa N, Hori T, Hatakeyama N, et al. Large-scale multiplex polymerase chain reaction assay for diagnosis of viral reactivations after allogeneic hematopoietic stem cell transplantation. J Med Virol 2015;87(8):1427–35.

16. Inazawa N, Hori T, Nojima M, et al. Virus reactivations after autologous hematopoietic stem cell transplantation detected by multiplex PCR assay. J Med Virol 2017;89(2):358–62.

17. Ward KN, White RP, Mackinnon S, et al. Human herpesvirus-7 infection of the CNS with acute myelitis in an adult bone marrow recipient. Bone Marrow Transplant 2002;30(12):983–5.

18. Yoshikawa T, Yoshida J, Hamaguchi M, et al. Human herpesvirus 7-associated meningitis and optic neuritis in a patient after allogeneic stem cell transplantation. J Med Virol 2003;70(3):440–3.

19. Holden SR, Vas AL. Severe encephalitis in a haematopoietic stem cell transplant recipient caused by reactivation of human herpesvirus 6 and 7. J Clin Virol 2007; 40(3):245–7.

20. Sanz J, Andreu R. Epstein-Barr virus-associated posttransplant lymphoproliferative disorder after allogeneic stem cell transplantation. Curr Opin Oncol 2014; 26(6):677–83.

21. Deauna-Limayo D, Rajabi B, Qiu W, et al. Kaposi sarcoma after non-myeloablative hematopoietic stem cell transplant: response to withdrawal of

immunosuppressant therapy correlated with whole blood human herpesvirus-8 reverse transcriptase-polymerase chain reaction levels. Leuk Lymphoma 2013; 54(10):2299–302.

22. Meyers JD. Treatment of herpesvirus infections in the immunocompromised host. Scand J Infect Dis Suppl 1985;47:128–36.

23. Dadwal SS, Ito JI. 5th edition. Herpes simplex virus infections, vol. 2. Sussex (England): Wiley Blackwell; 2016.

24. Ho Dy, Arvin AM. Varicella zoster virus infections, vol. 2. Sussex (England): Wiley Blackwell; 2016.

25. Dalloul A, Oksenhendler E, Chosidow O, et al. Severe herpes virus (HSV-2) infection in two patients with myelodysplasia and undetectable NK cells and plasmacytoid dendritic cells in the blood. J Clin Virol 2004;30(4):329–36.

26. Young JA, Logan BR, Wu J, et al, Blood and Marrow Transplant Clinical Trials Network Trial 0201. Infections after transplantation of bone marrow or peripheral-blood stem cells from unrelated donors. Biol Blood Marrow Transplant 2016;22(2):359–70.

27. Kakiuchi S, Tsuji M, Nishimura H, et al. Association of the emergence of acyclovir-resistant herpes simplex virus type 1 with prognosis in hematopoietic stem cell transplantation patients. J Infect Dis 2017;215(6):865–73.

28. Dvorak CC, Cowan MJ, Horn B, et al. Development of herpes simplex virus stomatitis during receipt of cidofovir therapy. Clin Infect Dis 2009;49(8):e92–5.

29. Frobert E, Burrel S, Ducastelle-Lepretre S, et al. Resistance of herpes simplex viruses to acyclovir: an update from a ten-year survey in France. Antiviral Res 2014;111:36–41.

30. Langston AA, Redei I, Caliendo AM, et al. Development of drug-resistant herpes simplex virus infection after haploidentical hematopoietic progenitor cell transplantation. Blood 2002;99(3):1085–8.

31. Erard V, Wald A, Corey L, et al. Use of long-term suppressive acyclovir after hematopoietic stem-cell transplantation: impact on herpes simplex virus (HSV) disease and drug-resistant HSV disease. J Infect Dis 2007;196(2):266–70.

32. Van der Beek MT, Laheij AM, Raber-Durlacher JE, et al. Viral loads and antiviral resistance of herpesviruses and oral ulcerations in hematopoietic stem cell transplant recipients. Bone Marrow Transplant 2012;47(9):1222–8.

33. McDonald GB, Sharma P, Hackman RC, et al. Esophageal infections in immunosuppressed patients after marrow transplantation. Gastroenterology 1985;88(5 Pt 1):1111–7.

34. Spencer GD, Shulman HM, Myerson D, et al. Diffuse intestinal ulceration after marrow transplantation: a clinicopathologic study of 13 patients. Hum Pathol 1986;17(6):621–33.

35. Naik HR, Chandrasekar PH. Herpes simplex virus (HSV) colitis in a bone marrow transplant recipient. Bone Marrow Transplant 1996;17(2):285–6.

36. Kingreen D, Nitsche A, Beyer J, et al. Herpes simplex infection of the jejunum occurring in the early post-transplantation period. Bone Marrow Transplant 1997;20(11):989–91.

37. Johnson JR, Egaas S, Gleaves CA, et al. Hepatitis due to herpes simplex virus in marrow-transplant recipients. Clin Infect Dis 1992;14(1):38–45.

38. Corey L, Spear PG. Infections with herpes simplex viruses (2). N Engl J Med 1986;314(12):749–57.

39. Ramsey PG, Fife KH, Hackman RC, et al. Herpes simplex virus pneumonia: clinical, virologic, and pathologic features in 20 patients. Ann Intern Med 1982; 97(6):813–20.

40. Romee R, Brunstein CG, Weisdorf DJ, et al. Herpes simplex virus encephalitis after allogeneic transplantation: an instructive case. Bone Marrow Transplant 2010;45(4):776–8.

41. Burnett JW, Laing JM, Aurelian L. Acute skin eruptions that are positive for herpes simplex virus DNA polymerase in patients with stem cell transplantation: a new manifestation within the erythema multiforme reactive dermatoses. Arch Dermatol 2008;144(7):902–7.

42. Green JA, Spruance SL, Wenerstrom G, et al. Post-herpetic erythema multiforme prevented with prophylactic oral acyclovir. Ann Intern Med 1985;102(5): 632–3.

43. Sable CA, Donowitz GR. Infections in bone marrow transplant recipients. Clin Infect Dis 1994;18(3):273–81 [quiz: 282–4].

44. Haanpaa M, Paavonen J. Transient urinary retention and chronic neuropathic pain associated with genital herpes simplex virus infection. Acta Obstet Gynecol Scand 2004;83(10):946–9.

45. Frobert E, Thouvenot D, Lina B, et al. Genotyping diagnosis of acyclovir resistant herpes simplex virus. Pathol Biol (Paris) 2007;55(10):504–11.

46. Fujii H, Kakiuchi S, Tsuji M, et al. Application of next-generation sequencing to detect acyclovir-resistant herpes simplex virus type 1 variants at low frequency in thymidine kinase gene of the isolates recovered from patients with hematopoietic stem cell transplantation. J Virol Methods 2018;251:123–8.

47. Locksley RM, Flournoy N, Sullivan KM, et al. Infection with varicella-zoster virus after marrow transplantation. J Infect Dis 1985;152(6):1172–81.

48. Onozawa M, Hashino S, Haseyama Y, et al. Incidence and risk of postherpetic neuralgia after varicella zoster virus infection in hematopoietic cell transplantation recipients: Hokkaido Hematology Study Group. Biol Blood Marrow Transplant 2009;15(6):724–9.

49. Boeckh M, Kim HW, Flowers ME, et al. Long-term acyclovir for prevention of varicella zoster virus disease after allogeneic hematopoietic cell transplantation–a randomized double-blind placebo-controlled study. Blood 2006;107(5):1800–5.

50. Offidani M, Corvatta L, Olivieri A, et al. A predictive model of varicella-zoster virus infection after autologous peripheral blood progenitor cell transplantation. Clin Infect Dis 2001;32(10):1414–22.

51. Koc Y, Miller KB, Schenkein DP, et al. Varicella zoster virus infections following allogeneic bone marrow transplantation: frequency, risk factors, and clinical outcome. Biol Blood Marrow Transplant 2000;6(1):44–9.

52. Safdar A, Rodriguez GH, De Lima MJ, et al. Infections in 100 cord blood transplantations: spectrum of early and late posttransplant infections in adult and pediatric patients 1996-2005. Medicine 2007;86(6):324–33.

53. David DS, Tegtmeier BR, O'Donnell MR, et al. Visceral varicella-zoster after bone marrow transplantation: report of a case series and review of the literature. Am J Gastroenterol 1998;93(5):810–3.

54. Nahass GT, Goldstein BA, Zhu WY, et al. Comparison of Tzanck smear, viral culture, and DNA diagnostic methods in detection of herpes simplex and varicellazoster infection. JAMA 1992;268(18):2541–4.

55. Kalpoe JS, Kroes AC, Verkerk S, et al. Clinical relevance of quantitative varicella-zoster virus (VZV) DNA detection in plasma after stem cell transplantation. Bone Marrow Transplant 2006;38(1):41–6.

56. Yamanishi K, Mori Y, Pellett PE. Human herpes virus 6 and 7. 6th edition. Philadelphia: Wolters Kluwer Health; 2013.

57. Zerr DM, Meier AS, Selke SS, et al. A population-based study of primary human herpesvirus 6 infection. N Engl J Med 2005;352(8):768–76.

58. Luppi M, Barozzi P, Morris C, et al. Human herpesvirus 6 latently infects early bone marrow progenitors in vivo. J Virol 1999;73(1):754–9.

59. Kondo K, Kondo T, Okuno T, et al. Latent human herpesvirus 6 infection of human monocytes/macrophages. J Gen Virol 1991;72(Pt 6):1401–8.

60. Olson AL, Dahi PB, Zheng J, et al. Frequent human herpesvirus-6 viremia but low incidence of encephalitis in double-unit cord blood recipients transplanted without antithymocyte globulin. Biol Blood Marrow Transplant 2014;20(6): 787–93.

61. Ogata M, Satou T, Kawano R, et al. Correlations of HHV-6 viral load and plasma IL-6 concentration with HHV-6 encephalitis in allogeneic stem cell transplant recipients. Bone Marrow Transplant 2010;45(1):129–36.

62. Ogata M, Kikuchi H, Satou T, et al. Human herpesvirus 6 DNA in plasma after allogeneic stem cell transplantation: incidence and clinical significance. J Infect Dis 2006;193(1):68–79.

63. Pellett PE, Ablashi DV, Ambros PF, et al. Chromosomally integrated human herpesvirus 6: questions and answers. Rev Med Virol 2012;22(3):144–55.

64. Hill JA, Sedlak RH, Zerr DM, et al. Prevalence of chromosomally integrated human herpesvirus 6 in patients with human herpesvirus 6-central nervous system dysfunction. Biol Blood Marrow Transplant 2015;21(2):371–3.

65. Lee SO, Brown RA, Razonable RR. Chromosomally integrated human herpesvirus-6 in transplant recipients. Transpl Infect Dis 2012;14(4):346–54.

66. Betts BC, Young JA, Ustun C, et al. Human herpesvirus 6 infection after hematopoietic cell transplantation: is routine surveillance necessary? Biol Blood Marrow Transplant 2011;17(10):1562–8.

67. Hill JA, Koo S, Guzman Suarez BB, et al. Cord-blood hematopoietic stem cell transplant confers an increased risk for human herpesvirus-6-associated acute limbic encephalitis: a cohort analysis. Biol Blood Marrow Transplant 2012; 18(11):1638–48.

68. Zerr DM. Human herpesvirus 6 and central nervous system disease in hematopoietic cell transplantation. J Clin Virol 2006;37(Suppl 1):S52–6.

69. Ogata M, Satou T, Kawano R, et al. Plasma HHV-6 viral load-guided preemptive therapy against HHV-6 encephalopathy after allogeneic stem cell transplantation: a prospective evaluation. Bone Marrow Transplant 2008;41(3):279–85.

70. Ishiyama K, Katagiri T, Hoshino T, et al. Preemptive therapy of human herpesvirus-6 encephalitis with foscarnet sodium for high-risk patients after hematopoietic SCT. Bone Marrow Transplant 2011;46(6):863–9.

71. Zerr DM, Fann JR, Breiger D, et al. HHV-6 reactivation and its effect on delirium and cognitive functioning in hematopoietic cell transplantation recipients. Blood 2011;117(19):5243–9.

72. Seeley WW, Marty FM, Holmes TM, et al. Post-transplant acute limbic encephalitis: clinical features and relationship to HHV6. Neurology 2007;69(2):156–65.

73. Ogata M, Satou T, Kadota J, et al. Human herpesvirus 6 (HHV-6) reactivation and HHV-6 encephalitis after allogeneic hematopoietic cell transplantation: a multicenter, prospective study. Clin Infect Dis 2013;57(5):671–81.

74. Ljungman P, Wang FZ, Clark DA, et al. High levels of human herpesvirus 6 DNA in peripheral blood leucocytes are correlated to platelet engraftment and disease in allogeneic stem cell transplant patients. Br J Haematol 2000;111(3): 774–81.

75. Dulery R, Salleron J, Dewilde A, et al. Early human herpesvirus type 6 reactivation after allogeneic stem cell transplantation: a large-scale clinical study. Biol Blood Marrow Transplant 2012;18(7):1080–9.

76. Seo S, Renaud C, Kuypers JM, et al. Idiopathic pneumonia syndrome after hematopoietic cell transplantation: evidence of occult infectious etiologies. Blood 2015;125(24):3789–97.

77. Le Bourgeois A, Labopin M, Guillaume T, et al. Human herpesvirus 6 reactivation before engraftment is strongly predictive of graft failure after double umbilical cord blood allogeneic stem cell transplantation in adults. Exp Hematol 2014; 42(11):945–54.

78. Boutolleau D, Agut H, Gautheret-Dejean A. Human herpesvirus 6 genome integration: a possible cause of misdiagnosis of active viral infection? J Infect Dis 2006;194(7):1019–20 [author reply: 1021–3].

79. Strenger V, Caselli E, Lautenschlager I, et al. Detection of HHV-6-specific mRNA and antigens in PBMCs of individuals with chromosomally integrated HHV-6 (ciHHV-6). Clin Microbiol Infect 2014;20(10):1027–32.

80. Chan PK, Li CK, Chik KW, et al. Risk factors and clinical consequences of human herpesvirus 7 infection in paediatric haematopoietic stem cell transplant recipients. J Med Virol 2004;72(4):668–74.

81. Rouce RH, Louis CU, Heslop HE. Epstein-Barr virus lymphoproliferative disease after hematopoietic stem cell transplant. Curr Opin Hematol 2014;21(6):476–81.

82. David M, Damania BA. Kaposi's sarcoma-associated herpesvirus. 6th edition 2013.

83. Styczynski J, van der Velden W, Fox CP, et al. Management of Epstein-Barr Virus infections and post-transplant lymphoproliferative disorders in patients after allogeneic hematopoietic stem cell transplantation: Sixth European Conference on Infections in Leukemia (ECIL-6) guidelines. Haematologica 2016;101(7): 803–11.

84. Brunstein CG, Weisdorf DJ, DeFor T, et al. Marked increased risk of Epstein-Barr virus-related complications with the addition of antithymocyte globulin to a non-myeloablative conditioning prior to unrelated umbilical cord blood transplantation. Blood 2006;108(8):2874–80.

85. Blaes AH, Cao Q, Wagner JE, et al. Monitoring and preemptive rituximab therapy for Epstein-Barr virus reactivation after anti-thymocyte globulin containing nonmyeloablative conditioning for umbilical cord blood transplantation. Biol Blood Marrow Transplant 2010;16(2):287–91.

86. Landgren O, Gilbert ES, Rizzo JD, et al. Risk factors for lymphoproliferative disorders after allogeneic hematopoietic cell transplantation. Blood 2009;113(20): 4992–5001.

87. Uhlin M, Wikell H, Sundin M, et al. Risk factors for Epstein-Barr virus-related post-transplant lymphoproliferative disease after allogeneic hematopoietic stem cell transplantation. Haematologica 2014;99(2):346–52.

88. Fox CP, Burns D, Parker AN, et al. EBV-associated post-transplant lymphoproliferative disorder following in vivo T-cell-depleted allogeneic transplantation: clinical features, viral load correlates and prognostic factors in the rituximab era. Bone Marrow Transplant 2014;49(2):280–6.

89. Kinch A, Oberg G, Arvidson J, et al. Post-transplant lymphoproliferative disease and other Epstein-Barr virus diseases in allogeneic haematopoietic stem cell transplantation after introduction of monitoring of viral load by polymerase chain reaction. Scand J Infect Dis 2007;39(3):235–44.

90. Weber T, Wickenhauser C, Monecke A, et al. Treatment of rare co-occurrence of Epstein-Barr virus-driven post-transplant lymphoproliferative disorder and hemophagocytic lymphohistiocytosis after allogeneic stem cell transplantation. Transpl Infect Dis 2014;16(6):988–92.
91. Dojcinov SD, Venkataraman G, Raffeld M, et al. EBV positive mucocutaneous ulcer-a study of 26 cases associated with various sources of immunosuppression. Am J Surg Pathol 2010;34(3):405–17.
92. Fryer JF, Heath AB, Wilkinson DE, et al. A collaborative study to establish the 1st WHO International Standard for Epstein-Barr virus for nucleic acid amplification techniques. Biologicals 2016;44(5):423–33.
93. Panagiotidis E, Quigley AM, Pencharz D, et al. (18)F-fluorodeoxyglucose positron emission tomography/computed tomography in diagnosis of post-transplant lymphoproliferative disorder. Leuk Lymphoma 2014;55(3):515–9.
94. Plancoulaine S, Abel L, van Beveren M, et al. Human herpesvirus 8 transmission from mother to child and between siblings in an endemic population. Lancet 2000;356(9235):1062–5.
95. Sergerie Y, Abed Y, Roy J, et al. Comparative evaluation of three serological methods for detection of human herpesvirus 8-specific antibodies in Canadian allogeneic stem cell transplant recipients. J Clin Microbiol 2004;42(6):2663–7.
96. Luppi M, Barozzi P, Schulz TF, et al. Bone marrow failure associated with human herpesvirus 8 infection after transplantation. N Engl J Med 2000;343(19):1378–85.
97. Luppi M, Barozzi P, Schulz TF, et al. Nonmalignant disease associated with human herpesvirus 8 reactivation in patients who have undergone autologous peripheral blood stem cell transplantation. Blood 2000;96(7):2355–7.
98. Bruno B, Sorasio R, Barozzi P, et al. Kaposi's sarcoma triggered by endogenous HHV-8 reactivation after non-myeloablative allogeneic haematopoietic transplantation. Eur J Haematol 2006;76(4):342–7.
99. Tomblyn M, Chiller T, Einsele H, et al. Guidelines for preventing infectious complications among hematopoietic cell transplantation recipients: a global perspective. Biol Blood Marrow Transplant 2009;15(10):1143–238.
100. Strasfeld L, Chou S. Antiviral drug resistance: mechanisms and clinical implications. Infect Dis Clin North Am 2010;24(2):413–37.
101. Avery RK. Antiviral resistance and implications for prophylaxis. New York: Springer; 2011.
102. Kim JH, Schaenman JM, Ho DY, et al. Treatment of acyclovir-resistant herpes simplex virus with continuous infusion of high-dose acyclovir in hematopoietic cell transplant patients. Biol Blood Marrow Transplant 2011;17(2):259–64.
103. Gilquin J, Weiss L, Kazatchkine MD. Genital and oral erosions induced by foscarnet. Lancet 1990;335(8684):287.
104. Martinez V, Molina JM, Scieux C, et al. Topical imiquimod for recurrent acyclovir-resistant HSV infection. Am J Med 2006;119(5):e9–11.
105. Sims CR, Thompson K, Chemaly RF, et al. Oral topical cidofovir: novel route of drug delivery in a severely immunosuppressed patient with refractory multidrug-resistant herpes simplex virus infection. Transpl Infect Dis 2007;9(3):256–9.
106. Available at: https://clinicaltrials.gov/ct2/show/NCT03073967. Accessed February 20, 2019.
107. El-Haddad D, El Chaer F, Vanichanan J, et al. Brincidofovir (CMX-001) for refractory and resistant CMV and HSV infections in immunocompromised cancer patients: A single-center experience. Antiviral Res 2016;134:58–62.
108. Liesegang TJ. Varicella zoster viral disease. Mayo Clin Proc 1999;74(10): 983–98.

109. Kawashima M, Nemoto O, Honda M, et al. Amenamevir, a novel helicase-primase inhibitor, for treatment of herpes zoster: a randomized, double-blind, valaciclovir-controlled phase 3 study. J Dermatol 2017;44(11):1219–27.

110. Pandit A, Leblebjian H, Hammond SP, et al. Safety of live-attenuated measles-mumps-rubella and herpes zoster vaccination in multiple myeloma patients on maintenance lenalidomide or bortezomib after autologous hematopoietic cell transplantation. Bone Marrow Transplant 2018;53(7):942–5.

111. Winston DJ, Mullane KM, Cornely OA, et al. Inactivated varicella zoster vaccine in autologous haemopoietic stem-cell transplant recipients: an international, multicentre, randomised, double-blind, placebo-controlled trial. Lancet 2018; 391(10135):2116–27.

112. Solomon T, Michael BD, Smith PE, et al. Management of suspected viral encephalitis in adults–Association of British Neurologists and British Infection Association National Guidelines. J Infect 2012;64(4):347–73.

113. Patriarca F, Medeot M, Isola M, et al. Prognostic factors and outcome of Epstein-Barr virus DNAemia in high-risk recipients of allogeneic stem cell transplantation treated with preemptive rituximab. Transpl Infect Dis 2013;15(3):259–67.

114. Rees L, Tizard EJ, Morgan AJ, et al. A phase I trial of Epstein-Barr virus gp350 vaccine for children with chronic kidney disease awaiting transplantation. Transplantation 2009;88(8):1025–9.

115. Elliott SL, Suhrbier A, Miles JJ, et al. Phase I trial of a CD8+ T-cell peptide epitope-based vaccine for infectious mononucleosis. J Virol 2008;82(3): 1448–57.

116. Schneider JW, Dittmer DP. Diagnosis and treatment of Kaposi sarcoma. Am J Clin Dermatol 2017;18(4):529–39.

Cytomegalovirus Infections of the Stem Cell Transplant Recipient and Hematologic Malignancy Patient

Anupam Pande, MD, MPH*, Erik R. Dubberke, MD, MSPH

KEYWORDS

- Cytomegalovirus • Stem cell transplant • Antiviral agents • Resistance

KEY POINTS

- CMV is a frequent cause of morbidity and mortality in stem cell transplant recipients and patients with hematologic malignancies.
- This article focuses on the risk factors for CMV infection, clinical manifestations of infection and disease, and its management.
- Resistant CMV is an emerging problem, and treatment options for common scenarios are discussed.

INTRODUCTION

Cytomegalovirus (CMV) infection is a frequent complication in immunocompromised patients with impaired cellular immunity, including recipients of hematopoietic stem cell transplant (HSCT) and those with hematologic malignancies. CMV disease has historically been a frequent cause of death after allogeneic HSCT.[1]

PATHOPHYSIOLOGY OF CYTOMEGALOVIRUS INFECTION

CMV is an icosahedral double-stranded DNA β herpesvirus. Its genome contains approximately 230 kilobase pairs organized into unique long (UL) and unique short segments that are flanked by inverted genomic repeats. Like all herpesviruses, CMV establishes latency after primary infection. Replication-competent virus remains present in infected cells; however, evidence of viral replication is undetectable until it is

Disclosure Statement: E.R. Dubberke has research support from Pfizer, Merck & Company, Rebiotix, Sanofi and serves as consultant for Pfizer, Merck and Company, Rebiotix, Sanofi, Synthetic Biologics, Valneva, and Aerobiotix.
Division of Infectious Disease, Department of Internal Medicine, Washington University School of Medicine, 4523 Clayton Avenue, Box #8051, Saint Louis, MO 63110-1093, USA
* Corresponding author.
E-mail address: apande@wustl.edu

Infect Dis Clin N Am 33 (2019) 485–500
https://doi.org/10.1016/j.idc.2019.02.008
0891-5520/19/© 2019 Elsevier Inc. All rights reserved.

id.theclinics.com

triggered to reactivate. Sites of latency include bone marrow stem cells of the myeloid lineage, such as $CD34^+$ and its progeny,[2] and peripheral blood mononuclear cells.[3] CMV infection is associated with a marked adaptive immunity response, which is necessary to control viral replication. $CD8^+$ and $CD4^+$ T cells respond to a large number of lytic and latency-associated antigens.[4] Innate immunity exerts a direct antiviral effect and induces adaptive immunity through the production of interferon-α, interferon-β, interleukin-12 (IL-12), and tumor necrosis factor.[5] Natural killer cells have been noted to expand during infection, but their role is less clear.[6]

CMV uses virion-associated and immediate-early proteins to effectively prevent host cell apoptosis and interferon-mediated pathways, and shuts off host cell protein synthesis in response to viral nucleic acid accumulation to evade host immune response.[7] Several CMV proteins also contribute to a blunting of cytotoxic T lymphocyte response by inhibiting major histocompatibility complex class 1–restricted antigen presentation.[8]

EPIDEMIOLOGY AND RISK FACTORS
Definitions

An important distinction in CMV diagnosis is that between CMV infection and CMV invasive disease.

- CMV infection is defined as isolation of CMV by culture or detection of viral protein or nucleic acid in the blood, body fluid, or tissue specimen in a patient without signs or symptoms of end-organ damage.[9] In an immunocompromised patient, infection is almost always from reactivation of latent CMV; although primary infection or reinfection can also occur.
- CMV invasive disease is defined as end-organ damage diagnosed by any of several tests including tissue viral culture, CMV-specific immunohistochemical staining, histopathology examination, or in situ hybridization accompanied by documented signs and symptoms associated with the end-organs involved.[9]
- Early CMV disease occurs typically within first 100 days of HSCT, and late CMV disease occurs after this period.

Risk Factors in Autologous Hematopoietic Stem Cell Transplant Recipients and Other Non-transplant Hematologic Malignancy Settings

Risk factors for CMV disease after autologous HSCT include $CD34^+$ selection, high-dose corticosteroids, and total body irradiation, or fludarabine as a part of the conditioning regimen.[10] Among those with hematologic malignancies, use of alemtuzumab and bortezomib has also been implicated.[11] Although CMV disease is rare in these populations, certain high-risk patients may merit routine surveillance and preemptive therapy. The National Comprehensive Cancer Network (NCCN) recommends weekly surveillance for at least 2 months after receipt of alemtuzumab.[12]

Risk Factors in Allogeneic Hematopoietic Stem Cell Transplant Recipients

CMV seropositivity in HSCT recipients is not only the main risk factor for CMV reactivation but also a surrogate marker for significant mortality after allogeneic HSCT (Fig. 1A).[13,14] The serologic status of the donor and the recipient is routinely assessed before allogeneic HSCT. With the use of irradiated or leukodepleted blood products, CMV D^-/R^- transplants carry a very low risk of CMV disease.[15] Primary infection may still occur if there is contact with another individual with active CMV infection. Among CMV D^+/R^- transplants, 20% to 30% will develop primary CMV infection without prophylaxis, most commonly caused by transmission of latent CMV via stem cell

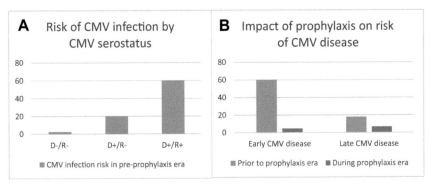

Fig. 1. Incidence rates of CMV infection in allogeneic HSCT recipients (*A*) depend on CMV serostatus of donor (D) and recipient (R). Rates reported are approximate and based on incidence ranges after routine use of CMV-seronegative or leukocyte-reduced blood products. The rates for autologous transplant are expected to be similar to the D⁻/R⁻ group. Incidence rates of CMV disease in allogeneic HSCT recipients across all donor and recipient serostatuses (*B*) decreased after introduction of antiviral prophylaxis, especially in the early post-transplant period. HSCT, hematopoietic stem cell transplant.

allograft.[13] In CMV-positive recipients, 60% to 70% will develop CMV infection after transplantation in the absence of prophylaxis.[14]

Other risk factors influencing development of CMV infection after allogeneic HSCT include older age, the use of steroids >1 mg/kg of body weight/d, ex vivo or in vivo T cell depletion, acute and chronic graft-versus-host disease (GVHD), use of total body irradiation, chemotherapy with fludarabine, alemtuzumab, or antithymocyte globulin, CD4⁺ lymphopenia, and use of mismatched (including haploidentical) or un-related donors.[16–21] Recipients of umbilical cord transplantation have similar risks of CMV infection, responses to antiviral therapy, and survival following CMV infection as recipients of either marrow or peripheral blood stem cells.[22]

Late CMV infection has similar risk factors, in addition to prolonged or repeated early CMV infection or disease and use of antivirals for CMV in the early post-transplant period.[23–25] The NCCN recommends weekly surveillance for 1 to 6 months after allogeneic HSCT and during treatment of GVHD.[12]

Incidence, Prevalence, and Time of Diagnosis

Specific CMV end-organ diseases have been reported with varying frequencies over time as CMV prophylaxis has evolved. Among those with hematologic malignancies, CMV disease was thought to be uncommon, but more recently contained frequencies of up to 12% have been reported when monitoring criteria were based on a clinically driven strategy in certain patients with lymphoma and myeloma.[11] After autologous HSCT, it was originally reported that approximately 40% of seropositive patients will develop detectable CMV infection.[14] However, clinically significant CMV disease is now rare after autologous HSCT, so much so that it was recommended to forgo CMV surveillance in seropositive patients.[26] As mentioned previously, after allogeneic HSCT, depending on donor and recipient serostatus, CMV was as common as 60% to 70%, but with introduction of prophylaxis and pre-emptive therapy strategies, prevalence of early CMV disease is 3% to 6% (**Fig. 1B**).[27] Similarly, incidence of late CMV disease used to be as high as 18% but is now reported to be 5% to 8%.[25,28] The incidence of CMV pneumonia in the early years of HSCT was around 10% to 35% after allogeneic HSCT and 1% to 6% after autologous HSCT.[29] CMV pneumonia used to be the most common manifestation of CMV disease, but is now superseded by CMV gastrointestinal (GI) disease.[30] The incidence of CMV central nervous system (CNS) disease is unknown because of its rarity, and the prevalence of CMV retinitis is estimated to be 1.4% after HSCT.[31]

CMV disease, especially pneumonia, used to be frequent in the early post-transplant period, but now most disease occurs in the late post-transplant period between 3 months and 1 year.[29,31,32] CMV GI disease can occur up to 2 years post transplant.[32] Late CMV disease has become more common than early CMV disease after the introduction of prophylaxis and pre-emptive therapy in the early post-HSCT period. Because CMV GI disease tends to occur later, this likely explains why it accounts for an increasing proportion of CMV disease.[25,28]

Outcomes

Although improved over time, CMV infection and disease is unequivocally associated with decreased overall survival and increased transplant-related mortality.[1,33] CMV pneumonia carries a very high mortality of 30% to 50%, even in the antiviral era.[34,35] CMV infection is also associated with bacterial and fungal infections.[32,34,36] Some studies have reported decreased relapse-related or non–relapse-related mortality in CMV-positive recipients if the donor is also CMV positive compared with those with CMV-negative donors.[14] However, this relative protective effect may be limited to low-risk transplant settings (reduced-intensity conditioning may result in lower incidence of CMV disease as opposed to those who received myeloablative conditioning, resulting in loss of recipient CMV-specific T cell function in D^-/R^+ allogeneic HSCT).[37]

DIAGNOSIS

Because of difficulty in making a diagnosis of CMV disease and inability to always obtain tissue to make a definitive diagnosis, categories of certainty have been developed for use in clinical trials, classifying disease as possible, probable, or proven (**Table 1**).[9]

Diagnostic Tests for Cytomegalovirus Infection

Tests for diagnosing CMV have evolved over time and continue to do so (**Fig. 2**). Viral culture is rarely performed today because this involves growing CMV in human fibroblastoid cell lines, a process that is slow, not reproducible, and not sensitive, making it an impractical test. The shell vial culture matter is a rapid culture method, involving identification of virus using monoclonal antibodies to the immediate-early antigen within 24 hours. Although sensitive and specific, this method is highly operator dependent.

The CMV antigenemia assay detects the CMV phosphoprotein 65 (pp65) in neutrophils, which correlates semiquantitatively with viral replication.[38] Today this test is infrequently used despite being inexpensive and rapid because it relies on the presence of an adequate neutrophil count. This test has for the most part been replaced by detection of CMV DNA using polymerase chain reaction (PCR) with quantification. Quantitative DNA detection techniques are highly sensitive and useful for prognostication.[39] The limitations of these tests include lack of standardization of the assay and variability depending on specimen type (plasma versus whole blood). Most centers now use an assay standardized to the lyophilized Merlin virus preparation with an assigned potency of 5×10^6 IU as recommended by the first World Health Organization (WHO) international standard for human CMV for nucleic acid amplification

Table 1
Criteria for categories of certainty of CMV disease

End-Organ Disease	Proven	Probable	Possible
Pneumonia	Clinical and radiographic criteria and CMV in lung tissue documented by virus isolation, rapid culture, histopathology, immunohistochemistry, or DNA hybridization	Clinical and radiographic criteria and detection of CMV by viral isolation, rapid culture of BAL fluid, or the quantitation of CMV DNA in BAL fluid	Clinical and radiographic criteria without meeting criteria for proven or probable disease
Gastrointestinal disease	Clinical symptoms and macroscopic mucosal lesions and CMV in upper or lower GI tissue documented by virus isolation, rapid culture, histopathology, immunohistochemistry, or DNA hybridization	Clinical symptoms and CMV in upper or lower GI tissue documented by virus isolation, rapid culture, histopathology, immunohistochemistry, or DNA hybridization	Clinical criteria without meeting criteria for proven or probable disease
Encephalitis/ventriculitis	Central nervous system symptoms plus detection of CMV in CNS tissue by virus isolation, rapid culture, immunohistochemical analysis, in situ hybridization, or (preferably) quantitative PCR	CNS symptoms plus detection of CMV in CSF without visible contamination of blood ("bloody tap") plus abnormal imaging results or evidence of encephalitis on electroencephalography	Not a recommended category
Retinitis	Typical ophthalmologic signs judged by an ophthalmologist experienced with the diagnosis of CMV retinitis	Not a recommended category	Not a recommended category
Other (eg, hepatitis, nephritis, myocarditis, cystitis)	Compatible clinical syndrome and CMV documented in tissue by histopathology, immunohistochemistry, virus isolation, rapid culture, or DNA hybridization	Not a recommended category	Not a recommended category

From Ljungman P, Boeckh M, Hirsch HH, et al. Definitions of cytomegalovirus infection and disease in transplant patients for use in clinical trials. Clin Infect Dis 2017;64(1):87–91; with permission.

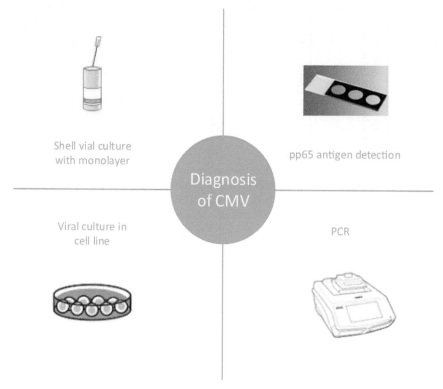

Fig. 2. The evolution of tests for diagnosis of CMV infection over time, starting bottom left and moving clockwise.

techniques.[40] Although this standard improved test commutability, significant interlaboratory and interassay variability still exists because of sequence variability, amplicon length, and nonencapsidated CMV genome fragments.[41]

Diagnosis of Cytomegalovirus Invasive Disease

Cytomegalovirus pneumonitis

Patients with CMV pneumonitis usually have pulmonary dysfunction manifesting with nonproductive cough, hypoxemia, tachypnea, fever, and characteristic bilateral, diffuse interstitial infiltrates on chest radiography (**Fig. 3**A).[23] Computed tomography (**Fig. 3**B) is more sensitive than plain radiography for diagnosing early disease.[42] Involvement can often be asymmetric, or sometimes in the form of focal airspace opacities, centrilobular nodules, and rarely in the form of nodules or focal consolidations.[23,43] However, clinical or radiologic findings are not specific enough to make a definitive diagnosis without identification of CMV in the blood and bronchoalveolar lavage (BAL) fluid or in lung biopsy specimens.[9] In addition, other competing diagnoses, especially those that often coexist with CMV pneumonitis and have similar presentations (*Pneumocystis jirovecii* pneumonia and lower respiratory tract infections with community respiratory viruses), must be excluded.[44] In general, CMV viremia by antigenemia assay or PCR is reliably present in cases of CMV pneumonia in HSCT recipients unlike other forms of CMV disease (especially GI disease).[30] The current gold standard for diagnosis of CMV is demonstrating

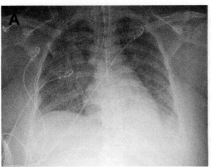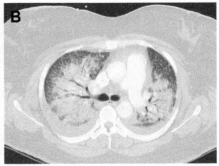

Fig. 3. Diffuse, bilateral, interstitial infiltrates on chest plain radiography (A) and computed tomography (B) of a patient with CMV pneumonitis; a common but nonspecific finding.

CMV intranuclear inclusions (owl's eye appearance) or detecting CMV using immunohistochemical staining or in situ hybridization in lung biopsy specimens.[20] However, lung biopsies are not always feasible in these patients because of rapidly progressive respiratory failure, thrombocytopenia, and other overall safety concerns. Hence, BAL fluid is frequently used to make a probable diagnosis.[9] Viral culture of BAL fluid is rarely performed for the reasons mentioned previously. Cytopathology to identify CMV inclusion bodies is specific but not sensitive enough, and sensitivity can be improved by using immunohistochemical staining.[45] Qualitative CMV PCR from BAL fluid has been shown to have a good negative predictive value but poor positive predictive value for the diagnosis of CMV pneumonia, as viral shedding is common even in the absence of end-organ disease; hence this test is not used as a criterion by current guidelines.[9,46] Quantitative PCR in the BAL fluid is a promising test, although a cutoff threshold to define CMV pneumonia is absent.

Gastrointestinal Cytomegalovirus disease

Patients with hematologic malignancies and HSCT recipients present with erosive or ulcerative lesions that can occur in any part of the GI tract from mouth to rectum; however, upper tract involvement is more common than in other populations.[47] Symptoms can be subtle and depend on infected site; with odynophagia, abdominal pain, bloody or watery diarrhea, and tenesmus being frequent. Allogeneic HSCT recipients often have concomitant GVHD, and distinction between these 2 entities often requires biopsy of the involved mucosal tissue. Because the histologic findings of GI CMV disease and GVHD are also similar, diagnosis heavily relies on identification of viral inclusions or immunohistochemical staining for CMV.[48] CMV viremia is infrequently detected in patients with GI CMV disease.[49] Often, patients have histologic evidence of CMV without macroscopic lesions on endoscopy; this is qualified as probable CMV disease.[9]

Cytomegalovirus central nervous system disease

Patients with hematologic malignancies and HSCT recipients rarely develop CNS CMV disease; however, when it occurs it manifests as ventriculitis and encephalitis with prominent cognitive dysfunction, confusion, mutism, cranial nerve palsies, and nystagmus.[50] Cerebral spinal fluid (CSF) shows lymphocyte-predominant pleocytosis.[50,51] Fluid-attenuated inversion recovery MRI of the brain demonstrates abnormal periventricular hyperintensity.[51] A positive CMV PCR in CSF makes the diagnosis highly probable.[52]

Cytomegalovirus retinitis

Presentation of CMV retinitis in patients with hematologic malignancies and in HSCT recipients is similar to that in patients with HIV, although it is much less frequent.[31] Diagnosis relies on clinical symptoms consistent with retinitis (blurring or loss of central vision, floaters, photopsia, and scotomata) and fundoscopic examination by an experienced ophthalmologist (perivascular exudates, white macular exudates, hemorrhages, and retinal detachment in later stages).[53] Symptoms may be minimal and the presentation can be indolent.[54] Retinitis is the only form of CMV disease that can be diagnosed without testing for CMV in a tissue sample; however, ocular fluid qualitative CMV PCR is useful if presentation is atypical or an experienced ophthalmologist is not available.[9] As with GI CMV disease, CMV viremia is uncommon with CMV retinitis.

Other manifestations of Cytomegalovirus end-organ disease

Rare manifestations of CMV disease in HSCT recipients include hepatitis, nephritis, cystitis, myocarditis, pancreatitis, bone marrow failure, and CMV syndrome. CMV syndrome is an acute mononucleosis-like illness seen with primary infection, usually not seen in patients with hematologic malignancies and HSCT recipients because of abnormal immune response to primary CMV infection.[9] Other diagnoses usually require histopathologic testing.

MANAGEMENT

Mechanisms of Antiviral Agents

The antiviral agents primarily used for the treatment of CMV infection and disease are ganciclovir and its oral prodrug valganciclovir, foscarnet, and cidofovir. Although all of these agents directly or indirectly inhibit the viral DNA polymerase UL54 (which incorporates 2-deoxyguanosine triphosphate into CMV DNA), only ganciclovir and its prodrug valganciclovir require activation by the phosphokinase UL97 (**Fig. 4**). Newer agents maribavir (oral UL97 inhibitor) and brincidofovir (oral, non-nephrotoxic lipid-conjugated nucleotide analog of cidofovir) showed initial promise but neither agent is likely to be used as monotherapy for CMV treatment.[55] Letermovir is an inhibitor of the viral terminase enzyme complex UL56, but is yet to be studied fully for treatment.

Antiviral Regimens

CMV infection and disease are usually treated with ganciclovir unless complicated by resistance, intolerance, or toxicity.[56] Induction dosing usually entails treatment with intravenous ganciclovir at 5 mg/kg every 12 hours adjusted for renal function for at least 3 to 4 weeks, but duration is frequently determined by resolution of viremia. This regimen is frequently followed by several weeks of maintenance dosing at 5 mg/kg daily adjusted for renal function, especially for GI disease and when immunosuppression cannot be effectively reduced or reversed. Valganciclovir, although not studied in management of CMV disease after HSCT, may be used in the treatment of non–life-threatening CMV infection and disease after resolution of initial high-level viremia if there are no concerns about oral absorption of the medication (eg, GI GVHD), based on a study performed in solid organ transplant recipients.[57] Valganciclovir is usually not recommended for induction in severe CMV disease because of the lack of evidence of efficacy. If foscarnet (90 mg/kg every 12 hours) or cidofovir (5 mg/kg once weekly) is used, principles of induction and maintenance dosing are similar to that with ganciclovir.

CMV retinitis is also treated in a similar fashion. Systemic therapy is usually successful for CMV retinitis; however, systemic toxicity may necessitate intraocular

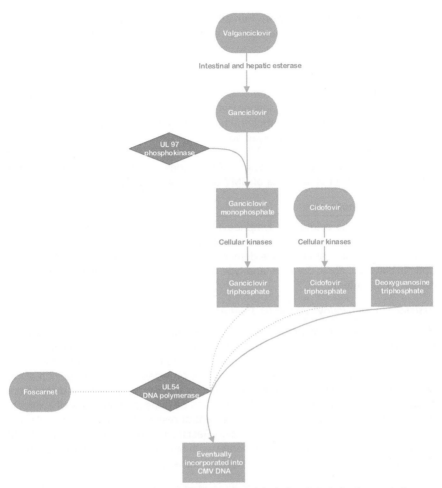

Fig. 4. Mechanisms of action of commonly used antivirals for CMV infection and disease.

ganciclovir or foscarnet.[31] Intraocular ganciclovir implants are not available in the United States.

For CMV CNS disease, there are no standard treatment recommendations because of its rarity; however, owing to significant mortality, variability of drug penetration despite inflammation of meninges, and the possibility of viral compartmentalization (unidentified resistance mutation) in the CSF, experts suggest dual therapy with ganciclovir and foscarnet, especially in treatment-experienced patients.[58]

Given the lack of a universally standardized assay for detection of viremia, there is no consensus on a threshold for treating viremia without end-organ disease. This aspect is discussed in further detail in the section on prevention of viral infections.

Toxicities

Ganciclovir and valganciclovir are associated with cytopenias, especially neutropenia in HSCT recipients, which often requires administration of growth factor.[27] These agents can also cause diarrhea and fever. Foscarnet and cidofovir are nephrotoxic; the former is known to cause electrolyte wasting. Foscarnet has also been associated with urethral or genital ulceration. Paresthesia and hallucinations are less common. Cidofovir may also cause neutropenia and diarrhea, and uveitis has also been observed.

Intravenous Immunoglobulin

Although the recommendation remains controversial, pooled intravenous immuno-globulin (IVIG) is used in the management of CMV pneumonia based on a few small studies that used historical controls demonstrating a survival benefit.[59,60] However, a recent retrospective review showed no added benefit.[33] CMV-specific immune glob-ulin can be used in place of pooled IVIG, but offers no added benefit in euvolemic pa-tients at a substantially higher cost.[61] There does not seem to be any definitive advantage of IVIG in other forms of CMV disease such as GI disease.[62]

Adoptive Immunotherapy

CMV pp65-specific cytotoxic T lymphocytes and $CD8^+$ T cells may be cultured from normal healthy donors and have been shown to be safe, with low risk of development of GVHD.[63–65] Some studies have demonstrated some benefit from this therapy, but optimal cell type, dose, duration, and type of patient who will benefit from this therapy remain to be determined.[66]

Resistant Cytomegalovirus and Its Treatment

Resistance is usually uncommon, except in the setting of accumulated drug exposure with intermittent antiviral use, recurrent viral reactivation, increasing host immune sup-pression, and/or reduced drug delivery. As pre-emptive therapy and prophylaxis be-comes the norm, blood and marrow transplant providers have become increasingly comfortable with administering first-line therapy for viremia. Infectious disease spe-cialists are more likely than in previous years to be consulted on cases of suspected resistance; hence, knowledge of management of resistant CMV is of particular rele-vance to the infectious disease specialist. Resistance should be suspected if CMV viral load increases after 2 weeks of therapy with or without worsening clinical disease (**Fig. 5**). It should be noted that in treatment-naive patients, no decrease or even a

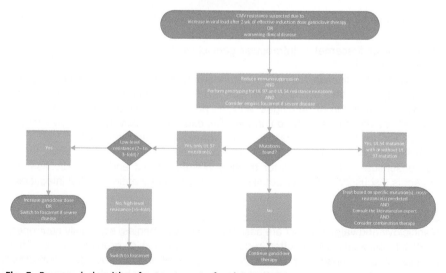

Fig. 5. Proposed algorithm for treatment of resistant CMV.

moderate increase in the viral load may occur in the first 2 weeks of therapy because of underlying immunosuppression.[38] When resistance after this initial period is suspected, immune suppression should be reduced if feasible and genotyping for UL97 and UL54 resistance mutations should be performed. An empiric change to foscarnet may be considered while awaiting genotype resistance testing if CMV disease is severe, progressive, and symptomatic. If no mutations are found, induction-dose ganciclovir should be continued. Ganciclovir resistance is usually due to mutations in the UL97 gene. Low-level (2- to 3-fold) UL97 resistance can be treated with a higher dose of ganciclovir therapy (up to double the conventional induction dose).[67] High-level (>5-fold) UL97 resistance requires foscarnet as long as it is not accompanied by a mutation in the UL54 gene.[68] Mutations in the UL54 gene confer resistance to ganciclovir, foscarnet, cidofovir, or combinations of these. Cross-resistance between foscarnet and ganciclovir rarely occurs, although most UL54 mutations that confer ganciclovir resistance also result in cidofovir resistance, which can be explained by their shared binding site (see **Fig. 4**).[68] Therapy for UL54 mutations should be guided by the nature of specific mutations present and by consulting an expert or referencing the literature on the subject. Often, sources recommend combination therapy and addition of leflunomide and/or one of the newer agents already mentioned.[27,69]

PREVENTION

CMV can be prevented by careful donor selection, use of CMV-seronegative blood products, and chemoprophylaxis with antiviral agents: currently, most commonly with valganciclovir. In sentinel studies from the 1980s and 1990s, prophylaxis with intravenous acyclovir significantly reduced the risk of both CMV infection (from 87% to 70%) and CMV disease (38% to 20%) in seropositive patients after allogeneic bone marrow transplantation, and was also associated with significantly improved survival.[70,71] Ganciclovir prophylaxis was shown to reduce risk of CMV infection and disease, but at the cost of significant neutropenia.[72,73] Later it was proved that CMV disease could also be prevented by administering pre-emptive antiviral therapy with ganciclovir after early detection of CMV viremia, particularly in the early post-transplant period.[74] Since then, valganciclovir has been increasingly used for prophylaxis, although data for valganciclovir are limited to its comparison with historical controls and to pre-emptive therapy, the latter becoming more popular over time at most transplant centers because of its similar efficacy at preventing disease and decreased risk of neutropenia.[75] Letermovir has been recently approved for prophylaxis for certain populations.[76] Nuances of prophylaxis and pre-emptive therapy are discussed in detail in a separate article. "Antimicrobial prophylaxis and preemptive approaches for the prevention of infections in the stem cell transplant recipient, with analogies to the hematologic malignancy patient" by Dionysios Neofytos, in this issue.

SUMMARY

Despite decreasing frequency of CMV infection and disease caused by prophylaxis and pre-emptive therapy, CMV continues to present a significant clinical challenge, causing a high burden of morbidity and mortality. Evolving diagnostic techniques and research advances have led to formulation of more refined criteria for the diagnosis of CMV disease. Diagnosis and treatment often require a multidisciplinary approach and consultation with transplant infectious disease specialists. Despite newer drugs being studied, ganciclovir still remains the drug of choice in treatment-naive patients. Epidemiology of CMV infection is continuing to change and will present new challenges in the future.

REFERENCES

1. Mori T, Kato J. Cytomegalovirus infection/disease after hematopoietic stem cell transplantation. Int J Hematol 2010;91(4):588–95.
2. Khaiboullina SF, Maciejewski JP, Crapnell K, et al. Human cytomegalovirus persists in myeloid progenitors and is passed to the myeloid progeny in a latent form. Br J Haematol 2004;126(3):410–7.
3. Larsson S, Söderberg-Nauclér C, Wang F, et al. Cytomegalovirus DNA can be detected in peripheral blood mononuclear cells from all seropositive and most seronegative healthy blood donors over time. Transfusion 1998;38:271–8.
4. Sylwester AW, Mitchell BL, Edgar JB, et al. Broadly targeted human cytomegalovirus-specific CD4+ and CD8+ T cells dominate the memory compartments of exposed subjects. J Exp Med 2005;202(5):673–85.
5. Smith C, Khanna R. Immune regulation of human herpesviruses and its implications for human transplantation. Am J Transplant 2013;13(s3):9–23.
6. Gumà M, Angulo A, Vilches C, et al. Imprint of human cytomegalovirus infection on the NK cell receptor repertoire. Blood 2004;104(12):3664–72.
7. Brinkmann MM, Dağ F, Hengel H, et al. Cytomegalovirus immune evasion of myeloid lineage cells. Med Microbiol Immunol 2015;204(3):367–82.
8. Basta S, Bennink JR. A survival game of hide and seek: cytomegaloviruses and MHC class I antigen presentation pathways. Viral Immunol 2003;16(3):231–42.
9. Ljungman P, Boeckh M, Hirsch HH, et al. Definitions of cytomegalovirus infection and disease in transplant patients for use in clinical trials. Clin Infect Dis 2017; 64(1):87–91.
10. Holmberg LA, Boeckh M, Hooper H, et al. Increased incidence of cytomegalovirus disease after autologous CD34-selected peripheral blood stem cell transplantation. Blood 1999;94(12):4029–36.
11. Marchesi F, Pimpinelli F, Ensoli F, et al. Cytomegalovirus infection in hematologic malignancy settings other than the allogeneic transplant. Hematol Oncol 2018; 36(2):381–91.
12. Baden LR, Swaminathan S, Angarone M, et al. Prevention and treatment of cancer-related infections, version 2.2016. J Natl Compr Canc Netw 2016;14(7): 882–913.
13. Ljungman P. The role of cytomegalovirus serostatus on outcome of hematopoietic stem cell transplantation. Curr Opin Hematol 2014;21(6):466–9.
14. Boeckh M, Nichols WG. The impact of cytomegalovirus serostatus of donor and recipient before hematopoietic stem cell transplantation in the era of antiviral prophylaxis and preemptive therapy. Blood 2004;103(6):2003–8.
15. Bowden RA, Slichter SJ, Sayers M, et al. A comparison of filtered leukocyte-reduced and cytomegalovirus (CMV) seronegative blood products for the prevention of transfusion-associated CMV infection after marrow transplant. Blood 1995;86(9):3598–604.
16. Ljungman P, Perez-Bercoff L, Jonsson J, et al. Risk factors for the development of cytomegalovirus disease after allogeneic stem cell transplantation. Haematologica 2006;91(1):78–83.
17. Cohen L, Yeshurun M, Shpilberg O, et al. Risk factors and prognostic scale for cytomegalovirus (CMV) infection in CMV-seropositive patients after allogeneic hematopoietic cell transplantation. Transpl Infect Dis 2015;17(4):510–7.
18. Styczynski J. Who is the patient at risk of CMV recurrence: a review of the current scientific evidence with a focus on hematopoietic cell transplantation. Infect Dis Ther 2018;7(1):1–16.

19. Dziedzic M, Sadowska-Krawczenko I, Styczynski J. Risk factors for cytomegalovirus infection after allogeneic hematopoietic cell transplantation in malignancies: proposal for classification. Anticancer Res 2017;37(12):6551–6.

20. Ariza-Heredia EJ, Nesher L, Chemaly RF. Cytomegalovirus diseases after hematopoietic stem cell transplantation: a mini-review. Cancer Lett 2014; 342(1):1–8.

21. Crocchiolo R, Bramanti S, Vai A, et al. Infections after T-replete haploidentical transplantation and high-dose cyclophosphamide as graft-versus-host disease prophylaxis. Transpl Infect Dis 2015;17(2):242–9.

22. Walker CM, van Burik JH, De For TE, et al. Cytomegalovirus infection after allogeneic transplantation: comparison of cord blood with peripheral blood and marrow graft sources. Biol Blood Marrow Transplant 2007;13(9):1106–15.

23. Travi G, Pergam SA. Cytomegalovirus pneumonia in hematopoietic stem cell recipients. J Intensive Care Med 2014;29(4):200–12.

24. Özdemir E, Saliba RM, Champlin RE, et al. Risk factors associated with late cytomegalovirus reactivation after allogeneic stem cell transplantation for hematological malignancies. Bone Marrow Transplant 2007;40(2):125–36.

25. Boeckh M, Leisenring W, Riddell SR, et al. Late cytomegalovirus disease and mortality in recipients of allogeneic hematopoietic stem cell transplants: importance of viral load and T-cell immunity. Blood 2003;101(2):407–14.

26. Bilgrami S, Aslanzadeh J, Feingold JM, et al. Cytomegalovirus viremia, viruria and disease after autologous peripheral blood stem cell transplantation: no need for surveillance. Bone Marrow Transplant 1999;24(1):69–73.

27. El Chaer F, Shah DP, Chemaly RF. How I treat resistant cytomegalovirus infection in hematopoietic cell transplantation recipients. Blood 2016;128(23):2624–37.

28. Asano-Mori Y, Kanda Y, Oshima K, et al. Clinical features of late cytomegalovirus infection after hematopoietic stem cell transplantation. Int J Hematol 2008;87(3): 310–8.

29. Kotloff RM, Ahya VN, Crawford SW. Pulmonary complications of solid organ and hematopoietic stem cell transplantation. Am J Respir Crit Care Med 2004;170(1): 22–48.

30. Green ML, Leisenring W, Stachel D, et al. Efficacy of a viral load-based, risk-adapted, preemptive treatment strategy for prevention of cytomegalovirus disease after hematopoietic cell transplantation. Biol Blood Marrow Transplant 2007;18(11):1687–99.

31. Crippa F, Corey L, Chuang EL, et al. Virological, clinical, and ophthalmologic features of cytomegalovirus retinitis after hematopoietic stem cell transplantation. Clin Infect Dis 2001;32(2):214–9.

32. van Burik JH, Lawatsch EJ, Defor TE, et al. Cytomegalovirus enteritis among hematopoietic stem cell transplant recipients. Biol Blood Marrow Transplant 2001; 679:674–9.

33. Erard V, Guthrie KA, Seo S, et al. Reduced mortality of cytomegalovirus pneumonia after hematopoietic cell transplantation due to antiviral therapy and changes in transplantation practices. Clin Infect Dis 2015;61(1):31–9.

34. van Burik JH, Carter SL, Freifeld AG, et al. Higher risk of cytomegalovirus and aspergillus infections in recipients of T cell-depleted unrelated bone marrow: analysis of infectious complications in patients treated with T cell depletion versus immunosuppressive therapy to prevent graft-versus-host disease. Biol Blood Marrow Transplant 2007;13(12):1487–98.

35. Boeckh M, Nichols WG, Papanicolaou G, et al. Cytomegalovirus in hematopoietic stem cell transplant recipients: current status, known challenges, and future strategies. Biol Blood Marrow Transplant 2003;9(9):543–58.

36. Nichols WG, Corey L, Gooley T, et al. High risk of death due to bacterial and fungal infection among cytomegalovirus (CMV)-seronegative recipients of stem cell transplants from seropositive donors: evidence for indirect effects of primary CMV infection. J Infect Dis 2002;185(3):273–82.

37. Ljungman P, Brand R, Hoek J, et al. Donor cytomegalovirus status influences the outcome of allogeneic stem cell transplant: a study by the European Group for Blood and Marrow Transplantation. Clin Infect Dis 2014;59(4):473–81.

38. Nichols WG, Corey L, Gooley T, et al. Rising pp65 antigenemia during preemptive anticytomegalovirus therapy after allogeneic hematopoietic stem cell transplantation: risk factors, correlation with DNA load, and outcomes. Blood 2001;97(4): 867–75.

39. Boeckh M, Huang M, Ferrenberg J, et al. Optimization of quantitative detection of cytomegalovirus DNA in plasma by real-time PCR. J Clin Microbiol 2004;42(3): 1142–8.

40. Fryer JF, Heath AB, Minor PD, Collaborative Study Group. A collaborative study to establish the 1st WHO International Standard for human cytomegalovirus for nucleic acid amplification technology. Biologicals 2016;44(5):242–51.

41. Naegele K, Lautenschlager I, Gosert R, et al. Cytomegalovirus sequence variability, amplicon length, and DNase-sensitive non-encapsidated genomes are obstacles to standardization and commutability of plasma viral load results. J Clin Virol 2018;104:39–47.

42. Maschmeyer G. Pneumonia in febrile neutropenic patients: radiologic diagnosis. Curr Opin Oncol 2001;13(4):229–35.

43. Gasparetto EL, Ono SE, Escuissato D, et al. Cytomegalovirus pneumonia after bone marrow transplantation: high resolution CT findings. Br J Radiol 2004;77: 724–7.

44. Yu Q, Jia P, Su L, et al. Outcomes and prognostic factors of non-HIV patients with *Pneumocystis jirovecii* pneumonia and pulmonary CMV co-infection: a retrospective cohort study. BMC Infect Dis 2017;17(1):392.

45. Tamm M, Traenkel P, Grilli B, et al. Pulmonary cytomegalovirus infection in immunocompromised patients. Chest 2001;119(3):838–43.

46. Ruutu P, Ruutu T, Volin L, et al. Cytomegalovirus is frequently isolated in bronchoalveolar lavage fluid of bone marrow transplant recipients without pneumonia. Ann Intern Med 1990;112(12):913–6.

47. Torres HA, Kontoyiannis DP, Bodey GP, et al. Gastrointestinal cytomegalovirus disease in patients with cancer: a two decade experience in a tertiary care cancer center. Eur J Cancer 2005;41(15):2268–79.

48. Liu A, Meyer E, Johnston L, et al. Prevalence of graft versus host disease and cytomegalovirus infection in patients post-haematopoietic cell transplantation presenting with gastrointestinal symptoms. Aliment Pharmacol Ther 2013;38(8): 955–66.

49. Ruell J, Barnes C, Mutton K, et al. Active CMV disease does not always correlate with viral load detection. Bone Marrow Transplant 2007;40(1):55–61.

50. Reddy SM, Winston DJ, Territo MC, et al. CMV central nervous system disease in stem-cell transplant recipients: an increasing complication of drug-resistant CMV infection and protracted immunodeficiency. Bone Marrow Transplant 2010;45(6): 979–84.

51. Ando T, Mitani N, Yamashita K, et al. Cytomegalovirus ventriculoencephalitis in a reduced- intensity conditioning cord blood transplant recipient. Transpl Infect Dis 2010;12(5):441–5.
52. Wolf DG, Lurain NS, Zuckerman T, et al. Emergence of late cytomegalovirus central nervous system disease in hematopoietic stem cell transplant recipients. Blood 2003;101(2):463–5.
53. Xhaard A, Robin M, Scieux C, et al. Increased incidence of cytomegalovirus retinitis after allogeneic hematopoietic stem cell transplantation. Transplantation 2007;83(1):80–3.
54. Jeon S, Lee WK, Lee Y, et al. Risk factors for cytomegalovirus retinitis in patients with cytomegalovirus viremia after hematopoietic stem cell transplantation. Ophthalmology 2012;119(9):1892–8.
55. Frange P, Leruez-Ville M. Maribavir, brincidofovir and letermovir: efficacy and safety of new antiviral drugs for treating cytomegalovirus infections. Med Mal Infect 2018. https://doi.org/10.1016/j.medmal.2018.03.006.
56. Meesing A, Razonable RR. New developments in the management of cytomegalovirus infection after transplantation. Drugs 2018;78(11):1085–103.
57. Åsberg A, Humar A, Rollag H, et al. Oral valganciclovir is noninferior to intravenous ganciclovir for the treatment of cytomegalovirus disease in solid organ transplant recipients. Am J Transplant 2007;7(9):2106–13.
58. Baghban A, Malinis M. Ganciclovir and foscarnet dual-therapy for cytomegalovirus encephalitis: a case report and review of the literature. J Neurol Sci 2018; 15(388):28–36.
59. Reed EC, Bowden RA, Dandliker PS, et al. Treatment of cytomegalovirus pneumonia with Ganciclovir and intravenous cytomegalovirus immunoglobulin in patients with bone marrow transplants. Ann Intern Med 1988;109(10):783–8.
60. Emanuel D, Cunningham I, Jules-Elysee K, et al. Cytomegalovirus pneumonia after bone marrow transplantation successfully treated with the combination of Ganciclovir and high-dose intravenous immune globulin. Ann Intern Med 1988; 109(10):777–82.
61. Ljungman P, Engelhard D, Link H, et al. Treatment of interstitial pneumonitis due to cytomegalovirus with ganciclovir and intravenous immune globulin: experience of European Bone Marrow Transplant Group. Clin Infect Dis 1992;14(4):831–5.
62. Ljungman P, Cordonnier C, Einsele H, et al. Use of intravenous immune globulin in addition to antiviral therapy in the treatment of CMV gastrointestinal disease in allogeneic bone marrow transplant patients: a report from the European Group for Blood and Marrow Transplantation (EBMT). Infectious Diseases Working Party of the EBMT. Bone Marrow Transplant 1998;21(5):473–6.
63. Bao L, Sun Q, Lucas KG. Rapid generation of CMV pp65-specific T cells for immunotherapy. J Immunother 2007;30(5):557–61.
64. Bao L, Cowan M, Dunham K, et al. Lymphocytes for stem cell transplant patients with refractory CMV infections. J Immunother 2013;35(3):293–8.
65. Neuenhahn M, Albrecht J, Odendahl M, et al. Transfer of minimally manipulated CMV-specific T cells from stem cell or third-party donors to treat CMV infection after allo-HSCT. Leukemia 2017;31(10):2161–71.
66. Blyth E, Withers B, Clancy L, et al. CMV-specific immune reconstitution following allogeneic stem cell transplantation. Virulence 2016;7(8):967–80.
67. West P, Schmiedeskamp M, Neeley H, et al. Use of high-dose ganciclovir for a resistant cytomegalovirus infection due to UL97 mutation. Transpl Infect Dis 2008;10(2):129–32.

68. Lurain NS, Chou S. Antiviral drug resistance of human cytomegalovirus. Clin Microbiol Rev 2010;23(4):689–712.

69. Boeckh M, Ljungman P. How we treat cytomegalovirus in hematopoietic cell transplant recipients. Blood 2009;113(23):5711–20.

70. Meyers JD, Reed EC, Shepp DH, et al. Acyclovir for prevention of cytomegalovirus infection and disease after allogeneic marrow transplantation. N Engl J Med 1988;318(2):70–5.

71. Prentice HG, Gluckman E, Powles RL, et al. Long-term survival in allogeneic bone marrow transplant recipients following acyclovir prophylaxis for CMV infection. Bone Marrow Transplant 1997;19(2):129–33.

72. Winston DJ, Ho WG, Bartoni K, et al. Ganciclovir prophylaxis of cytomegalovirus infection and disease in allogeneic bone marrow transplant recipients: results of a placebo-controlled, double-blind trial. Ann Intern Med 1993;118(3):179–84.

73. Goodrich JM, Bowden RA, Fisher L, et al. Ganciclovir prophylaxis to prevent cytomegalovirus disease after allogeneic marrow transplant. Ann Intern Med 1993;118(3):173–8.

74. Boeckh BM, Gooley TA, Myerson D, et al. Cytomegalovirus pp65 antigenemia-guided early treatment with ganciclovir versus ganciclovir at engraftment after allogeneic marrow transplantation: a randomized double-blind study. Blood 1996;88(10):4063–71.

75. Boeckh M, Nichols W, Chemaly R, et al. Valganciclovir for the prevention of complications of late cytomegalovirus infection after allogeneic hematopoietic cell transplantation: a randomized controlled trial. Ann Intern Med 2015;162(1):1–10.

76. Marty F, Ljungman P, Chemaly R, et al. Letermovir prophylaxis for cytomegalovirus in hematopoietic-cell transplantation. N Engl J Med 2017;377(25):2433–44.

Infections with DNA Viruses, Adenovirus, Polyomaviruses, and Parvovirus B19 in Hematopoietic Stem Cell Transplant Recipients and Patients with Hematologic Malignancies

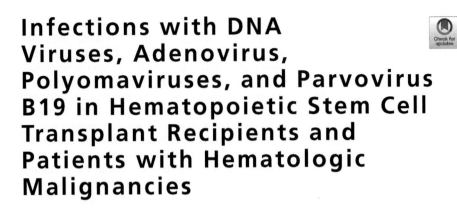

Karam M. Obeid, MD

KEYWORDS

- Adenovirus • BK virus • JC virus • Polyomavirus • Parvovirus B19
- Hematopoietic stem cell transplant • Hematologic malignancies • Therapy

KEY POINTS

- DNA viruses, other than the more common cytomegalovirus, play a role in the post-hematopoietic stem cell transplant (HCT) period resulting in major morbidity and mortality in these patients.
- These viruses include adenovirus, parvovirus B19, and polyomaviruses mainly BK and JC viruses.
- Hemorrhagic cystitis, gastroenteritis, pneumonitis, hepatitis, encephalitis, and disseminated disease are few of the clinical complications of these viruses.
- This review summarizes the diseases associated with these viruses in the post-HCT period, the approach to HCT recipients with these viral infections and therapeutic options available, and the impact of these viral infections on the morbidity and mortality of HCT recipients.

ADENOVIRUS

Overview

Adenovirus (ADV) is a large, nonenveloped, double-stranded DNA (dsDNA) virus that was first isolated in 1953 in human adenoid tissue-–derived cell cultures.[1] Subsequently, 7 species (A–G) and approximately 100 serotypes of ADV were identified; only half of these serotypes are infectious to humans.[2–4] Infections with different serotypes

Disclosure: No financial disclosure and no conflict of interest.
Division of Infectious Diseases and International Medicine, University of Minnesota, 420 Delaware Street SE, MMC250, Minneapolis, MN 55455, USA
E-mail address: kmobeid@umn.edu

Infect Dis Clin N Am 33 (2019) 501–521
https://doi.org/10.1016/j.idc.2019.02.005
0891-5520/19/

id.theclinics.com

occur in childhood throughout the year but mostly from fall to spring.[2] Different serotypes have different organ tropism and lead to serotype-specific immunity[3]; ADV then remains latent in hosts' cells such as in the adenoids and tonsils. Of the 50+ serotypes infecting humans, only a few are associated with infections in immunocompromised patients; these include serotypes 1, 2, and 5 of species C, type 31 of species A, and rarely serotypes 11, 34, 35 belonging to species B.[5] In allogeneic hematopoietic stem cell transplant recipients (Allo-HCT), ADV infections are either due to the reactivation of a latent virus, or as a primary infection due to a certain ADV serotype circulating in the community.[6] Nosocomial infections and outbreaks have been described in bone marrow transplant wards.[5,6] Donor-derived primary infections from contaminated cells are extremely rare, because ADV is rarely recovered from the peripheral mononuclear stem cells.[6,7] The incidence of ADV infections in Allo-HCT recipients ranges from as low as 2.5% to as high as 20%, with higher rates reported among the pediatric and the T-cell depleted (TCD) Allo-HCT recipients.[2,6] **Table 1** summarizes the reported rates of ADV viremia and disease in adult, pediatric, TCD, and replete T-cell (RTC) Allo-HCT.

Syndromes Associated with Adenovirus Infections in Allogeneic Hematopoietic Stem Cell Transplant Recipients

Although ADV infection in Allo-HCT recipients might be asymptomatic, it may progress to ADV disease with end-organ damage. ADV disease is usually defined as the detection of the virus in one organ in the case of localized infection, or in more than one organ in disseminated disease in a patient with signs and symptoms of infection.[2,8,9] The role of ADV viremia in the diagnosis of ADV disease is unclear; however, a rising viral load in patients who are unable to tolerate invasive procedures may substitute for the detection of ADV in the involved organ.[8,9] Syndromes associated with the ADV disease in Allo-HCT recipients include ADV colitis, pneumonitis, hepatitis, nephritis, hemorrhagic cystitis (HC), encephalitis, or multiorgan disease due to a viremic spread.[9–17] The presentation of ADV disease in this population might be atypical on occasions, with reports of encephalitis mimicking posterior reversible encephalopathy, which is usually associated with calcineurin inhibitors,[12] or ADV fulminant hepatitis as opposed to the more common and less severe ADV hepatitis.[10,13] Among viral-induced HC, ADV was the culprit in 10% to 77% of these cases, with a trend of higher rates of ADV-associated HC among the pediatric population.[14,15,17] In Allo-HCT recipients, coinfection with more than one serotype, each serotype involving a different organ system, has been reported.[3,16,18] ADV infection is less well described among patients with hematologic malignancies (HMs). A 2014 report suggests a possible link between ADV infection and subsequent mantle cell lymphoma.[19]

Risk Factors of Adenovirus Infections in Allogeneic Hematologic Stem Cell Transplant Recipients

Although the incidence of ADV infections among adult Allo-HCT recipients is low, it seems to be higher in the pediatric population. In Allo-HCT recipients, with the exception of HC and gastroenteritis/diarrhea, ADV infections causing end-organ damage are associated with a high mortality rate of 20% to 44%.[8,20,21] In an all-adult, all-TCD Allo-HCT recipients study by Lee and colleagues,[20] a clinically significant viremia (defined ≥10,000 copies/mL) occurred in 8% of patients, one-third of them progressed to ADV disease, and the overall mortality rate was 44%. Given the rarity of the disease, albeit with high mortality, preventive measures need to be successful yet cost-effective. There are currently no available large randomized studies to evaluate the benefit of a preemptive approach with routine surveillance for ADV in blood (viremia),

Table 1
Adenovirus viremia and disease in allogeneic hematopoietic stem cell recipients; incidence, risk factors, and prevention in recently published studies

Reference	Study Design, Sample Size, and Population	Ex Vivo, In Vivo, or ST (% of Patients)	Frequency of Monitoring	Viremia (Cutoff of Initiating Therapy)	Disease	Risk Factors for ADV Viremia	Risk Factors for ADV Disease	Comment	Recommendations
Pediatric									
Rustia et al,[8] 2016[a]	Retrospective, 140	Alemtuzumab or ATG (82.2%)	Weekly	11% of ADV alone (≥1000 copies/mL)	NA for ADV (17% of all CMV, EBV, ADV)	Risk factors for combined CMV, EBV, and ADV: donor and recipient CMV + serostatus, pre-Allo-HCT viremia, alemtuzumab	Risk factors for combined CMV, EBV, ADV diseases: Pre-Allo-HCT viremia	Survival of patients with ADV viremia was significantly lower than that of CMV	Weekly monitoring for ADV for all patients
Hiwarkar et al,[23] 2013[a]	Retrospective, 278	Alemtuzumab or ATG (56%)	Twice a week	15% (≥1000 copies/mL)	NA	Pre-Allo-HCT ADV infection[b] and aGVHD.	NA	Survival was worse for CMV and ADV viremia and worse if ADV viremia was ≥1000 copies/mL vs <1000 copies/mL, CMV and ADV viremia predicted higher mortality	Weekly monitoring of ADV for high-risk patients

(continued on next page)

Table 1
(continued)

Reference	Study Design, Sample Size, and Population	Ex Vivo, In Vivo, or ST (% of Patients)	Frequency of Monitoring	Viremia (Cutoff of Initiating Therapy)	Disease	Risk Factors for ADV Viremia	Risk Factors for ADV Disease	Comment	Recommendations
Shönberger et al,[25] 2010[a]	Prospective, 40	ATG 60% for GVHD prophylaxis otherwise RTC	Weekly	2.5% (1 copy/μg) (only 1 patient with ADV viremia)	None	NA (only 1 patient with ADV viremia)	NA (only 1 patient with ADV viremia)	In HLA-matched and RTC HCT, ADV viremia is rare	Not related to ADV
Srinivasan et al,[22] 2015	Retrospective, 71 with stool samples available due to diarrhea	TCD 44% without mentioning if it was ex vivo or in vivo	On stool samples previously stored due to diarrhea, and weekly on blood	15% in patients with diarrhea, 28% in patients with diarrhea and ADV in stool, and 60% if ADV load in stool >10^6 copies/g	All had diarrhea (colitis/enteritis)	NA	NA		ADV of >10^6 copies/g in stool predicts viremia and can allow earlier initiation of antiviral therapy
Adults									
Yilmaz et al,[2] 2013	Retrospective, 2879	NA	No routine screening	NA	2.5%	NA	Risk factors for disseminated ADV cord HCT, male, and ALC $\leq$200/mm^3	Survival was shorter in disseminated ADV infection	Strategies for early diagnosis and intervention are essential

								This study	Not specific to ADV
Huang et al,[18] 2017[a]	Prospective observational, 156	Ex vivo TCD 100%	Weekly with no cutoff for therapy for ADV viremia	7%	4%	Seropositive CMV recipients were at high risk for combination of CMV, EBV, HHV6, and ADV viremia	NA	This study evaluated CMV, EBV, HHV6, and ADV	Not specific to ADV
Lee et al,[20] 2016	Prospective observational, 215	Alemtuzumab 100% TCD	Weekly	8% (10,000 copies/mL)	3% (33% of viremic patients)	No risk factors identified	NA	ADV disease followed an early-onset viremia at a median +29 d. Mortality rate in viremic patients is 44%, ADV attributed mortality 22%	In TCD Allo-HCT, ADV viremia is still rare but associated with disease if occurred early post-HCT and associated with high mortality; monitor for viremia and treat especially the first 2 mo post-HCT
Adults and pediatric									
Ramsay et al,[9] 2017	Retrospective, 733, including Auto-HCT, also included a few pediatric patients	NA	Every other week 2005–2006 then only if symptomatic until 2015	3%	6%, 23% of these were disseminated infection (1.4% of total patients)	NA	NA	Viremia occurred in 36% of ADV disease, 100% of disseminated disease; mortality rate with disseminated infection 30%	Disseminated disease is rare but with high mortality

(continued on next page)

Table 1
(continued)

Reference	Study Design, Sample Size, and Population	Ex Vivo, In Vivo, or ST (% of Patients)	Frequency of Monitoring	Viremia (Cutoff of Initiating Therapy)	Disease	Risk Factors for ADV Viremia	Risk Factors for ADV Disease	Comment	Recommendations
Lee et al,[24] 2013	Observational, 624	64% TCD	No routine surveillance	7% (4% RTC and 8% TCD)	2% (93% of them TCD)	Young age and aGVHD	aGVHD		TCD recipients with aGVHD are high risk for ADV infection and monitoring for ADV viremia needs to be further studied
Symeonidis et al,[21] 2007	Retrospective, 687	73% TCD	No routine surveillance	NA	9% (8% adults and 13% pediatric)	NA	None for adults, aGVHD and MUD in pediatric		Clinical trials for the management of ADV infection are needed

Abbreviations: ADV, adenovirus; aGVHD, acute graft versus host disease; ALC, absolute lymphocytes count; Allo-HCT, allogeneic hematopoietic stem cell transplant; ATG, antithymocyte globulin rabbit; Auto-HCT, autologous hematopoietic stem cell transplant; CMV, cytomegalovirus; EBV, Epstein-Barr virus; HHV6, human herpesvirus 6; MUD, matched unrelated donor; NA, not available; RTC, replete T-cell; ST, serotherapy with either alemtuzumab or antithymocyte globulin rabbit; TCD, T-cell depleted.
[a] Study included monitoring viruses other than adenovirus viremia.
[b] Detection of AVD from nasopharyngeal aspirate or stool or blood.

stool, conjunctival, or nasopharyngeal swabs and initiating therapy when the ADV is detected. In addition to the lack of an effective therapy, the viral load (VL) at which to consider initiating such therapy is not well defined. Among Allo-HCT recipients with a diarrheal illness, ADV viremia was detected when the stool VL reached 10^6 copies/g.[22] Screening the stool of Allo-HCT recipients with diarrheal illness risks missing few ADV infections, because neither a diarrheal illness nor viremia are obligatory findings in an ADV disease. In a 2017 study by Ramsay and colleagues,[9] viremia occurred only in 17 of 43 Allo-HCT recipients with ADV disease (40%); 7 of these viremic patients (41%) had only a localized infection and the remainder (10 of 17, 59%) had disseminated disease. We can conclude that not all Allo-HCT recipients with ADV disease will have viremia, especially those with a localized disease; however, a few patients with a localized disease and almost all patients with a disseminated disease will have ADV viremia.

Because ADV disease is rare yet associated with high mortality, it seems sensible to screen for ADV viremia among high-risk patients. A few questions remain to be answered: which Allo-HCT recipient should be considered at high risk for ADV disease? When to start the screening and for how long? Last, how to treat ADV viremia? Based on retrospective and observational studies listed and summarized in **Table 1**, it seems that a preexisting ADV infection documented by the isolation of ADV from a tissue, swab, or blood/plasma samples, acute graft versus host disease (aGVHD), pediatric patients, and ex vivo or in vivo TCD Allo-HCT recipients are considered high risk for ADV infections.[2,8,9,18,20–25] In addition, low absolute lymphocytes count (ALC ≤200 cells/mL) and cord HCT are significant risks for disseminated ADV infection.[2] In these high-risk patients, ADV viremia and disease usually occur within the first +100 days after Allo-HCT.[8,18,20] However, RTC Allo-HCT recipients may experience ADV infections beyond +100 days (median of +135 days). The time from ADV viremia to disease is relatively short, especially in high-risk patients, with a median time as short as 11 days.[20] Although it may make sense to initiate antiviral therapy as soon as the viremia is detected, many additional factors play a role in that decision, most importantly the availability and safety of these antivirals. Cidofovir (CDV) is used for the treatment of ADV infection but its use is fraught with significant adverse events including renal failure and optic neuritis. Brincidofovir (BCV) is an oral antiviral that seems to be better tolerated, but is currently available only as an investigational drug for compassionate use. Physicians may choose a higher threshold of VL to initiate a toxic antiviral medication, compared with a lower threshold when a safer antiviral is available. Additional information regarding the treatment of ADV infections is detailed in the "Treatment" section. An alternative to the screening for ADV viremia is to monitor for ADV-specific quantitative CD8 and/or CD4 cell immune response; patients with low levels of such ADV-specific immunity are at increased risk for disease and deserve either close clinical monitoring or empiric therapy.[26]

In summary, recipients of a TCD Allo-HCT with aGVHD, ALC ≤200 cells/mL, and cord HCT may benefit from weekly surveillance for ADV viremia during the first 100 days following HCT. Physicians then may choose to either closely monitor these patients for signs or symptoms of ADV or to preemptively initiate antiviral therapy if the VL is greater than a predetermined threshold, such as ≥10,000 copies/mL. Antiviral therapy can be initiated at lower levels (ie, >1000 copies/mL) with rising VL if the available antivirals are felt to be tolerated and/or safe.

Treatment

It has been reported that ribavirin and ganciclovir have activity against ADV; many of these studies and case reports, however, were limited to ADV-associated HC, and failed to show significant improvement with more severe infections.[27,28] Although no randomized trials are available, case series and other small studies reported a success rate between 70% and 100% when intravenous CDV, at dosages that range between 1 mg/kg thrice a week and 5 mg/kg per week, has been used to treat severe ADV infections mainly among pediatric HCT recipients.[29–32] It seems that the success rate depends on early detection and prompt initiation of therapy, which also may help shortening the course of therapy and avoiding toxic side effects.[32] Conversely, clinical success may depend on the need for a longer duration of therapy, which results in adverse events, mainly nephrotoxicity, occurring in up to 50% of patients.[30] The median duration of CDV was 60 days in one study[31] and up to 8 months in another.[29] After such prolonged therapy, it is believed that the role of CDV may be limited to partially controlling the infection until the immune system is reconstituted and the viral infection is eventually cleared.[33]

BCV is a lipid conjugate of CDV that has better oral bioavailability, higher intracellular concentration, and is not associated with nephrotoxicity owing to the lack of its uptake by the renal tubules.[34–36] BCV, however, is currently available only through an expanded access program. Among immunocompromised patients who failed CDV for the treatment of severe ADV infections, BCV has been successfully used as a salvage therapy.[35,36] In a small (48 Allo-HCT recipients), randomized, multicenter, phase II trial that compared placebo with 2 different dosages oral BCV (100 mg twice a week or 200 mg weekly for adults and 2 mg/kg twice a week or 4 mg/kg per week for pediatric patients) for the treatment of ADV viremia, there were no statistically significant differences in treatment failure among all 3 groups.[34] However, there was a trend to better outcomes in a subpopulation of high-risk patients (defined as haploidentical HCT, cord HCT, total or partial TCD, severe GVHD, and <6 months after HCT) who received twice-weekly dosing when compared with placebo ($P = .09$). In this study, treatment failure was defined as a combination of lack of worsening of viremia by ≥1 log and/or progression from viremia to definite or probable disease. In this study, the lack of significant findings might be due to the small number of patients. Another caveat to this study is that these patients were being monitored routinely for ADV viremia; hence, therapy was initiated early and promptly after viremia was detected.

Immunosuppressive therapies offered to prevent GVHD following HCT weaken the viral-specific T-cell response to viral infections; hence, reconstituting this form of immunity plays an important role in the prevention and treatment of viral infections. This reconstitution might be accomplished by decreasing or eliminating the immunosuppressive therapy, which may not be feasible; the other option would be to infuse these viral-specific T cells to susceptible HCT recipients. Viral-specific T cells are collected either from the donor or from a pool of healthy donors (third-party donors); they are then expanded by ex vivo cultures following stimulation by viral antigens.[37] In the case of ADV, these viral antigens are hexon and penton.[38] Very limited information is available regarding the use and outcomes of ADV-specific T cells. In a study evaluating viral-specific T-cell therapy, only 1 patient had ADV infection and was successfully treated with ADV-specific T cells.[39] In another study, 7 patients were treated for ADV infections and the success rate was 70%.[38] Interestingly, and in spite of the partial HLA matching to recipients, GVHD was not a significant adverse event following the viral-specific T-cell therapies in these studies.[37–39]

Plasma exchange has also been reported to decrease the VL and to help with ADV therapy in 1 patient with ADV encephalitis; however, in this patient, the clinical and virological response coincided with the use of CDV and the recovery of the lymphocyte count.[40]

In summary, there is still no known effective therapy for ADV infections. CDV might help if initiated early; however, is associated with significant adverse events, specifically nephrotoxicity. BCV might be an alternative to CDV, but further studies are needed and it is not readily available. ADV-specific T-cell therapy is promising, but it was reported in only 8 patients.

POLYOMAVIRUSES
Overview

Polyomaviruses (PyV) are small, nonenveloped, dsDNA viruses that include BK virus (BKV), JC virus (JCV), KI virus (KIV), WU virus (WUV), MC virus (MCV), TC virus (TCV), and simian virus 40 (SV40), among others.[41,42] Whereas JCV and BKV exclusively infect humans, SV40 was found in monkeys and humans and demonstrated oncogenic behaviors in animal models and possibly humans.[43] Primary infections related to PyV usually occur during childhood and are asymptomatic. Following the primary infection, the virus remains latent only to reactivate among immunocompromised patients, such as in patients with HM or AIDS, or solid organ transplant recipients, and HCT recipients. The clinical implications of PyV infections are not yet known, with the exception of infections due to JCV and BKV. Rahiala and colleagues[41] found that half of the pediatric Allo-HCT recipients experienced PyV viremia, JCV and BKV accounting for 12% and 77% of these viremias, respectively. Given their clinical significance, this discussion will address only JCV-related and BKV-related infections.

JC Virus

Based on serologic testing, 50% to 90% of the general population is infected with JCV, with most of the primary infections occurring during the first decade of life.[44,45] The route of transmission is not clearly identified, but is believed to be via the respiratory and/or oral-fecal routes. Following primary infection, the virus then hibernates in multiple cells for which it is trophic. The virus has been detected in brain, lungs, liver, kidneys, bladder, prostate, and CD34[+] progenitor cells that differentiate to lymphocytic lineage, specifically B cells.[44] In immunocompetent individuals, the JCV may reactivate occasionally and result in intermittent shedding; however, this reactivation may result in serious diseases in immunocompromised patients. Progressive multifocal leukoencephalopathy (PML) is the most common manifestation of JCV infection among immunocompromised patients. Although 85% of PML cases are currently described in patients with AIDS, it was actually first described in patients with chronic lymphocytic leukemia (CLL) in 1958.[46] Since then, PML has been described in multiple other HMs, mostly lymphoproliferative diseases (LPDs) such as Hodgkin lymphoma and non-Hodgkin lymphoma, in addition to CLL. It is thought that the chemotherapeutic agents used to treat these LPDs, including the alkylating agents (ie, cyclophosphamide) and purine nucleoside analogues (ie, fludarabine), are strongly associated with PML.[47] T-cell immunity is of utmost importance to protect against the reactivation of JCV; however, this type of immunity is inherently deficient in patients with LPD, especially when treated with agents such as fludarabine, leading to diseases similar to those seen in patients with AIDS, such as PML and *Pneumocystis jirovecii* pneumonia (PCP).[48]

Although JCV is isolated from multiple tissues, reactivation and replication of latent virus occurs in the central nervous system (CNS) of immunocompromised patients. It is thought that after an immunocompromising state, dissemination occurs through the B cells, with strong tropism to the CNS. Nuclear factor-1 (NF-1), a much-needed family of DNA-binding proteins, is abundant in the CNS oligodendrocytes and astrocytes and facilitates JCV transcription and replication, leading to the demyelinating process responsible for PML.[47,49] In addition to LPD, PML has been also described in other immunocompromising conditions, including among autologous-HCT (Auto-HCT) and Allo-HCT recipients. The incidence is rare, and the information about PML in the HCT recipients is scarce and available in only a few case series and reports.[45,47,50–54] In HCT recipients, PML usually occurs in patients who were heavily treated with either an alkylating or purine nucleoside analogue agent before the Auto-HCT or Allo-HCT.[47]

MRI findings of PML are relatively distinct, with hyperintense signals involving the white matter in T2 and fluid-attenuated inversion recovery images. Atypical MRI findings with subtle mass effect or gray matter involvement have been described in the HCT recipients.[52] The detection of JCV by polymerase chain reaction (PCR) in the cerebrospinal fluid (CSF) is an alternative diagnostic method to the more invasive (yet gold standard) of brain biopsy. The sensitivity of JCV PCR in the CSF ranges between 74% and 93% and specificity between 96% and 99%; hence, a negative JCV PCR should not totally exclude the diagnosis of PML, and a brain biopsy may still be needed for a definitive diagnosis. Brain biopsy allows for the detection of the enlarged nuclei of the oligodendrocytes and possibly identifying the viral inclusions, and also allows for the in situ hybridization studies to identify the JCV DNA in tissues.[47,52]

Although PML is the major clinical syndrome related to JCV infection among immunocompromised patients, JCV viruria and HC have been described in HCT recipients with rates of 10% to 14% and 0% to 9%, respectively.[55,56]

BK Virus

BKV is another PyV that is, classified into 4 subtypes (I–IV) and many subgroups with specific geographic distribution. The most common subtypes isolated from humans are subtype I followed by IV. As in all PyV, 90% of children are seropositive by the first decade of life.[57,58] Serious infections occur in immunocompromised patients and are usually due to the reactivation of primary infections; however, nosocomial transmission has been reported.[58] BKV was first isolated in the urine of a kidney transplant recipient in 1971, and this infection resulted in a ureteric stenosis.[59] In addition to ureteral stenosis, BKV infection also may result in allograft nephropathy following renal transplantation. In HCT recipients on the other hand, HC is the most common syndrome associated with BKV infection. BKV has also been associated with gastrointestinal bleed,[60] encephalitis,[61] and pneumonia.[62]

When discussing BKV infection in HCT recipients, it is important to differentiate among HC, BKV viruria, and BKV-associated HC. BKV viruria may occur in 7% of healthy individuals[63] and in 25% to 100% of HCT recipients.[56,57,64] HC occurs in 16% to 62% of HCT recipients[55,57,65–69] and it could be either drug-induced or due to viral infections. HC is usually a drug-induced complication following the conditioning regimen, usually cyclophosphamide-induced when it occurs early after HCT, and to be due to a viral illness if occurs late after HCT (see earlier chapters). Some investigators define early and late HC as that occurring <+7 and ≥+7 day post-HCT, respectively. Others define early and late HC when it occurs before or after engraftment, respectively.[57,67,70] HC is classified into 4 grades: grade 0: no hematuria, grade I: microscopic hematuria, grade II: macroscopic hematuria, grade III: hematuria with blood clots, and grade IV: hematuria and blood clots resulting in obstructive uropathy.[66,67] BKV-associated HC occurs in 11% to 55% of HCT recipients.[55,65,67,68] Although BKV-associated HC may result in increasing morbidity and a longer hospital stay, no correlation with overall survival has been identified in several studies.[55,56,65–67] Two studies, however, showed that BKV-associated HC was an independent risk factor for declining kidney function and worse survival following receipt of Allo-HCT.[64,69] Identifying risk factors predictive of BKV-associated HC conferred conflicting and differing results, reflecting the nonhomogenized populations included in these studies. It seems that myeloablative (MA) conditioning regimen, unrelated donors, haploidentical and cord HCT, and HLA mismatch should be considered risk factors for BKV-associated HC.[65,67,68,70] BKV viremia and viruria did not predict BKV-associated HC, with a very low positive predictive value of 14% and 39% for a viruria with a VL of 1×10^7 and a viremia with a VL of 1×10^3, respectively.[69] In other studies, the timing of the viremia (occurring at/or beyond 45 days after the conditioning therapy) and the viruria (preceding the HCT) were more predictive of BKV-associated HC than the mere detection of viremia and/or viruria.[57,70] Only one study showed that severe GVHD and mucositis predicted PyV viruria and HC among Auto-HCT and Allo-HCT recipients.[56] Several factors limit the value of screening for BKV-associated HC in HCT recipients, including the following: (1) the lack of effective therapy, (2) conflicting evidence regarding the value of BKV viremia or viruria in predicting BKV-associated HC, (3) no unified cutoff for BKV viremia and/or viruria that would predict BKV-associated HC, (4) no agreed on HCT cohort that would benefit from such screening, and (5) no strong evidence that BKV-associated HC is associated with worse outcomes. Hence, the European Conference of Infections in Leukemia recommends against the routine screening for BKV in urine or plasma/blood.[71]

Treatment

No active antivirals against PyV are available at the time of writing this review. The replication of the PyV depends on the host rather than the viral DNA polymerase. As such, antiviral agents known to treat other DNA viruses, such as ganciclovir, are ineffective. CDV is a nucleotide analogue that bypasses the viral kinase and uses the host's cellular kinase for its phosphorylation; however, as is the case with ganciclovir, CDV is an inhibitor of the viral not the host's DNA polymerase. Cytosine arabinoside (Ara-C), a nucleoside analogue that inhibits human DNA polymerase, has been used but it is significantly cytotoxic, and its effectiveness has not been reproducible in clinical studies.[72]

Treatment for JC virus–associated progressive multifocal leukoencephalopathy

CDV and Ara-C have successfully halted JCV replication in in vitro studies using a fetal brain cell line.[72,73] Several limitations, however, prevent the use of these agents in clinical settings, mainly their cytotoxicity and nephrotoxicity, in addition to their significant poor penetration of the blood brain barrier (BBB). Given its lipid derivative structure, BCV is thought to cross the BBB efficiently, and with its improved safety profile it becomes an attractive option for PyV-related infections. In an in vitro study, BCV was more effective than CDV in treating JCV-infected fetal cell lines, sparing the noninfected host cells.[72] We have to emphasize that to date, there are no clinical trials evaluating BCV for the treatment of PML.

Treatment of BK virus–associated hemorrhagic cystitis

CDV has been used with limited success, and the recovery of the immune system remains a prerequisite condition for the resolution of symptoms. One study showed that the intravenous CDV at high dose of 5 mg/kg per week (in addition to oral probenecid to decrease its nephrotoxicity), with or without intravesicular instillation, was successful only when the recovery of the immune system was achieved.[74] To bypass the nephrotoxicity associated with the higher doses of CDV, lower doses of intravenous CDV of 0.5 to 1.0 mg/kg week without probenecid have been used with resolution of hematuria and declining VL in 70% and 75% of patients, respectively.[75] In in vitro studies, BCV was effective in treating urothelial BKV-infected cells[76]; however, BCV effectiveness was limited when it was used against high-density cellular viral infections, suggesting that its optimal efficiency is achieved when given early in the course of infection and/or for prophylaxis.[76] Given the limited safe and effective options to treat BKV-related HC, adjunctive modalities have been sought, with hyperbaric oxygen therapy showing some success when started early after the diagnosis of HC.[77] Because the recovery of the virus-specific T-cell immunity is essential to control the viral infections, a donor or third-party–derived BKV-specific T cells, stimulated using the BKV VP1 and large T antigens, are used to treat BKV infections in limited number of HCT recipients with complete resolution of hematuria in all treated patients.[38]

Summary of potential therapies for PyV-associated infections is available in **Table 2**.

PARVOVIRUS B19
Overview

Parvovirus B19 (PvB19) is a nonenveloped, single-stranded DNA (ssDNA) virus (unlike the other dsDNA viruses discussed previously in this review). Its seroprevalence among preschool children, young adults, and elderly individuals is estimated to be 15%, 50%, and 85%, respectively.[78] The mode of transmission is usually through the respiratory tract. PvB10 ssDNA was detected in 18% and 1% of Allo-HCT products and standard blood products, respectively.[79] Transmissions through the transfusion of blood products and Auto-HCT and Allo-HCT have been described.[79–82] After the primary infection, specific immunoglobulin (Ig)M antibodies contribute to the clearance of viremia; IgM antibodies develop 10 days after the acute infection and last for approximately 2 to 3 months.[83,84] IgG antibodies develop 15 days after acute infections; however, only IgG antibodies directed against the capsid proteins VP1 and VP2 are considered neutralizing antibodies that confer lifelong immunity. IgG antibodies against nonstructural protein NS1 have low neutralizing immunity and are usually associated with longer duration of viremia, and extramedullary manifestation (ie, myocarditis, polyarthritis) even among immunocompetent patients.[83] In immunocompromised patients, IgM and IgG antibodies may not develop, or are detected late during the course of infection without the capability to neutralize the virus, which in turn results in chronic infection, long-term viremia, and inability to prevent reinfections.[83,84]

The most common manifestations following acute primary infection with PvB19 is erythema infectiosum in children and polyarthropathy in adults; myocarditis and glomerulonephritis also have been described.[85,86] Anemia is the mainstay manifestation of PvB19 infection owing to its special predilection to infect the erythroid progenitor cells expressing the P antigen. The P antigen facilitates the entry of the virus into the cell with subsequent viral replication leading to cellular lysis and pure red blood cell anemia (PRA). This phenomenon is best described in patients with underlying hemolytic anemia following the acute infection with PvB19 and is usually transient requiring supportive care. In immunocompromised patients, however, the infection can be chronic and is associated with persistent viremia and chronic PRA. Ninety-nine percent of immunocompromised patients with PvB19 infection will develop PRA.[87] Leukopenia and thrombocytopenia also may occur in 38% and 21% of these patients, respectively; hence, pancytopenia may also occur in this population.[87,88] PvB19-associated bone marrow suppression is confirmed by the presence of aplastic anemia and the detection of the PvB19 in the blood by PCR, or in the bone marrow either by PCR or by the presence of the giant pronormoblasts with intranuclear inclusions.[83,87]

Table 2
Characterizations of adenovirus, JC virus, BK virus, and parvovirus B19 infections in immunocompromised patients

Characteristics	ADV	JCV	BKV	Parvovirus B19
Most common syndrome(s)	Gastroenteritis/diarrhea, conjunctivitis, upper respiratory infection	PML	HC	Pure red blood cell anemia
Less common syndrome(s)	Encephalitis, pneumonitis, hepatitis, HC, and disseminated disease	HC	Encephalitis, pneumonia, gastroenteritis with bleed	Leukopenia, thrombocytopenia, pancytopenia
Most vulnerable population(s)	Allo-HCT	LPD	HCT	Immunocompromised patients in general including with HM and HCT
Risk factors	Allo-HCT with aGVHD and/or TCD, pediatric patients	LPD treated with alkylating and purine nucleoside analogue	Conflicting reports, but possibly cord HCT, haploidentical HCT, MA, unrelated donors, HLA mismatch, late occurrence of viremia, severe GVHD and mucositis, CMV infection, and BKV viruria before transplantation Viruria of 10^7 and viremia of 10^3	Any immunocompromised state

(continued on next page)

Table 2
(continued)

Characteristics	ADV	JCV	BKV	Parvovirus B19
Mode of infection	Reactivation, acute/primary	Reactivation	Reactivation	Primary/acute, blood products, donor-related, reactivation
Screening	Recommended in high-risk population	Not known	Not recommended in most studies	
Treatment	No approved drugs, CDV is sometimes used	No approved drugs, decrease immunosuppressants; intravesicular or IV CDV, ?BCV, HBO, and adoptive specific T cells are sometimes used	No approved drugs, decrease immunosuppressants. ?BCV, HBO, and adoptive specific Tcells are sometimes used	Decrease immunosuppressants, IVIG
Prognosis	Poor with disseminated disease and with end-organ damage other than HC and gastroenteritis/diarrhea	Poor with PML	HC is inconsequential, could be associated with decline of kidney function and higher mortality	

Abbreviations: ADV, adenovirus; aGVHD, acute graft versus host disease; Allo-HCT, allogeneic hematopoietic stem cell transplant; BCV, brincidofovir; BKV, BK virus; CDV, cidofovir; CMV, cytomegalovirus; HBO, hyperbaric oxygen therapy; HC, hemorrhagic cystitis; HM, hematologic malignancies; IV, intravenous; IVIG, intravenous immunoglobulins; JCV, JC virus; LPD, lymphoproliferative disease; MA, myeloablative; PML, progressive multifocal leukoencephalopathy; TCD, T-cell depleted.

Characteristics of Parvovirus B19 Infections in Hematopoietic Stem Cell Transplantation Recipients and Patients with Hematologic Malignancy

PvB19 infection has been described in Allo-HCT and Auto-HCT recipients as well as patients with HM.[80–82,87,89–95] Anemia and other cytopenias are inherently common among HCT recipients and patients with HM, and are usually attributed to the underlying disease; this results in the lack of testing for PvB19 infection and subsequent underestimation of the infection rate. The PvB19 infection rate is reported to be between 4% and 72% depending on the underlying disease and the populations being evaluated with lowest rates in Auto-HCT and the highest in hematological diseases.[84,89,91,95,96] As in other immunocompromised patients, the most common presentation is PRA; however, fever, rash, arthralgia, leukopenia, thrombocytopenia, and pancytopenia have been described.[81,87,92–94] The hematological manifestations of PvB19 infection with prolonged PRA and other cytopenias, in patients whose underlying disease is characterized by the same manifestations, present a unique challenge in managing these patients. PvB19-associated PRA, thrombocytopenia, and leukopenia may lead physicians to erroneously attribute these manifestations to a refractory or relapsed underlying HM, delay subsequent rounds of much-needed chemotherapy, and more transfusions of blood products.[87,90,91] Because of these implications, some advocate for the routine screening for PvB19 viremia to be able intervene early during the course of infection.

Treatment

Antivirals active against PvB19 are not available. Because humoral immunity, through the neutralizing effect of the IgG antibodies, plays a major role in the protection against and the eradication of PvB19 infection, intravenous immunoglobulin (IVIG) is considered a viable option against PvB19 infections in these immunocompromised patients.[80,83,93,94] High-dose IVIG, up to 1 g/kg weekly in divided doses, then less frequently until the resolution of symptoms or viremia, have been used[80,94]; however, lower doses at 100 to 400 mg/kg have also been successfully used,[83,93] likely due to the high rate of seropositivity for PvB19 among the general population, which makes specific IgG readily available in pooled IVIG preparations.

In conclusion, infections due to the DNA viruses, ADV, JCV, BKV, and PvB19, in Auto-HCT and Allo-HCT recipients and patients with HM, are associated with significant diseases that interfere with patients' recovery and survival. Treating physicians are faced with multiple dilemmas managing patients with suspected infections due to these viruses including the lack of clear guidance regarding testing for these viruses and more importantly the lack of effective therapy against these viruses. **Table 2** summarizes the characterizations of the diseases associated with these viruses and provides an insight to the currently available and suggested diagnostic and therapeutic approaches.

REFERENCES

1. Rowe WP, Huebner RJ, Gilmore LK, et al. Isolation of a cytopathogenic agent from human adenoids undergoing spontaneous degeneration in tissue culture. Proc Soc Exp Biol Med 1953;84(3):570–3.
2. Yilmaz M, Chemaly RF, Han XY, et al. Adenoviral infections in adult allogeneic hematopoietic SCT recipients: a single center experience. Bone Marrow Transplant 2013;48(9):1218–23.

3. Lo AA, Lo EC, Rao MS, et al. Concurrent acute necrotizing adenovirus hepatitis and enterocolitis in an adult patient after double cord blood stem cell transplant for refractory Crohn's disease. Int J Surg Pathol 2015;23(5):404–8.

4. Lee YJ, Prockop SE, Papanicolaou GA. Approach to adenovirus infections in the setting of hematopoietic cell transplantation. Curr Opin Infect Dis 2017;30(4): 377–87.

5. Mattner F, Sykora KW, Meissner B, et al. An adenovirus type F41 outbreak in a pediatric bone marrow transplant unit: analysis of clinical impact and preventive strategies. Pediatr Infect Dis J 2008;27(5):419–24.

6. Leruez-Ville M, Chardin-Ouachee M, Neven B, et al. Description of an adenovirus A31 outbreak in a paediatric haematology unit. Bone Marrow Transplant 2006; 38(1):23–8.

7. Flomenberg P, Gutierrez E, Piaskowski V, et al. Detection of adenovirus DNA in peripheral blood mononuclear cells by polymerase chain reaction assay. J Med Virol 1997;51(3):182–8.

8. Rustia E, Violago L, Jin Z, et al. Risk factors and utility of a risk-based algorithm for monitoring cytomegalovirus, Epstein-Barr virus, and adenovirus infections in pediatric recipients after allogeneic hematopoietic cell transplantation. Biol Blood Marrow Transplant 2016;22(9):1646–53.

9. Ramsay ID, Attwood C, Irish D, et al. Disseminated adenovirus infection after allogeneic stem cell transplant and the potential role of brincidofovir - Case series and 10 year experience of management in an adult transplant cohort. J Clin Virol 2017;96:73–9.

10. Nakazawa H, Ito T, Makishima H, et al. Adenovirus fulminant hepatic failure: disseminated adenovirus disease after unrelated allogeneic stem cell transplantation for acute lymphoblastic leukemia. Intern Med 2006;45(16): 975–80.

11. Inoue N, Isomoto H, Yamaguchi N, et al. Adenovirus-related gastric lesion in a patient with a bone marrow transplant. Endoscopy 2010;42(Suppl 2):E328–9.

12. Claveau JS, LeBlanc R, Ahmad I, et al. Cerebral adenovirus endotheliitis presenting as posterior reversible encephalopathy syndrome after allogeneic stem cell transplantation. Bone Marrow Transplant 2017;52(10):1457–9.

13. Kawashima N, Muramatsu H, Okuno Y, et al. Fulminant adenovirus hepatitis after hematopoietic stem cell transplant: retrospective real-time PCR analysis for adenovirus DNA in two cases. J Infect Chemother 2015;21(12):857–63.

14. Bil-Lula I, Ussowicz M, Rybka B, et al. Hematuria due to adenoviral infection in bone marrow transplant recipients. Transplant Proc 2010;42(9):3729–34.

15. Nakazawa Y, Saito S, Yanagisawa R, et al. Recipient seropositivity for adenovirus type 11 (AdV11) is a highly predictive factor for the development of AdV11-induced hemorrhagic cystitis after allogeneic hematopoietic SCT. Bone Marrow Transplant 2013;48(5):737–9.

16. Abe T, Furukawa T, Masuko M, et al. Sequential adenovirus infection of type 14 hemorrhagic cystitis and type 35 generalized infection after cord blood transplantation. Int J Hematol 2009;90(3):421–5.

17. Hayden RT, Gu Z, Liu W, et al. Risk factors for hemorrhagic cystitis in pediatric allogeneic hematopoietic stem cell transplant recipients. Transpl Infect Dis 2015;17(2):234–41.

18. Huang YT, Kim SJ, Lee YJ, et al. Co-infections by double-stranded DNA viruses after ex vivo T cell-depleted, CD34(+) selected hematopoietic cell transplantation. Biol Blood Marrow Transplant 2017;23(10):1759–66.

19. Kosulin K, Rauch M, Ambros PF, et al. Screening for adenoviruses in haematological neoplasia: high prevalence in mantle cell lymphoma. Eur J Cancer 2014; 50(3):622–7.

20. Lee YJ, Huang YT, Kim SJ, et al. Adenovirus viremia in Adult CD34(+) selected hematopoietic cell transplant recipients: low incidence and high clinical impact. Biol Blood Marrow Transplant 2016;22(1):174–8.

21. Symeonidis N, Jakubowski A, Pierre-Louis S, et al. Invasive adenoviral infections in T-cell-depleted allogeneic hematopoietic stem cell transplantation: high mortality in the era of cidofovir. Transpl Infect Dis 2007;9(2):108–13.

22. Srinivasan A, Klepper C, Sunkara A, et al. Impact of adenoviral stool load on adenoviremia in pediatric hematopoietic stem cell transplant recipients. Pediatr Infect Dis J 2015;34(6):562–5.

23. Hiwarkar P, Gaspar HB, Gilmour K, et al. Impact of viral reactivations in the era of pre-emptive antiviral drug therapy following allogeneic haematopoietic SCT in paediatric recipients. Bone Marrow Transplant 2013;48(6):803–8.

24. Lee YJ, Chung D, Xiao K, et al. Adenovirus viremia and disease: comparison of T cell-depleted and conventional hematopoietic stem cell transplantation recipients from a single institution. Biol Blood Marrow Transplant 2013;19(3):387–92.

25. Schonberger S, Meisel R, Adams O, et al. Prospective, comprehensive, and effective viral monitoring in children undergoing allogeneic hematopoietic stem cell transplantation. Biol Blood Marrow Transplant 2010;16(10):1428–35.

26. Guerin-El Khourouj V, Dalle JH, Pedron B, et al. Quantitative and qualitative CD4 T cell immune responses related to adenovirus DNAemia in hematopoietic stem cell transplantation. Biol Blood Marrow Transplant 2011;17(4):476–85.

27. Nakazawa Y, Suzuki T, Fukuyama T, et al. Urinary excretion of ganciclovir contributes to improvement of adenovirus-associated hemorrhagic cystitis after allogeneic bone marrow transplantation. Pediatr Transplant 2009;13(5):632–5.

28. Chen FE, Liang RH, Lo JY, et al. Treatment of adenovirus-associated haemorrhagic cystitis with ganciclovir. Bone Marrow Transplant 1997;20(11):997–9.

29. Hoffman JA, Shah AJ, Ross LA, et al. Adenoviral infections and a prospective trial of cidofovir in pediatric hematopoietic stem cell transplantation. Biol Blood Marrow Transplant 2001;7(7):388–94.

30. Ljungman P, Ribaud P, Eyrich M, et al. Cidofovir for adenovirus infections after allogeneic hematopoietic stem cell transplantation: a survey by the Infectious Diseases Working Party of the European Group for Blood and Marrow Transplantation. Bone Marrow Transplant 2003;31(6):481–6.

31. Yusuf U, Hale GA, Carr J, et al. Cidofovir for the treatment of adenoviral infection in pediatric hematopoietic stem cell transplant patients. Transplantation 2006; 81(10):1398–404.

32. Neofytos D, Ojha A, Mookerjee B, et al. Treatment of adenovirus disease in stem cell transplant recipients with cidofovir. Biol Blood Marrow Transplant 2007;13(1): 74–81.

33. Brown AEC, Cohen MN, Tong SH, et al. Pharmacokinetics and safety of intravenous cidofovir for life-threatening viral infections in pediatric hematopoietic stem cell transplant recipients. Antimicrob Agents Chemother 2015;59(7):3718–25.

34. Grimley MS, Chemaly RF, Englund JA, et al. Brincidofovir for asymptomatic adenovirus viremia in pediatric and adult allogeneic hematopoietic cell transplant recipients: a randomized placebo-controlled phase II trial. Biol Blood Marrow Transplant 2017;23(3):512–21.

35. Hiwarkar P, Amrolia P, Sivaprakasam P, et al. Brincidofovir is highly efficacious in controlling adenoviremia in pediatric recipients of hematopoietic cell transplant. Blood 2017;129(14):2033–7.

36. Florescu DF, Pergam SA, Neely MN, et al. Safety and efficacy of CMX001 as salvage therapy for severe adenovirus infections in immunocompromised patients. Biol Blood Marrow Transplant 2012;18(5):731–8.

37. Naik S, Nicholas SK, Martinez CA, et al. Adoptive immunotherapy for primary immunodeficiency disorders with virus-specific T lymphocytes. J Allergy Clin Immunol 2016;137(5):1498–505.e1.

38. Tzannou I, Papadopoulou A, Naik S, et al. Off-the-shelf virus-specific T cells to treat BK virus, human herpesvirus 6, cytomegalovirus, Epstein-Barr virus, and adenovirus infections after allogeneic hematopoietic stem-cell transplantation. J Clin Oncol 2017;35(31):3547–57.

39. Withers B, Blyth E, Clancy LE, et al. Long-term control of recurrent or refractory viral infections after allogeneic HSCT with third-party virus-specific T cells. Blood Adv 2017;1(24):2193–205.

40. Nishikawa T, Nakashima K, Fukano R, et al. Successful treatment with plasma exchange for disseminated cidofovir-resistant adenovirus disease in a pediatric SCT recipient. Bone Marrow Transplant 2012;47(8):1138–9.

41. Rahiala J, Koskenvuo M, Sadeghi M, et al. In children with allogeneic hematopoietic stem cell transplantation. Pediatr Transplant 2016;20(3):424–31.

42. Hu JH, Li SY, Yang MF, et al. Incidence, risk factors and the effect of polyomavirus infection in hematopoietic stem cell transplant recipients. J Int Med Res 2017; 45(2):762–70.

43. Fisher SG, Weber L, Carbone M. Cancer risk associated with simian virus 40 contaminated polio vaccine. Anticancer Res 1999;19(3B):2173–80.

44. Monaco MC, Atwood WJ, Gravell M, et al. JC virus infection of hematopoietic progenitor cells, primary B lymphocytes, and tonsillar stromal cells: implications for viral latency. J Virol 1996;70(10):7004–12.

45. Kharfan-Dabaja MA, Ayala E, Greene J, et al. Two cases of progressive multifocal leukoencephalopathy after allogeneic hematopoietic cell transplantation and a review of the literature. Bone Marrow Transplant 2007;39(2):101–7.

46. Astrom KE, Mancall EL, Richardson EP. Progressive multifocal leukoencephalopathy—a hitherto unrecognized complication of chronic lymphatic leukaemia and Hodgkins disease. Brain 1958;81(1):93–&.

47. D'Souza A, Wilson J, Mukherjee S, et al. Progressive multifocal leukoencephalopathy in chronic lymphocytic leukemia: a report of three cases and review of the literature. Clin Lymphoma Myeloma Leuk 2010;10(1):E1–9.

48. Obeid KM, Aguilar J, Szpunar S, et al. Risk factors for Pneumocystis jirovecii pneumonia in patients with lymphoproliferative disorders. Clin Lymphoma Myeloma Leuk 2012;12(1):66–9.

49. Monaco MC, Sabath BF, Durham LC, et al. JC virus multiplication in human hematopoietic progenitor cells requires the NF-1 class D transcription factor. J Virol 2001;75(20):9687–95.

50. Buckanovich RJ, Liu G, Stricker C, et al. Nonmyeloablative allogeneic stem cell transplantation for refractory Hodgkin's lymphoma complicated by interleukin-2 responsive progressive multifocal leukoencephalopathy. Ann Hematol 2002; 81(7):410–3.

51. Carson KR, Evens AM, Richey EA, et al. Progressive multifocal leukoencephalopathy after rituximab therapy in HIV-negative patients: a report of 57 cases from

the Research on Adverse Drug Events and Reports project. Blood 2009;113(20): 4834–40.

52. Kaufman GP, Aksamit AJ, Klein CJ, et al. Progressive multifocal leukoencephalopathy: a rare infectious complication following allogeneic hematopoietic cell transplantation (HCT). Eur J Haematol 2014;92(1):83–7.

53. Di Pauli F, Berger T, Walder A, et al. Progressive multifocal leukoencephalopathy complicating untreated chronic lymphatic leukemia: case report and review of the literature. J Clin Virol 2014;60(4):424–7.

54. Steurer M, Clausen J, Gotwald T, et al. Progressive multifocal leukoencephalopathy after allogeneic stem cell transplantation and posttransplantation rituximab. Transplantation 2003;76(2):435–6.

55. Schneidewind L, Neumann T, Knoll F, et al. Are the polyomaviruses BK and JC associated with opportunistic infections, graft-versus-host disease, or worse outcomes in adult patients receiving their first allogeneic stem cell transplantation with low-dose alemtuzumab? Acta Haematol 2017;138(1):3–9.

56. Peterson L, Ostermann H, Fiegl M, et al. Reactivation of polyomavirus in the genitourinary tract is significantly associated with severe GvHD and oral mucositis following allogeneic stem cell transplantation. Infection 2016;44(4):483–90.

57. Holler K, Fabeni L, Herling M, et al. Dynamics of BKPyV reactivation and risk of hemorrhagic cystitis after allogeneic hematopoietic stem cell transplantation. Eur J Haematol 2017;99(2):133–40.

58. Kato J, Mori T, Suzuki T, et al. Nosocomial BK polyomavirus infection causing hemorrhagic cystitis among patients with hematological malignancies after hematopoietic stem cell transplantation. Am J Transplant 2017;17(9):2428–33.

59. Gardner SD, Field AM, Coleman DV, et al. New human papovavirus (Bk) isolated from urine after renal transplantation. Lancet 1971;1(7712):1253–7.

60. Koskenvuo M, Lautenschlager I, Kardas P, et al. Diffuse gastrointestinal bleeding and BK polyomavirus replication in a pediatric allogeneic haematopoietic stem cell transplant patient. J Clin Virol 2015;62:72–4.

61. da Silva RL, Ferreira I, Teixeira G, et al. BK virus encephalitis with thrombotic microangiopathy in an allogeneic hematopoietic stem cell transplant recipient. Transpl Infect Dis 2011;13(2):161–7.

62. Akazawa Y, Terada Y, Yamane T, et al. Fatal BK virus pneumonia following stem cell transplantation. Transpl Infect Dis 2012;14(6):E142–6.

63. Egli A, Infanti L, Dumoulin A, et al. Prevalence of polyomavirus BK and JC infection and replication in 400 healthy blood donors. J Infect Dis 2009;199(6):837–46.

64. Abudayyeh A, Hamdi A, Lin H, et al. Symptomatic BK virus infection is associated with kidney function decline and poor overall survival in allogeneic hematopoietic stem cell recipients. Am J Transplant 2016;16(5):1492–502.

65. Ruggeri A, Roth-Guepin G, Battipaglia G, et al. Incidence and risk factors for hemorrhagic cystitis in unmanipulated haploidentical transplant recipients. Transpl Infect Dis 2015;17(6):822–30.

66. Oshrine B, Bunin N, Li YM, et al. Kidney and bladder outcomes in children with hemorrhagic cystitis and BK virus infection after allogeneic hematopoietic stem cell transplantation. Biol Blood Marrow Transplant 2013;19(12):1702–7.

67. Dosin G, Aoun F, El Rassy E, et al. Viral-induced hemorrhagic cystitis after allogeneic hematopoietic stem cell transplant. Clin Lymphoma Myeloma Leuk 2017;17(7):438–42.

68. Ghosh A, Tan TT, Linn YC, et al. What we learned from plasma BK-virus monitoring in allogeneic hematopoietic transplant recipients. Transplantation 2016; 100(4):E17–8.

69. Cesaro S, Tridello G, Pillon M, et al. A prospective study on the predictive value of plasma BK virus-DNA load for hemorrhagic cystitis in pediatric patients after stem cell transplantation. J Pediatric Infect Dis Soc 2015;4(2):134–42.

70. Silva LD, Patah PA, Saliba RM, et al. Hemorrhagic cystitis after allogeneic hematopoietic stem cell transplants is the complex result of BK virus infection, preparative regimen intensity and donor type. Haematologica 2010;95(7):1183–90.

71. Cesaro S, Dalianis T, Hanssen Rinaldo C, et al. ECIL guidelines for the prevention, diagnosis and treatment of BK polyomavirus-associated haemorrhagic cystitis in haematopoietic stem cell transplant recipients. J Antimicrob Chemother 2018; 73(1):12–21.

72. Jiang ZG, Cohen J, Marshall LJ, et al. Hexadecyloxypropyl-cidofovir (CMX001) suppresses JC virus replication in human fetal brain SVG cell cultures. Antimicrob Agents Chemother 2010;54(11):4723–32.

73. Hou J, Major EO. The efficacy of nucleoside analogs against JC virus multiplication in a persistently infected human fetal brain cell line. J Neurovirol 1998;4(4): 451–6.

74. Koskenvuo M, Dumoulin A, Lautenschlager I, et al. BK polyomavirus-associated hemorrhagic cystitis among pediatric allogeneic bone marrow transplant recipients: treatment response and evidence for nosocomial transmission. J Clin Virol 2013;56(1):77–81.

75. Ganguly N, Clough LA, DuBois LK, et al. Low-dose cidofovir in the treatment of symptomatic BK virus infection in patients undergoing allogeneic hematopoietic stem cell transplantation: a retrospective analysis of an algorithmic approach. Transpl Infect Dis 2010;12(5):406–11.

76. Tylden GD, Hirsch HH, Rinaldo CH. Brincidofovir (CMX001) inhibits BK polyomavirus replication in primary human urothelial cells. Antimicrob Agents Chemother 2015;59(6):3306–16.

77. Savva-Bordalo J, Vaz CP, Sousa M, et al. Clinical effectiveness of hyperbaric oxygen therapy for BK-virus-associated hemorrhagic cystitis after allogeneic bone marrow transplantation. Bone Marrow Transplant 2012;47(8):1095–8.

78. Sundin M, Lindblom A, Orvell C, et al. Persistence of human parvovirus B19 in multipotent mesenchymal stromal cells expressing the erythrocyte P antigen: implications for transplantation. Biol Blood Marrow Transplant 2008;14(10):1172–9.

79. Plentz A, Hahn J, Knoll A, et al. Exposure of hematologic patients to parvovirus B19 as a contaminant of blood cell preparations and blood products. Transfusion 2005;45(11):1811–5.

80. Arnold DM, Neame PB, Meyer RM, et al. Autologous peripheral blood progenitor cells are a potential source of parvovirus B19 infection. Transfusion 2005;45(3): 394–8.

81. Wasak-Szulkowska EW, Grabarczyk P, Rzepecki P. Pure red cell aplasia due to parvovirus B19 infection transmitted probably through hematopoietic stem cell transplantation. Transpl Infect Dis 2008;10(3):201–5.

82. Flunker G, Peters A, Wiersbitzky S, et al. Persistent parvovirus B19 infections in immunocompromised children. Med Microbiol Immunol 1998;186(4):189–94.

83. Karrasch M, Schmidt V, Hammer A, et al. Chronic persistent parvovirus B19 bone marrow infection resulting in transfusion-dependent pure red cell aplasia in multiple myeloma after allogeneic haematopoietic stem cell transplantation and severe graft versus host disease. Hematology 2017;22(2):93–8.

84. Jain A, Jain P, Kumar A, et al. Incidence and progression of Parvovirus B19 infection and molecular changes in circulating B19V strains in children with haematological malignancy: a follow up study. Infect Genet Evol 2018;57:177–84.

85. Molina KM, Garcia X, Denfield SW, et al. Parvovirus B19 myocarditis causes significant morbidity and mortality in children. Pediatr Cardiol 2013;34(2):390–7.
86. Obeid KM, Effendi AR, Khatib R. Association of parvovirus B19 infection with glomerulonephritis in an immunocompetent host: a case report. Scand J Infect Dis 2009;41(11–12):890–2.
87. Eid AJ, Brown RA, Patel R, et al. Parvovirus B19 infection after transplantation: a review of 98 cases. Clin Infect Dis 2006;43(1):40–8.
88. Muir K, Todd WT, Watson WH, et al. Viral-associated haemophagocytosis with parvovirus-B19-related pancytopenia. Lancet 1992;339(8802):1139–40.
89. Atay D, Akcay A, Erbey F, et al. The impact of alternative donor types on viral infections in pediatric hematopoietic stem cell transplantation. Pediatr Transplant 2018. [Epub ahead of print].
90. Jitschin R, Peters O, Plentz A, et al. Impact of parvovirus B19 infection on paediatric patients with haematological and/or oncological disorders. Clin Microbiol Infect 2011;17(9):1336–42.
91. Lindblom A, Heyman M, Gustafsson I, et al. Parvovirus B19 infection in children with acute lymphoblastic leukemia is associated with cytopenia resulting in prolonged interruptions of chemotherapy. Clin Infect Dis 2008;46(4):528–36.
92. Graeve JLA, Dealarcon PA, Naides SJ. Parvovirus-B19 infection in patients receiving cancer-chemotherapy—the expanding spectrum of disease. Am J Pediatr Hematol Oncol 1989;11(4):441–4.
93. Koda Y, Mori T, Kato J, et al. Persistent parvovirus B19 infection resulting in red cell aplasia after allogeneic hematopoietic stem cell transplantation. Transpl Infect Dis 2013;15(6):E239–42.
94. Itala M, Kotilainen P, Nikkari S, et al. Pure red cell aplasia caused by B19 parvovirus infection after autologous blood stem cell transplantation in a patient with chronic lymphocytic leukemia. Leukemia 1997;11(1):171.
95. Inazawa N, Hori T, Nojima M, et al. Virus reactivations after autologous hematopoietic stem cell transplantation detected by multiplex PCR assay. J Med Virol 2017;89(2):358–62.
96. Gustafsson I, Kaldensjo T, Lindblom A, et al. Evaluation of parvovirus B19 infection in children with malignant or hematological disorders. Clin Infect Dis 2010; 50(10):1426–7.

Respiratory Virus Infections of the Stem Cell Transplant Recipient and the Hematologic Malignancy Patient

Lauren Fontana, DO*, Lynne Strasfeld, MD

KEYWORDS

- Respiratory virus infection • Hematopoietic stem cell transplant • RSV • Influenza
- Parainfluenza • Human metapneumovirus • Rhinovirus • Coronavirus

KEY POINTS

- The morbidity and associated complications of respiratory virus infections are greater in hematopoietic stem cell transplant recipients and patients with hematologic malignancy than in immunocompetent individuals, with severity of illness related to the degree of immunosuppression.
- Molecular microbiologic testing is the gold standard for diagnosis, allowing differentiation of what are largely overlapping clinical syndromes.
- Most of the respiratory viruses, apart from influenza and in some circumstances respiratory syncytial virus and adenovirus, are managed supportively.
- Prevention is key and should focus on vaccination for influenza, avoidance of ill contacts, and compliance with principles of infection control.

Respiratory virus infections (RVIs) are increasingly recognized as a cause of significant morbidity and mortality in recipients of hematologic stem cell transplant (HCT) and patients with hematologic malignancy (HM).[1,2] With now widespread use of molecular diagnostics, the epidemiology and spectrum of clinical disease of these infections can be better characterized. Apart from influenza, the currently available antivirals are limited in efficacy and/or associated with potential for toxicity, thus emphasizing the importance of prevention strategies. This article provides a review of the epidemiology, clinical characteristics, management, and prevention of RVIs in HCT recipients and HM patients.

No disclosures.
Division of Infectious Disease, Department of Medicine, Oregon Health and Science University, 3181 Southwest Sam Jackson Park Road, Mail Code L457, Portland, OR 97239, USA
* Corresponding author.
E-mail address: fontanla@ohsu.edu

EPIDEMIOLOGY AND TRANSMISSION

The reported incidence of RVIs (**Table 1**) is wide ranging, a consequence of variation in screening parameters, study population, and testing methodology. Seasonal trends and peaks in patients with HM and HCT recipients mirror those of the community RVI activity, with sometimes significant year-to-year variability in disease incidence and severity (**Fig. 1**). Older studies relied on less sensitive methods, such as viral culture and direct fluorescent antigen, likely underestimating the incidence of RVI.

Although influenza and respiratory syncytial virus (RSV) typically have a defined seasonality, many of the other viruses can occur throughout the year and in overlapping time frames (see **Fig. 1**). This makes use of broad-range diagnostic strategies like multiplex polymerase chain reaction (PCR) critical, because it is often difficult to differentiate the virus type based on season or clinical presentation.

Respiratory viruses are transmitted by direct contact, fomite, or aerosolized droplet nuclei. Enveloped viruses, such as RSV, parainfluenza virus (PIV), coronavirus (CoV), rhinovirus, and influenza A/B, can remain viable on fomites from 2 hours to 72 hours.[31] Transmission can occur through direct contact with infectious material and indirectly through fomites or inhalation of particles.

CLINICAL PRESENTATION

Clinical presentation is nonspecific and variable in severity, with the spectrum of illness ranging from pauci-symptomatic to respiratory failure. Clinical syndromes are categorized as upper respiratory tract infection (URTI), with rhinorrhea, nasal congestion, sinusitis, headache, otitis media, sore throat, malaise and/or fever, and lower respiratory tract infection (LRTI), with localized or diffuse pneumonia.[9] Although RVI in the immunocompetent host typically is acute and self-limited, the presentation in HCT recipients in particular can be atypical, severe, and protracted. A majority present with fever and cough, but fever can be absent in approximately a third of the cases.[7] Normal findings on chest auscultation with LRTI are present with greater frequency in the immunocompromised population.[32]

Table 1
Incidence of viral infections, rate of lower respiratory tract infection at diagnosis, and mortality rates for respiratory viral infections

Respiratory Virus	Incidence (%)	Lower Respiratory Tract Infection at Diagnosis (%)	Mortality (%)[c]
Influenza A/B	1.3–40[1,3–9,a]	7–44[2–8,10,a]	8–28[1–3,5,7,8,10,a]
PIV	3–27[4,6,11,12,a]	7–50[2,4,5,8,13–15,a]	10–50[1,2,6,8,12,14,a]
RSV	1–50[1,3,4,6,16,17,a]	14–70[2–5,a]	11–47[3,5,6,8,17,18,a]
HMPV	2–11[1–4,19,20,b]	5–41[2,4,8,20,21,b]	6–40[2,19–21,b]
Adenovirus	1–30[1,2,4,8,22–24,a]	14–42[2,3,22,23,a]	14–73[2,8,22,23,a]
Rhinovirus	2–34[1,2,4,8,25,a]	<5–27[2,4,8,26,a]	<5–41[2,26,27,a]
CoV	3–23[1,2,4,25,28,b]	<5[2,4,8,b]	<5–54[2,28,b]
Bocavirus	1–3[2,25,29,30,b]	0[2,8,25,30,b]	Not reported[25,29,30,d]

[a] Studies are a combination of PCR and traditional laboratory methods (eg, culture, direct fluorescent antibody, and enzyme immunoassay).
[b] PCR-based studies.
[c] Includes all-cause and attributable mortality with variable timeframe to death.
[d] One mortality in a coinfected patient attributed to enterovirus/rhinovirus infection.

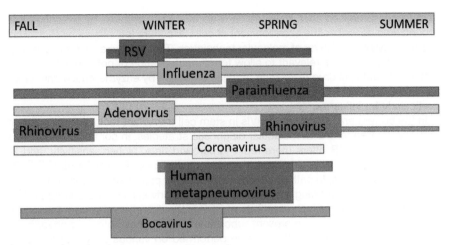

Fig. 1. Northern hemisphere seasonality trends.

There is considerable overlap in radiographic findings for the RVIs and between RVIs and other infectious and noninfectious entities, on plain film and CT imaging of the chest. Radiographic abnormalities include diffuse bilateral ground-glass infiltrates, small multifocal nodules, bronchial vascular thickening, and/or airspace consolidation.[33–36] A majority of immunocompromised patients have radiographic studies performed and a little more than half have a radiographic abnormality at the time of diagnosis.[32] Several studies in the radiology literature have proposed specific imaging features typifying particular RVIs. For example, a retrospective study of CT findings in HCT recipients found that those infected with RSV were more likely to have an airway-centric pattern of disease with tree-in-bud opacities and bronchial wall thickening with or without consolidation. Adenovirus appeared as multifocal consolidation or ground-glass opacities without inflammatory airway findings.[37] Although these features may be suggestive, they are not highly specific.

Progression from URTI to LRTI occurs with variable frequency (see **Table 1**), dependent on RVI type and host factors, and is associated with an increased likelihood of a fatal outcome. The viruses most frequently associated with LRTI include influenza virus, PIV, RSV, and human metapneumovirus (HMPV). Risk factors associated with the development of LRTI include older age, lymphopenia, early post-transplant infection, myeloablative conditioning regimen, unmatched donor status, and conditions, such as graft-versus-host disease (GVHD), necessitating increased immunosuppression.[2,5] Variations in host immune status, through modulation of molecular and cellular response to infection, provide explanation for differences in clinical manifestation. For example, RSV elicits a strong neutrophilic response in the respiratory tract that corresponds with disease severity, whereas CD8[+] T cells play a protective role in promoting viral clearance.[38]

LABORATORY DIAGNOSIS

Given that the clinical presentations of the various RVIs are nonspecific, microbiologic testing is required, which in turn can inform patient-specific treatment decisions, isolation precautions, and epidemiologic investigation. Serologic testing has limited application given that reinfection is common over time and because humoral responses to viral infections are often not detectable or significantly impaired in the immunocompromised host. Reliance on viral culture is hampered by prolonged turn-around time as well as the abandonment of cell vial culture techniques by clinical laboratories, typically in favor of molecular techniques. That said, viral culture does allow for strain typing and is relevant to allow for characterization of point mutations associated with antiviral drug resistance. Antigen detection by enzyme-based immunoassays are available for some respiratory viruses but lack sufficient sensitivity, particularly for influenza.[39,40]

In the current era, diagnosis of RVIs in stem cell transplant recipients and patients with HM is often reliant on molecular diagnostic strategies. In comparison with other methodologies, PCR offers more rapid turnaround time, higher sensitivity, and the ability to test for multiple viruses in a single test with multiplex platforms.[39,41,42] The ability to detect multiple pathogens based on specific primers has revolutionized molecular diagnostics, allowing for panel-based testing driven by clinical syndrome.[43] An important caveat of the high sensitivity of PCR is the detection of virus in the asymptomatic patient, which can represent subclinical infection, asymptomatic shedding, or a false-positive test result. PCR can be performed on various specimen types (eg, nasopharyngeal [NP] washes or swabs, oropharyngeal swab, and bronchoalveolar lavage [BAL] samples). The positive and negative predictive values of NP specimens were 86% and 94%, respectively, when compared with BAL specimens, in a study of paired NP and BAL PCR testing in HCT and HM patients with LRTI.[44] Various studies have used quantitative viral load on respiratory and other specimens as a correlate of disease severity to predict outcomes and to gauge response to treatment.[45,46] That said, the practical clinical applications of quantitative PCR are limited at this time. One important exception to this is adenovirus infection, in which case viremia can predict risk for disseminated and end-organ disease as well as survival.[47] Although not yet the realm of routine clinical diagnostics, next-generation sequencing techniques, such as whole-genome sequencing, hold potential for better informing RVI outbreak investigations (for example, in the health care setting) than traditional PCR-based diagnostic platforms.[48]

COMPLICATIONS AND OUTCOMES

Coinfection and alloimmune lung syndromes have been associated with RVIs in HCT recipients and have additional impact on morbidity and mortality, beyond the direct and attributable risk of respiratory tract infection. Coinfection with other viruses and superinfection with bacteria or fungi are well described in HCT recipients with RVI.[3,11,13,18,49] RVI seems to be an important risk factor for the development of invasive aspergillosis in allogeneic HCT, although it is difficult to parse out the contribution of viral infection from the milieu of immunosuppression.[50] Late airflow decline occurs in a significant proportion of HCT recipients with RVI in the first 100 days after transplant, particularly in those affected by RSV and PIV infection.[51] There is a strong association between RVI after HCT and the development of what are termed alloimmune lung syndromes (eg, idiopathic pneumonia syndrome, bronchiolitis obliterans syndrome, and bronchiolitis obliterans organizing pneumonia), which in turn are associated with increased mortality.[52] It is postulated that RVI in the early post-transplant period makes the lungs a target for alloimmunity.

Outcome of RVI in HCT recipients is often multifactorial in nature, related to both the direct respiratory impact of infection and the aforementioned complications that contribute to morbidity and mortality risk. Mortality rates vary among the different respiratory viruses and dependent on clinical presentation as well as underlying host factors. Risk factors for increased mortality include LRTI, mismatched allogeneic HCT, infection in the pre-engraftment phase (eg, health care–associated infection during the index transplant hospitalization), high-dose steroids at time of LRTI infection, oxygen requirement, and mechanical ventilation.[4,53–55] Mortality has been demonstrated to be particularly high for RVI outbreaks in the health care setting, likely a consequence of the high-risk nature of this patient segment and perhaps due to delays in diagnosis in this setting.[54,56,57] Detection of RVI in the immediate pretransplant period is associated with both LRTI and with decreased survival at 100 days, with mortality greatest in symptomatic patients.[54,58]

The 14-day overall mortality was noted to be 12% (6 of 49 with RVI) in a large contemporary multicenter prospective cohort study of allogeneic HCT recipients with diverse infections.[59] Although this represents crude and not attributable mortality, short-term outcomes, as opposed to long-term outcomes, are more likely to be related to direct effects of viral infection. Attributable mortality for RVIs is highest in those with LRTI.[2,60] PIV, RSV, adenovirus, HMPV, and influenza are the viruses that most often present with LRTI, and in turn have the highest mortality rate (see **Table 1**). There have been attempts to develop severity scoring systems to predict risk of LRTI, progression of URTI to LRTI, and mortality after RVI in HCT recipients.[61]

MANAGEMENT

Management of RVI consists of supportive care and, when available and applicable, prompt initiation of antiviral therapy. Although a significant need, demonstration of clinical benefit in relevant host populations has been a challenge to new antiviral drug development. The use of adjuvant steroids is not advised, because high-dose steroids generally are associated with increased risk of progression to LRTI, prolonged viral shedding, and increased mortality.[9,21,45,53,62–64] As such, consideration should be given to decreasing the steroid dose whenever feasible to less than 1 mg per/kg/d.

The identification of RVIs in the immediate pretransplant setting raises difficult management questions. Given the risk for increased complications and mortality, conditioning and transplant ideally should be delayed until the RVI is treated and/or there is clinical improvement.[58] That said, the decision to delay transplant requires careful consideration, acknowledging both risk for relapse or progression of underlying disease and/or issues related to donor availability.

PREVENTION

Transmission of RVIs in the health care setting is well documented.[9,56,57,65,66] Health care–associated outbreaks highlight the importance of monitoring patients and visitors for signs and/or symptoms of RVI. Symptomatic patients should be isolated and tested and ill visitors and health care workers excluded from contact with vulnerable populations. Strict compliance with infection control procedures, including isolation precautions and use of relevant personal protective equipment and hand hygiene, is critical to preventing spread of RVI. There are several guidelines available (eg, Centers for Disease Control and Prevention guidelines) that outline specific recommendations regarding isolation strategies.[67] Patients with suspected or documented RVI should be placed on droplet and contact precautions.[62] Specific isolation protocols for patients with RVI vary from institution to institution. Patient education on avoiding ill contacts and on hand hygiene and influenza vaccination for patients and their close contacts are important interventions to decrease risk for acquisition of RVI.

Prolonged shedding of RVI occurs not infrequently in this host population. Shedding for more than 12 weeks for greater than 10% of allogeneic recipients with either human rhinovirus (HRV) or human CoV (HCoV) infection was reported in 1 study.[25] Prolonged asymptomatic shedding poses great challenges for infection prevention, with uncertainty regarding the degree of risk for transmission from asymptomatic shedders. Many centers opt to maintain isolation precautions until signs and symptoms have resolved and repeat respiratory virus testing is confirmed to be negative.

VIRUS SPECIFICS: OUTCOMES AND TREATMENT
Influenza A/B

Influenza is a single-stranded enveloped RNA virus belonging to the Orthomyxoviridae family. Influenza A is divided into subtypes based on surface proteins, hemagglutinins, and neuraminidases, with antigenic drifts and shifts resulting from minor and major changes in hemagglutinins and neuraminidases, respectively. Influenza B is less prone to antigenic variation.[68]

The incidence of infection in HCT recipients and HM patients is driven by the activity of influenza in the community (see **Table 1**). The development of LRTI is associated with allogeneic HCT status, longer duration of symptoms prior to presentation, neutropenia, lymphopenia, and respiratory coinfection.[3,5,61,69] Risk factors associated with increased mortality include older age, LRTI, hypoxemia, mechanical ventilation, lymphopenia, neutropenia, and delayed antiviral therapy.[45,57,69,70] Disease severity and outcomes can vary based on the circulating strain, as exemplified by the 2009 H1N1 influenza pandemic, which resulted in greater illness severity and higher morality than seasonal influenza. LRTI occurred in 30% to 40% of patients, and the 30-day mortality rate for H1N1 among HCT recipients in 2009 was approximately 22%.[10]

Early recognition and treatment decreases the risk of progression to LRTI and improves survival.[7,9,45] Antiviral treatment should be given as early as possible,[7] regardless of the time from symptom onset to presentation in this patient population. Delayed administration has been shown to increase progression to LRTI and is associated with worse outcomes than early administration.[45,71] Neuraminidase inhibitors (NAIs) are the first-line agents for treatment of influenza A or influenza B. The currently available NAIs in the United States include oral oseltamivir, inhaled zanamivir, and intravenous peramivir. The standard dose of oseltamivir for treatment of influenza is 75 mg twice daily for 5 days. There are no data to support the use of high-dose oseltamivir rather than standard dose.[71] The optimal treatment duration in the HCT and HM population is not clear, and prospective trials to address this important question are needed. A longer duration of treatment (eg, 10 days) can be considered given the prolonged shedding and the risk for reactivation after remission, particularly with occurrence of infection in the pre-engraftment period.[72] The potential benefit of a longer course of antiviral therapy must be balanced against the concern and risk for emergence of resistance in this population. From the era of pandemic H1N1 in 2009, the preponderance of patients with emergence of oseltamivir-resistant virus (H275Y mutation, conferring cross-resistance to peramivir but not to zanamivir) were severely immunocompromised, mainly in HM patients and HCT recipients.[73–75]

There are several novel agents in development for treatment of influenza, although not much data is available in HCT recipients or HM patients. The NAI laninamivir octanoate is efficacious against oseltamivir-resistant strains and currently is used in Japan but is not yet Food and Drug Administration approved.[76–78] S-033188, a selective inhibitor of influenza cap-dependent endonuclease, was recently Food and Drug Administration approved for uncomplicated influenza, including resistant strains, but has not yet been studied in complicated influenza or in this patient population.[79]

DAS181, a recombinant sialidase fusion protein with demonstrated activity against both influenza[80] and PIV,[81] has completed phase II study in immunocompetent adults with influenza.[82] DAS181 seems a potential alternative for NAI-resistant influenza.[83] Favipiravir, a viral polymerase inhibitor, is approved in Japan for use against NAI-resistant influenza. Data from a phase II clinical trials of favipiravir for uncomplicated influenza in healthy adults in the United States are forthcoming (https://clinicaltrials.gov/ct2/show/NCT02008344, https://clinicaltrials.gov/ct2/show/NCT02026349).

Adjunctive corticosteroids are generally not advised for the management of influenza. Data from a retrospective study of 143 HCT recipients with seasonal influenza on no, low-dose (<1 mg/kg/d), or high-dose (≥1 mg/kg/d) steroids, largely for management of GVHD, demonstrated no significant difference in development of LRTI, hypoxemia, need for mechanical ventilation, or death but a trend toward a lower risk of LRTI in the group on low-dose steroids.[84] Although modest doses of steroids, if indicated for another cause, such as GVHD, may be continued after careful weighing of risks and benefits, steroids should not be started specifically for management of influenza infection.

Given the significant morbidity associated with influenza infection, oseltamivir chemoprophylaxis (75 mg daily for 10–14 days postexposure or for the duration of the exposure in an outbreak setting) should be strongly considered for high-risk patients in the context of a relevant exposure or an outbreak.[71,85] A caution regarding the broad use of prophylaxis is the report of development of oseltamivir-resistant influenza infection in an HM patient after oseltamivir (75 mg twice per day for 7 days) for prophylaxis after an exposure and then subsequent induction chemotherapy, with confirmed transmission of oseltamivir-resistant virus to 3 other patients on the unit.[66]

Although immune response to vaccination is suboptimal, particularly in HCT recipients and HM patients, vaccination is the cornerstone of prevention of influenza infection and its attendant complications. Receipt of influenza vaccine has been associated not only with a decreased risk for influenza infection in HCT recipients but also with a decrease in influenza severity and complications if infection occurs despite vaccination.[7] In a 5-year prospective observational study, allogeneic HCT recipients who received trivalent inactivated influenza vaccination had a significantly lower prevalence of virologically confirmed influenza infection (36% of vaccinated compared with 51% of nonvaccinated recipients; odds ratio [OR] 0.39), a decreased risk for progression to LRTI (OR 0.12) and a lower likelihood of influenza-related hospitalization compared with the nonvaccinated state.[29] All individuals greater than 6 months of age without contraindication, including HCT recipients and HM patients, should receive the influenza vaccination annually. Vaccination at less than 6 months post-transplant has been demonstrated to result in poor immune response,[86] and 2 doses of the influenza vaccine does not confer superior immunity compared with 1 dose.[87] As such, standard-dose inactivated influenza vaccination is strongly recommended for HCT recipients greater than or equal to 6 months post-transplant[88] and as early as 3 months to 4 months after transplant in patients without GVHD or otherwise requiring immune suppression[89] or during community outbreaks.[90] Live attenuated influenza vaccine is not recommended for HCT recipients or other immunocompromised hosts or for their close contacts.[90] Pretransplant vaccination (≥2 weeks prior to conditioning) is recommended largely as a strategy to provide early post-transplant protection, although acknowledging seroprotection declines rapidly in the post-transplant setting.[91] Given the vulnerability of this population and the suboptimal response to vaccination in the setting of immune compromise, vaccination of close contacts and health care workers is a critical arm of prevention.[90,92] HM patients receiving intensive chemotherapy or who have received anti–B-cell antibodies (eg, rituximab) in the preceding 6 months are unlikely to respond to influenza vaccination.[90]

Strategies to improve immune response to influenza vaccination include use of higher antigen dose and adjuvanted vaccines. In a large study of nonimmunocompromised adults greater than or equal to 65 years of age, high-dose trivalent vaccine resulted in significantly higher seroprotection rates and better protection against laboratory-confirmed influenza infection than standard-dose vaccine.[93] A phase I study comparing high-dose to standard-dose trivalent inactivated vaccine in adult HCT recipients demonstrated a higher rate of seroprotective titers in the high-dose group.[94] Small studies of adjuvanted vaccines and multidose vaccination have shown some promise, with improved immunogenicity to certain influenza strains, decreased hospital admission, and reduced mortality.[95–97]

Parainfluenza

PIVs are negative-sense, single-stranded, enveloped RNA viruses in the Paramyxoviridae family. There are 4 distinct serotypes, which include serotypes 1 and 3 in the *Respirovirus* genus and serotypes 2 and 4 in the *Rubulavirus* genus.

Epidemiologic and clinical features for each of the PIV serotypes vary widely. Although PIV2 and PIV3 circulate yearly, PIV1 has a biennial pattern. The incidence of symptomatic PIV in adult and pediatric HCT recipients is 3% to 27% (see **Table 1**). The reported incidence of PIV infection in HCT recipients may be falsely low due a larger percentage of asymptomatic or subclinical infections compared with other RVIs.[15,54] PIV3 is the predominant serotype associated with infection in HM patients and HCT recipients.[11,14,54] Multiple studies have demonstrated PIV3, in comparison to the other serotypes, to be associated with more severe infection, increased risk for progression to LRTI, and higher mortality.[12,54] PIV3 infection is associated with a 1.3-fold increase in mortality, after adjustment for age, CMV serostatus, donor type, and underlying disease.[12]

In a large systematic review of 28 studies of PIV infection in HM patients and HCT recipients, LRTI occurred in 36% and 39% of patients, respectively. Risk factors for LRTI included allogeneic HCT, early post-transplant infection, lymphopenia, neutropenia, and use of steroids during the URTI phase.[14] A retrospective study of 540 HCT recipients spanning 2 decades found an association of progression from URTI to LRTI with PIV3 serotype infection, presence of monocytopenia, greater than 1 mg/kg steroids prior to diagnosis, and copathogen detection. No patients who lacked all of these risk factors progressed to LRTI, whereas the progression risk increased to greater than 30% if 3 or more risk factors were present.[64] The need for mechanical ventilation in those with LRTI was 43% and survival from onset of mechanical ventilation was 23%. Although overall mortality with PIV LRTI is high after transplant, mortality decreases with time from transplant.[11] PIV-associated mortality is widely variable but is reported to be as high as 50% in those with copathogens (see **Table 1**).[12]

There is currently no licensed antiviral agent for the treatment of PIV infection. Despite data supporting in vitro PIV activity, numerous retrospective studies have shown lack of benefit of aerosolized or systemic ribavirin, with or without intravenous immunoglobulin (IVIG), in improving outcomes from an established LRTI or in preventing progression from URTI to LRTI[12,14,64] or in decreasing viral shedding.[12] There are few reports of successful treatment of HCT recipients with serious PIV infection with the investigational agent DAS181,[98–100] and data from a phase 2 study, including HCT recipients and HM patients, are forthcoming (https://clinicaltrials.gov/ct2/show/NCT01644877?cond=das181&rank=9).

Respiratory Syncytial Virus

RSV is a single-stranded, enveloped, negative-sense RNA virus within the Pneumoviridae family, as is HMPV. Two antigenic subtypes (A and B) circulate seasonally, either simultaneously or alternately.

RSV arguably is one of the respiratory virus infections associated with the highest disease severity and mortality risk in HCT recipients. Age, lymphopenia, neutropenia, myeloablative conditioning regimens, pre-engraftment infection or recent HCT, use of marrow or cord blood as graft source, mismatched or unrelated donor, GVHD, high-dose steroids, delayed diagnosis, and detection of viral RNA in serum all have been associated with RSV LRTI or RSV-associated mortality.[2,3,5,60,101-104] Attempts have been made to develop an immunodeficiency score index for RSV-infected HCT recipients to quantify the risk for LRTI and mortality[105] and to assist in decision making for initiating antiviral therapy.

The treatment of RSV infection in HCT recipients remains an area of significant controversy. The absence of high-quality prospective data, the toxicity and cost of available therapies, and the heterogeneity of host factors all contribute to uncertainty regarding the best approach to RSV management.[106] The preponderance of existing literature draws on single-center retrospective studies, with their inherent biases and limitations.

Ribavirin, a guanosine analog, is available in aerosolized, intravenous, and oral forms. Important toxicities include myelosuppression and, with the aerosolized form, bronchospasm.[107] Aerosolized ribavirin is both extremely costly in light of its orphan drug status[108] and complicated to administer given it is a potential teratogen, requiring use of personal protective equipment and a special air flow environment. Palivizumab, an RSV-specific recombinant monoclonal antibody, or polyclonal IVIG has been used in combination with ribavirin, although their contribution to RSV treatment is controversial and difficult to quantify[60,103,104] and their cost substantial, particularly for palivizumab. RSV monotherapy with palivizumab is neither supported by the literature nor recommended.[109] RSV-specific IVIG is no longer available.

Historically, numerous publications have demonstrated a benefit of aerosolized ribavirin (alone or with antibody-based therapy) for RSV, with a decrease rate of progression from URTI to LRTI and a decrease in mortality.[60,103,104] These studies, however, are severely limited on the basis of their single-center retrospective study design. A randomized controlled multicenter trial of aerosolized ribavirin for RSV URTI in HCT recipients was discontinued because of slow accrual, with failure to meet statistical significance for the primary endpoint of progression to LRTI.[46] A trend toward decreasing viral load over time was observed in the group assigned to ribavirin. Definitive prospective data regarding the use of aerosolized ribavirin for RSV infection in this population are lacking and unlikely to be forthcoming.

Systemic ribavirin, by oral or intravenous route and with or without antibody-based therapy, has been explored as a less toxic alternative to nebulized ribavirin for the treatment of RSV, with small case series demonstrating tolerability and suggesting potential efficacy.[110-112] There are more recent retrospective data comparing oral ribavirin with aerosolized ribavirin, providing increasing evidence to support the use of oral ribavirin as a safe, cost-effective, and potentially efficacious alternative to aerosolized ribavirin for HCT recipients and other severely immunocompromised hosts with RSV infection.[113,114]

RSV treatment decisions are complicated, taking into account host factors that inform the risk of progression to LRTI, disease severity at presentation, drug toxicity and side-effect profile, and cost. Although the available literature supports the use of ribavirin for high-risk patients with RSV infection, there are profound limitations in generalizing treatment algorithms from uncontrolled studies. To this end, a small case series described low morbidity (19% progression to LRTI) and no mortality in 32 pediatric HCT recipients with RSV infection who were managed without ribavirin and with maintenance IVIG with or without palivizumab.[115]

Several small molecule antiviral agents are in early phase development or under study for RSV infection.[116] Membrane fusion and RNA synthesis are important drug targets. GS-5806 (presatovir), a novel oral fusion protein inhibitor, showed promise in an early phase clinical trial but failed to demonstrate a reduction in nasal RSV viral load or symptom duration in lung transplant recipients.[117] Similarly, ALN-RSV01 (asvasiran), a small interfering RNA targeting RSV replication, has not progressed due to limited impact on viral parameters and lack of improvement in symptomatic patients.[118,119] ALS-8176 (lumicitabine), an RNA polymerase inhibitor, was associated with a reduction in viral load and clinical severity compared with placebo in a phase II RSV challenge study in healthy adults,[120] although the role of this and other agents awaits clarification in target populations. There are a few investigational agents in phase II study in HCT recipients, namely ALX-0171, a nanobody fusion inhibitor (https://clinicaltrials.gov/ct2/show/NCT03418571 and https://clinicaltrials.gov/ct2/show/NCT03468829)[1,16] and PC786, a non-nucleoside RSV L protein polymerase inhibitor (https://clinicaltrials.gov/ct2/show/study/NCT03715023). No RSV vaccine is currently available, although clinical trials are ongoing.

Adenovirus

Adenoviruses are a family of nonenveloped, double-stranded DNA viruses with more than 60 described serotypes categorized into 7 subgroups or species (A through G). Certain serotypes are associated with particular clinical syndromes, reflecting virus-specific tissue tropism for cellular receptors. Adenoviruses are nonenveloped viruses and can survive for extended periods on environmental surfaces and are resistant to killing by quaternary ammonium compounds, disinfectants widely used in the health care setting. Transmission can occur via aerosolized droplets or fomites as with other RVIs as well as by fecal-oral spread or through exposure to infected tissue or blood products.[121] Infection in HCT recipients and other severely immunocompromised hosts can be a consequence of new acquisition or reactivation of endogenous infection.

The spectrum of clinical disease in HCT recipients is broad, including URTI and/or LRTI, enterocolitis, hepatitis, nephritis, hemorrhagic cystitis, and meningoencephalitis.[22,121] Respiratory tract infection is caused most often by subgroups A, B, and C. The incidence is generally higher in the pediatric population.[47,122,123] Disseminated disease occurs in up to 10% to 20% of patients and is associated with allogeneic HCT, receipt of a T-cell–depleted graft, infection in the early post-transplant period, presence of GVHD, use of systemic steroids, and lymphopenia.[23,24,121,124] The presence of viremia as well as the height of the viral load is a meaningful predictor of risk for invasive and disseminated disease as well as mortality.[40,47,122,125] Overall mortality for all syndromes can be high, especially so for patients with pneumonia or disseminated disease, particularly in recipients of T cell-depleted grafts.[22,40,126]

Monitoring with PCR and preemptive antiviral treatment is advocated by some experts and supported by several studies in high-risk HCT recipients, notably in the pediatric population.[47,126,127] That said, other studies, including a prospective study in adult and pediatric non–T-cell–depleted recipients and a retrospective study in pediatric recipients of various graft types and conditioning regimens, have failed to demonstrate a benefit of monitoring and preemptive treatment.[128,129]

Currently, there are no antivirals that have a formal indication for adenovirus infection. Cidofovir, a nucleotide analog that inhibits DNA polymerase, is active against all serotypes of adenovirus, with both in vitro and animal data demonstrating virologic and clinical activity, respectively.[121] The human data supporting cidofovir for treatment of adenovirus infection in HCT recipients draw largely on retrospective studies demonstrating lower mortality rates in treated compared with untreated patients.[122,126] Pharmacologic disadvantages of cidofovir include active excretion of the unchanged drug in urine with resultant nephrotoxicity and low bioavailability, with limited concentration of the active phosphorylated compound in infected cells.[126] Furthermore, toxicities of cidofovir are often dose limiting—mainly nephrotoxicity, myelosuppression, and ocular toxicity. Brincidofovir, an oral lipid ester of cidofovir with improved bioavailability and a better safety profile, is an investigational agent under study for the treatment of adenovirus infection in HCT recipients. Although uncontrolled series have suggested efficacy and tolerability of brincidofovir in treating adenovirus viremia and disease in HCT recipients,[130,131] a randomized placebo-controlled phase II trial failed to meet the primary endpoint of reduction in treatment failure and demonstrated a signal for diarrhea in the group assigned to brincidofovir.[132] Although there are in vitro data to suggest that ribavirin has activity against adenovirus, in vivo data have not borne out clinical utility.[22,133] Clearance of viremia and survival are highly associated with lymphocyte reconstitution.[134] With this in mind, adoptive T-cell transfer of adenovirus-specific donor T cells remains an area of active investigation.[122] That said, despite well over a decade of work on adenovirus-specific cytotoxic T lymphocytes, this approach is far from routine for clinical application. In concert with consideration of antiviral treatment of serious adenovirus infection in HCT recipients, decrease in immune suppression as able also should be entertained.[124]

Human Metapneumovirus

HMPV, a large enveloped negative-sense RNA virus, is within the Pneumoviridae family, as is RSV. HMPV is a recently described viral infection, identified in 2001 with aid of molecular techniques.[135]

The reported incidence of HMPV has increased over time, in concert with improved molecular diagnostic capabilities. Knowledge of the disease spectrum continues to evolve, with increasing recognition of HMPV as a cause of RVI in the immunocompromised host population. A prospective study of URTI and LRTI in HM patients and HCT recipients with retrospective analysis for HMPV demonstrated an overall incidence of 9% with LRTI in 41% and death in 14% overall and in one-third of those with LRTI.[20] A retrospective study spanning a decade identified 118 cases of HMPV in HCT recipients. LRTI occurred in 25% overall, and progression to LRTI was as high as 60% in those with steroid dose greater than or equal to 1 mg/kg and lymphopenia at time of presentation with URTI.[21] A recent systematic review of the literature similarly found a low overall virus-associated mortality rate (6%), but substantially higher mortality (27%) for those with LRTI.[2,19]

Although there are in vitro data[136] and a few case series or case reports describing use of ribavirin with or without IVIG,[137,138] the preponderance of data, all retrospective in nature, fails to demonstrate a protective effect of ribavirin and/or IVIG in preventing HMPV LRTI and mortality.[21,139] An early but perhaps promising area of HMPV drug discovery research is the novel use of small interfering RNAs.[140]

Bocavirus

Human bocavirus (HBoV) is a small DNA virus within the Parvoviridae family. HBoV was first described in 2005 by molecular virus screening of NP aspirates from hospitalized children with LRTI.[141] Although studies in immunocompetent children with LRTI have demonstrated an incidence as high as 19%, data from the HCT population indicate infrequent infection. A prospective single-center study from Spain spanning 30 months found HBoV in only 6 of 192 (3%) virologically documented RVI episodes in 79 consecutive allogeneic HCT recipients. Interestingly, 5 of the 6 had coinfection with another respiratory virus. Disease severity was not substantial, with only 1 case of LRTI, which was believed likely caused by enterovirus/rhinovirus and no deaths from respiratory failure in the 6 affected patients.[28] Viral dissemination has been documented in transplant recipients, with detection of HBoV in blood and stool.[142] Given the frequency of coinfection and the mild disease severity, many questions remain regarding the pathogenic potential of HBoV in HCT recipients and other immunocompromised hosts.[143] Mode of transmission for HBoV is not well characterized. There is no specific antiviral treatment of HBoV infection.

Coronaviruses

CoVs are positive-sense, single-stranded, enveloped RNA viruses in the Coronaviridae family. CoVs are widespread among birds and animals. CoV in the alpha and beta genera have been associated with human infection: alpha-CoVs include HCoV-229E and HCoV-NL63, and beta-CoVs include HCoV-HKU1, HCoV-OC43, Middle East respiratory syndrome CoV, and severe acute respiratory syndrome CoV. HCoV-229E, HCoV-NL63, HCoV-HKU1, and HCoV-OC43 cocirculate during the nonsummer months.

A prospective surveillance study in HCT recipients detected HCoV in more than 10% of patients in the first year post-transplant, with approximately half of patients asymptomatic and with infrequent development of LRTI,[25] suggesting infection is common but typically not severe. Not surprisingly, prospective and retrospective studies of symptomatic cohorts point to higher but variable morbidity and mortality.[28,30,144] As with other RVIs, copathogen detection with HCoV is frequent,[28,30] making interpretation of attributable mortality complicated. That said, there are well-documented cases of severe and even fatal HCoV LRTI in HM patients and HCT recipients.[145,146] There is no specific antiviral treatment of CoV infection.

Rhinovirus

HRVs are small, single-stranded RNA viruses, members of the Picornaviridae family, genus *Enterovirus*. Rhinoviruses are classified into 3 species based on capsid features and sequencing: A, B, and C. Rhinoviruses circulate year-round, although with some seasonal clustering by species.[27] In contemporary studies that use molecular diagnostic techniques, rhinovirus is the most frequently detected RVI in HM patients and HCT recipients.[1,2,4,8,25,27] It is important to recognize the limitation of the current diagnostic platforms in the inability to differentiate between rhinovirus and enterovirus.

Clinical presentation is highly variable. In the reported literature, most patients have URTI, although a sizable minority have LRTI. In a large contemporary study of symptomatic HM patients with HRV infection, approximately 30% presented with LRTI.[27] Only 5% of those who presented at the URTI stage progressed to LRTI within 30 days, suggesting that symptomatic LRTI is uncommon. As with all RVIs and for HRV especially, it is likely that many studies overestimate the LRTI rate because they fail to account for the greater tendency of patients to seek medical care in the setting of more severe illness. Although some studies have found an association between HRV severity and LRTI and species type,[147] this is not a consistent finding.[27] Coinfection is common, particularly with LRTI, which makes interpretation of attributable morbidity and mortality challenging.[26,27,148] In a large retrospective study of approximately 700 HCT recipients with HRV infection spanning more than 2 decades, the overall 90-day mortality in the 128 subjects with LRTI was 41% and was significantly associated with low monocyte count, oxygen requirement at diagnosis, and steroid dose greater than 1 mg/kg/d before diagnosis; survival was not affected by the presence of copathogens.[26] As with other RVIs, early post-transplant infection is associated with greater disease severity.[149] There is no specific antiviral treatment of HRV infection.

REFERENCES

1. Paulsen GC, Danziger-Isakov L. Respiratory viral infections in solid organ and hematopoietic stem cell transplantation. Clin Chest Med 2017;38(4):707–26.
2. Renaud C, Campbell AP. Changing epidemiology of respiratory viral infections in hematopoietic cell transplant recipients and solid organ transplant recipients. Curr Opin Infect Dis 2011;24(4):333–43.
3. Martino R, Porras RP, Rabella N, et al. Prospective study of the incidence, clinical features, and outcome of symptomatic upper and lower respiratory tract infections by respiratory viruses in adult recipients of hematopoietic stem cell transplants for hematologic malignancies. Biol Blood Marrow Transplant 2005; 11(10):781–96.
4. D'Angelo CR, Kocherginsky M, Pisano J, et al. Incidence and predictors of respiratory viral infections by multiplex PCR in allogeneic hematopoietic cell transplant recipients 50 years and older including geriatric assessment. Leuk Lymphoma 2016;57(8):1807–13.
5. Ljungman P, Ward KN, Crooks BN, et al. Respiratory virus infections after stem cell transplantation: a prospective study from the Infectious Diseases Working Party of the European Group for Blood and Marrow Transplantation. Bone Marrow Transplant 2001;28(5):479–84.
6. Chemaly RF, Ghosh S, Bodey GP, et al. Respiratory viral infections in adults with hematologic malignancies and human stem cell transplantation recipients: a retrospective study at a major cancer center. Medicine (Baltimore) 2006;85(5): 278–87.
7. Kumar D, Ferreira VH, Blumberg E, et al. A 5-year prospective multicenter evaluation of influenza infection in transplant recipients. Clin Infect Dis 2018;67(9): 1322–9.
8. Shah DP, Ghantoji SS, Mulanovich VE, et al. Management of respiratory viral infections in hematopoietic cell transplant recipients. Am J Blood Res 2012;2(4): 203–18.
9. Chemaly RF, Shah DP, Boeckh MJ. Management of respiratory viral infections in hematopoietic cell transplant recipients and patients with hematologic malignancies. Clin Infect Dis 2014;59(Suppl 5):S344–51.
10. Reid G, Huprikar S, Patel G, et al. A multicenter evaluation of pandemic influenza A/H1N1 in hematopoietic stem cell transplant recipients. Transpl Infect Dis 2013;15(5):487–92.
11. Ustun C, Slaby J, Shanley RM, et al. Human parainfluenza virus infection after hematopoietic stem cell transplantation: risk factors, management, mortality, and changes over time. Biol Blood Marrow Transplant 2012;18(10):1580–8.
12. Nichols WG, Corey L, Gooley T, et al. Parainfluenza virus infections after hematopoietic stem cell transplantation: risk factors, response to antiviral therapy, and effect on transplant outcome. Blood 2001;98(3):573–8.

13. Nichols WG, Gooley T, Boeckh M. Community-acquired respiratory syncytial virus and parainfluenza virus infections after hematopoietic stem cell transplantation: the Fred Hutchinson Cancer Research Center experience. Biol Blood Marrow Transplant 2001;7(Suppl):11S–5S.

14. Shah DP, Shah PK, Azzi JM, et al. Parainfluenza virus infections in hematopoietic cell transplant recipients and hematologic malignancy patients: a systematic review. Cancer Lett 2016;370(2):358–64.

15. Peck AJ, Englund JA, Kuypers J, et al. Respiratory virus infection among hematopoietic cell transplant recipients: evidence for asymptomatic parainfluenza virus infection. Blood 2007;110(5):1681–8.

16. Ljungman P. Respiratory virus infections in stem cell transplant patients: the European experience. Biol Blood Marrow Transplant 2001;7(Suppl):5S–7S.

17. Khanna N, Widmer AF, Decker M, et al. Respiratory syncytial virus infection in patients with hematological diseases: single-center study and review of the literature. Clin Infect Dis 2008;46(3):402–12.

18. Campbell AP, Chien JW, Kuypers J, et al. Respiratory virus pneumonia after hematopoietic cell transplantation (HCT): associations between viral load in bronchoalveolar lavage samples, viral RNA detection in serum samples, and clinical outcomes of HCT. J Infect Dis 2010;201(9):1404–13.

19. Shah DP, Shah PK, Azzi JM, et al. Human metapneumovirus infections in hematopoietic cell transplant recipients and hematologic malignancy patients: a systematic review. Cancer Lett 2016;379(1):100–6.

20. Williams JV, Martino R, Rabella N, et al. A prospective study comparing human metapneumovirus with other respiratory viruses in adults with hematologic malignancies and respiratory tract infections. J Infect Dis 2005;192(6):1061–5.

21. Seo S, Gooley TA, Kuypers JM, et al. Human metapneumovirus infections following hematopoietic cell transplantation: factors associated with disease progression. Clin Infect Dis 2016;63(2):178–85.

22. La Rosa AM, Champlin RE, Mirza N, et al. Adenovirus infections in adult recipients of blood and marrow transplants. Clin Infect Dis 2001;32(6):871–6.

23. Yilmaz M, Chemaly RF, Han XY, et al. Adenoviral infections in adult allogeneic hematopoietic SCT recipients: a single center experience. Bone Marrow Transplant 2013;48(9):1218–23.

24. Ramsay ID, Attwood C, Irish D, et al. Disseminated adenovirus infection after allogeneic stem cell transplant and the potential role of brincidofovir - case series and 10 year experience of management in an adult transplant cohort. J Clin Virol 2017;96:73–9.

25. Milano F, Campbell AP, Guthrie KA, et al. Human rhinovirus and coronavirus detection among allogeneic hematopoietic stem cell transplantation recipients. Blood 2010;115(10):2088–94.

26. Seo S, Waghmare A, Scott EM, et al. Human rhinovirus detection in the lower respiratory tract of hematopoietic cell transplant recipients: association with mortality. Haematologica 2017;102(6):1120–30.

27. Jacobs SE, Lamson DM, Soave R, et al. Clinical and molecular epidemiology of human rhinovirus infections in patients with hematologic malignancy. J Clin Virol 2015;71:51–8.

28. Pinana JL, Madrid S, Perez A, et al. Epidemiologic and clinical characteristics of coronavirus and bocavirus respiratory infections after allogeneic stem cell transplantation: a prospective single-center study. Biol Blood Marrow Transplant 2018;24(3):563–70.

29. Pinana JL, Perez A, Montoro J, et al. Clinical effectiveness of influenza vaccination after allogeneic hematopoietic stem cell transplantation: a cross-sectional prospective observational study. Clin Infect Dis 2018. [Epub ahead of print].

30. Ogimi C, Waghmare AA, Kuypers JM, et al. Clinical significance of human coronavirus in bronchoalveolar lavage samples from hematopoietic cell transplant recipients and patients with hematologic malignancies. Clin Infect Dis 2017; 64(11):1532–9.

31. Boone SA, Gerba CP. Significance of fomites in the spread of respiratory and enteric viral disease. Appl Environ Microbiol 2007;73(6):1687–96.

32. Memoli MJ, Athota R, Reed S, et al. The natural history of influenza infection in the severely immunocompromised vs nonimmunocompromised hosts. Clin Infect Dis 2014;58(2):214–24.

33. Franquet T, Rodriguez S, Martino R, et al. Thin-section CT findings in hematopoietic stem cell transplantation recipients with respiratory virus pneumonia. AJR Am J Roentgenol 2006;187(4):1085–90.

34. Minnema BJ, Husain S, Mazzulli T, et al. Clinical characteristics and outcome associated with pandemic (2009) H1N1 influenza infection in patients with hematologic malignancies: a retrospective cohort study. Leuk Lymphoma 2013; 54(6):1250–5.

35. Kanne JP, Godwin JD, Franquet T, et al. Viral pneumonia after hematopoietic stem cell transplantation: high-resolution CT findings. J Thorac Imaging 2007; 22(3):292–9.

36. Shiley KT, Van Deerlin VM, Miller WT Jr. Chest CT features of community-acquired respiratory viral infections in adult inpatients with lower respiratory tract infections. J Thorac Imaging 2010;25(1):68–75.

37. Miller WT Jr, Mickus TJ, Barbosa E Jr, et al. CT of viral lower respiratory tract infections in adults: comparison among viral organisms and between viral and bacterial infections. AJR Am J Roentgenol 2011;197(5):1088–95.

38. Russell CD, Unger SA, Walton M, et al. The human immune response to respiratory syncytial virus infection. Clin Microbiol Rev 2017;30(2):481–502.

39. Kuypers J, Campbell AP, Cent A, et al. Comparison of conventional and molecular detection of respiratory viruses in hematopoietic cell transplant recipients. Transpl Infect Dis 2009;11(4):298–303.

40. Ganzenmueller T, Buchholz S, Harste G, et al. High lethality of human adenovirus disease in adult allogeneic stem cell transplant recipients with high adenoviral blood load. J Clin Virol 2011;52(1):55–9.

41. Zitterkopf NL, Leekha S, Espy MJ, et al. Relevance of influenza a virus detection by PCR, shell vial assay, and tube cell culture to rapid reporting procedures. J Clin Microbiol 2006;44(9):3366–7.

42. Xu M, Qin X, Astion ML, et al. Implementation of filmarray respiratory viral panel in a core laboratory improves testing turnaround time and patient care. Am J Clin Pathol 2013;139(1):118–23.

43. Ramanan P, Bryson AL, Binnicker MJ, et al. Syndromic panel-based testing in clinical microbiology. Clin Microbiol Rev 2018;31(1) [pii:e00024-17].

44. Hakki M, Strasfeld LM, Townes JM. Predictive value of testing nasopharyngeal samples for respiratory viruses in the setting of lower respiratory tract disease. J Clin Microbiol 2014;52(11):4020–2.

45. Choi SM, Boudreault AA, Xie H, et al. Differences in clinical outcomes after 2009 influenza A/H1N1 and seasonal influenza among hematopoietic cell transplant recipients. Blood 2011;117(19):5050–6.

46. Boeckh M, Englund J, Li Y, et al. Randomized controlled multicenter trial of aerosolized ribavirin for respiratory syncytial virus upper respiratory tract infection in hematopoietic cell transplant recipients. Clin Infect Dis 2007;44(2):245–9.

47. Lee YJ, Chung D, Xiao K, et al. Adenovirus viremia and disease: comparison of T cell-depleted and conventional hematopoietic stem cell transplantation recipients from a single institution. Biol Blood Marrow Transplant 2013;19(3):387–92.

48. Houlihan CF, Frampton D, Ferns RB, et al. Use of whole-genome sequencing in the investigation of a nosocomial influenza virus outbreak. J Infect Dis 2018; 218(9):1485–9.

49. Hardak E, Avivi I, Berkun L, et al. Polymicrobial pulmonary infection in patients with hematological malignancies: prevalence, co-pathogens, course and outcome. Infection 2016;44(4):491–7.

50. Martino R, Pinana JL, Parody R, et al. Lower respiratory tract respiratory virus infections increase the risk of invasive aspergillosis after a reduced-intensity allogeneic hematopoietic SCT. Bone Marrow Transplant 2009;44(11):749–56.

51. Erard V, Chien JW, Kim HW, et al. Airflow decline after myeloablative allogeneic hematopoietic cell transplantation: the role of community respiratory viruses. J Infect Dis 2006;193(12):1619–25.

52. Versluys AB, Rossen JW, van Ewijk B, et al. Strong association between respiratory viral infection early after hematopoietic stem cell transplantation and the development of life-threatening acute and chronic alloimmune lung syndromes. Biol Blood Marrow Transplant 2010;16(6):782–91.

53. Renaud C, Xie H, Seo S, et al. Mortality rates of human metapneumovirus and respiratory syncytial virus lower respiratory tract infections in hematopoietic cell transplantation recipients. Biol Blood Marrow Transplant 2013;19(8):1220–6.

54. Kakiuchi S, Tsuji M, Nishimura H, et al. Human parainfluenza virus type 3 infections in patients with hematopoietic stem cell transplants: the mode of nosocomial infections and prognosis. Jpn J Infect Dis 2018;71(2):109–15.

55. Fisher BT, Danziger-Isakov L, Sweet LR, et al. A multicenter consortium to define the epidemiology and outcomes of inpatient respiratory viral infections in pediatric hematopoietic stem cell transplant recipients. J Pediatr Infect Dis Soc 2017;7(4):275–82.

56. Maziarz RT, Sridharan P, Slater S, et al. Control of an outbreak of human parainfluenza virus 3 in hematopoietic stem cell transplant recipients. Biol Blood Marrow Transplant 2010;16(2):192–8.

57. Espinosa-Aguilar L, Green JS, Forrest GN, et al. Novel H1N1 influenza in hematopoietic stem cell transplantation recipients: two centers' experiences. Biol Blood Marrow Transplant 2011;17(4):566–73.

58. Campbell AP, Guthrie KA, Englund JA, et al. Clinical outcomes associated with respiratory virus detection before allogeneic hematopoietic stem cell transplant. Clin Infect Dis 2015;61(2):192–202.

59. Schuster MG, Cleveland AA, Dubberke ER, et al. Infections in Hematopoietic cell transplant recipients: results from the organ transplant infection project, a multicenter, prospective, cohort study. Open Forum Infect Dis 2017;4(2):ofx050.

60. Shah JN, Chemaly RF. Management of RSV infections in adult recipients of hematopoietic stem cell transplantation. Blood 2011;117(10):2755–63.

61. Kmeid J, Vanichanan J, Shah DP, et al. Outcomes of influenza infections in hematopoietic cell transplant recipients: application of an immunodeficiency scoring index. Biol Blood Marrow Transplant 2016;22(3):542–8.

62. Waghmare A, Englund JA, Boeckh M. How I treat respiratory viral infections in the setting of intensive chemotherapy or hematopoietic cell transplantation. Blood 2016;127(22):2682–92.

63. Damlaj M, Bartoo G, Cartin-Ceba R, et al. Corticosteroid use as adjunct therapy for respiratory syncytial virus infection in adult allogeneic stem cell transplant recipients. Transpl Infect Dis 2016;18(2):216–26.

64. Seo S, Xie H, Leisenring WM, et al. Risk factors for parainfluenza virus lower respiratory tract disease after hematopoietic cell transplantation. Biol Blood Marrow Transplant 2018;25(1):163–71.

65. Hoellein A, Hecker J, Hoffmann D, et al. Serious outbreak of human metapneumovirus in patients with hematologic malignancies. Leuk Lymphoma 2016;57(3): 623–7.

66. Chen LF, Dailey NJ, Rao AK, et al. Cluster of oseltamivir-resistant 2009 pandemic influenza A (H1N1) virus infections on a hospital ward among immunocompromised patients–North Carolina, 2009. J Infect Dis 2011;203(6): 838–46.

67. Siegel JD, Rhinehart E, Jackson M, et al, Health Care Infection Control Practices Advisory Committee. 2007 guideline for isolation precautions: preventing transmission of infectious agents in health care settings. Am J Infect Control 2007; 35(10 Suppl 2):S65–164.

68. Ariza-Heredia EJ, Chemaly RF. Influenza and parainfluenza infection in hematopoietic stem cell and solid organ transplant recipients. In: Ljungman P, Snydman D, Boeckh M, editors. Transplant infections. Fourth Edition. Cham (Switzerland): Springer International Publishing; 2016. p. 563–80.

69. Nichols WG, Guthrie KA, Corey L, et al. Influenza infections after hematopoietic stem cell transplantation: risk factors, mortality, and the effect of antiviral therapy. Clin Infect Dis 2004;39(9):1300–6.

70. Ljungman P, de la Camara R, Perez-Bercoff L, et al. Outcome of pandemic H1N1 infections in hematopoietic stem cell transplant recipients. Haematologica 2011;96(8):1231–5.

71. Uyeki TM, Bernstein HH, Bradley JS, et al. Clinical practice guidelines by the infectious diseases Society of America: 2018 update on diagnosis, treatment, chemoprophylaxis, and institutional outbreak management of seasonal influenza. Clin Infect Dis 2019;68(6):895–902.

72. Machado CM, Boas LS, Mendes AV, et al. Use of Oseltamivir to control influenza complications after bone marrow transplantation. Bone Marrow Transplant 2004; 34(2):111–4.

73. Centers for Disease Control and Prevention (CDC). Oseltamivir-resistant novel influenza A (H1N1) virus infection in two immunosuppressed patients - Seattle, Washington, 2009. MMWR Morb Mortal Wkly Rep 2009;58(32):893–6.

74. Tramontana AR, George B, Hurt AC, et al. Oseltamivir resistance in adult oncology and hematology patients infected with pandemic (H1N1) 2009 virus, Australia. Emerg Infect Dis 2010;16(7):1068–75.

75. Graitcer SB, Gubareva L, Kamimoto L, et al. Characteristics of patients with oseltamivir-resistant pandemic (H1N1) 2009, United States. Emerg Infect Dis 2011;17(2):255–7.

76. Kashiwagi S, Watanabe A, Ikematsu H, et al. Long-acting neuraminidase inhibitor laninamivir octanoate as post-exposure prophylaxis for influenza. Clin Infect Dis 2016;63(3):330–7.

77. Watanabe A, Chang SC, Kim MJ, et al. Long-acting neuraminidase inhibitor laninamivir octanoate versus oseltamivir for treatment of influenza: a double-blind, randomized, noninferiority clinical trial. Clin Infect Dis 2010;51(10):1167–75.

78. Watanabe A. A randomized double-blind controlled study of laninamivir compared with oseltamivir for the treatment of influenza in patients with chronic respiratory diseases. J Infect Chemother 2013;19(1):89–97.

79. Hayden FG, Sugaya N, Hirotsu N, et al. Baloxavir marboxil for uncomplicated influenza in adults and adolescents. N Engl J Med 2018;379(10):913–23.

80. Belser JA, Lu X, Szretter KJ, et al. DAS181, a novel sialidase fusion protein, protects mice from lethal avian influenza H5N1 virus infection. J Infect Dis 2007; 196(10):1493–9.

81. Moscona A, Porotto M, Palmer S, et al. A recombinant sialidase fusion protein effectively inhibits human parainfluenza viral infection in vitro and in vivo. J Infect Dis 2010;202(2):234–41.

82. Moss RB, Hansen C, Sanders RL, et al. A phase II study of DAS181, a novel host directed antiviral for the treatment of influenza infection. J Infect Dis 2012; 206(12):1844–51.

83. Triana-Baltzer GB, Sanders RL, Hedlund M, et al. Phenotypic and genotypic characterization of influenza virus mutants selected with the sialidase fusion protein DAS181. J Antimicrob Chemother 2011;66(1):15–28.

84. Boudreault AA, Xie H, Leisenring W, et al. Impact of corticosteroid treatment and antiviral therapy on clinical outcomes in hematopoietic cell transplant patients infected with influenza virus. Biol Blood Marrow Transplant 2011;17(7):979–86.

85. Vu D, Peck AJ, Nichols WG, et al. Safety and tolerability of oseltamivir prophylaxis in hematopoietic stem cell transplant recipients: a retrospective case-control study. Clin Infect Dis 2007;45(2):187–93.

86. Machado CM, Cardoso MR, da Rocha IF, et al. The benefit of influenza vaccination after bone marrow transplantation. Bone Marrow Transplant 2005;36(10): 897–900.

87. Karras NA, Weeres M, Sessions W, et al. A randomized trial of one versus two doses of influenza vaccine after allogeneic transplantation. Biol Blood Marrow Transplant 2013;19(1):109–16.

88. Ljungman P, Cordonnier C, Einsele H, et al. Vaccination of hematopoietic cell transplant recipients. Bone Marrow Transplant 2009;44(8):521–6.

89. Avetisyan G, Aschan J, Hassan M, et al. Evaluation of immune responses to seasonal influenza vaccination in healthy volunteers and in patients after stem cell transplantation. Transplantation 2008;86(2):257–63.

90. Rubin LG, Levin MJ, Ljungman P, et al. 2013 IDSA clinical practice guideline for vaccination of the immunocompromised host. Clin Infect Dis 2014;58(3): e44–100.

91. Ambati A, Boas LS, Ljungman P, et al. Evaluation of pretransplant influenza vaccination in hematopoietic SCT: a randomized prospective study. Bone Marrow Transplant 2015;50(6):858–64.

92. Frenzel E, Chemaly RF, Ariza-Heredia E, et al. Association of increased influenza vaccination in health care workers with a reduction in nosocomial influenza infections in cancer patients. Am J Infect Control 2016;44(9):1016–21.

93. DiazGranados CA, Dunning AJ, Kimmel M, et al. Efficacy of high-dose versus standard-dose influenza vaccine in older adults. N Engl J Med 2014;371(7): 635–45.

94. Halasa NB, Savani BN, Asokan I, et al. Randomized double-blind study of the safety and immunogenicity of standard-dose trivalent inactivated influenza

vaccine versus high-dose trivalent inactivated influenza vaccine in adult hematopoietic stem cell transplantation patients. Biol Blood Marrow Transplant 2016;22(3):528–35.

95. Ambati A, Einarsdottir S, Magalhaes I, et al. Immunogenicity of virosomal adjuvanted trivalent influenza vaccination in allogeneic stem cell transplant recipients. Transpl Infect Dis 2015;17(3):371–9.

96. Natori Y, Humar A, Lipton J, et al. A pilot randomized trial of adjuvanted influenza vaccine in adult allogeneic hematopoietic stem cell transplant recipients. Bone Marrow Transplant 2017;52(7):1016–21.

97. de Lavallade H, Garland P, Sekine T, et al. Repeated vaccination is required to optimize seroprotection against H1N1 in the immunocompromised host. Haematologica 2011;96(2):307–14.

98. Chalkias S, Mackenzie MR, Gay C, et al. DAS181 treatment of hematopoietic stem cell transplant patients with parainfluenza virus lung disease requiring mechanical ventilation. Transpl Infect Dis 2014;16(1):141–4.

99. Waghmare A, Wagner T, Andrews R, et al. Successful treatment of parainfluenza virus respiratory tract infection with DAS181 in 4 immunocompromised children. J Pediatr Infect Dis Soc 2015;4(2):114–8.

100. Salvatore M, Satlin MJ, Jacobs SE, et al. DAS181 for treatment of parainfluenza virus infections in hematopoietic stem cell transplant recipients at a single center. Biol Blood Marrow Transplant 2016;22(5):965–70.

101. Seo S, Campbell AP, Xie H, et al. Outcome of respiratory syncytial virus lower respiratory tract disease in hematopoietic cell transplant recipients receiving aerosolized ribavirin: significance of stem cell source and oxygen requirement. Biol Blood Marrow Transplant 2013;19(4):589–96.

102. Kim YJ, Guthrie KA, Waghmare A, et al. Respiratory syncytial virus in hematopoietic cell transplant recipients: factors determining progression to lower respiratory tract disease. J Infect Dis 2014;209(8):1195–204.

103. Shah DP, Ghantoji SS, Shah JN, et al. Impact of aerosolized ribavirin on mortality in 280 allogeneic haematopoietic stem cell transplant recipients with respiratory syncytial virus infections. J Antimicrob Chemother 2013;68(8):1872–80.

104. Waghmare A, Campbell AP, Xie H, et al. Respiratory syncytial virus lower respiratory disease in hematopoietic cell transplant recipients: viral RNA detection in blood, antiviral treatment, and clinical outcomes. Clin Infect Dis 2013;57(12): 1731–41.

105. Shah DP, Ghantoji SS, Ariza-Heredia EJ, et al. Immunodeficiency scoring index to predict poor outcomes in hematopoietic cell transplant recipients with RSV infections. Blood 2014;123(21):3263–8.

106. Griffiths C, Drews SJ, Marchant DJ. Respiratory syncytial virus: infection, detection, and new options for prevention and treatment. Clin Microbiol Rev 2017; 30(1):277–319.

107. Whimbey E, Champlin RE, Englund JA, et al. Combination therapy with aerosolized ribavirin and intravenous immunoglobulin for respiratory syncytial virus disease in adult bone marrow transplant recipients. Bone Marrow Transplant 1995; 16(3):393–9.

108. Chemaly RF, Aitken SL, Wolfe CR, et al. Aerosolized ribavirin: the most expensive drug for pneumonia. Transpl Infect Dis 2016;18(4):634–6.

109. de Fontbrune FS, Robin M, Porcher R, et al. Palivizumab treatment of respiratory syncytial virus infection after allogeneic hematopoietic stem cell transplantation. Clin Infect Dis 2007;45(8):1019–24.

110. Gueller S, Duenzinger U, Wolf T, et al. Successful systemic high-dose ribavirin treatment of respiratory syncytial virus-induced infections occurring pre-engraftment in allogeneic hematopoietic stem cell transplant recipients. Transpl Infect Dis 2013;15(4):435–40.

111. Marcelin JR, Wilson JW, Razonable RR, Mayo Clinic Hematology/Oncology and Transplant Infectious Diseases Services. Oral ribavirin therapy for respiratory syncytial virus infections in moderately to severely immunocompromised patients. Transpl Infect Dis 2014;16(2):242–50.

112. Gorcea CM, Tholouli E, Turner A, et al. Effective use of oral ribavirin for respiratory syncytial viral infections in allogeneic haematopoietic stem cell transplant recipients. J Hosp Infect 2017;95(2):214–7.

113. Foolad F, Aitken SL, Shigle TL, et al. Oral versus aerosolized ribavirin for the treatment of respiratory syncytial virus infections in hematopoietic cell transplantation recipients. Clin Infect Dis 2018. [Epub ahead of print].

114. Trang TP, Whalen M, Hilts-Horeczko A, et al. Comparative effectiveness of aerosolized versus oral ribavirin for the treatment of respiratory syncytial virus infections: a single-center retrospective cohort study and review of the literature. Transpl Infect Dis 2018;20(2):e12844.

115. El-Bietar J, Nelson A, Wallace G, et al. RSV infection without ribavirin treatment in pediatric hematopoietic stem cell transplantation. Bone Marrow Transplant 2016;51(10):1382–4.

116. Brendish NJ, Clark TW. Antiviral treatment of severe non-influenza respiratory virus infection. Curr Opin Infect Dis 2017;30(6):573–8.

117. Gottlieb JTF, Haddad T. A phase 2b randomized controlled trial of presatovir, an oral RSV fusion inhibitor, for the treatment of respiratory syncytial virus (RSV) in lung transplant (LT) recipients. J Heart Lung Transplant 2018;37(4):S155.

118. DeVincenzo J, Lambkin-Williams R, Wilkinson T, et al. A randomized, double-blind, placebo-controlled study of an RNAi-based therapy directed against respiratory syncytial virus. Proc Natl Acad Sci U S A 2010;107(19):8800–5.

119. Gottlieb J, Zamora MR, Hodges T, et al. ALN-RSV01 for prevention of bronchiolitis obliterans syndrome after respiratory syncytial virus infection in lung transplant recipients. J Heart Lung Transplant 2016;35(2):213–21.

120. DeVincenzo JP, McClure MW, Symons JA, et al. Activity of oral ALS-008176 in a respiratory syncytial virus challenge study. N Engl J Med 2015;373(21):2048–58.

121. Ison MG. Adenovirus infections in transplant recipients. Clin Infect Dis 2006;43(3):331–9.

122. Lee YJ, Prockop SE, Papanicolaou GA. Approach to adenovirus infections in the setting of hematopoietic cell transplantation. Curr Opin Infect Dis 2017;30(4):377–87.

123. Bruno B, Gooley T, Hackman RC, et al. Adenovirus infection in hematopoietic stem cell transplantation: effect of ganciclovir and impact on survival. Biol Blood Marrow Transplant 2003;9(5):341–52.

124. Chakrabarti S, Mautner V, Osman H, et al. Adenovirus infections following allogeneic stem cell transplantation: incidence and outcome in relation to graft manipulation, immunosuppression, and immune recovery. Blood 2002;100(5):1619–27.

125. Schilham MW, Claas EC, van Zaane W, et al. High levels of adenovirus DNA in serum correlate with fatal outcome of adenovirus infection in children after allogeneic stem-cell transplantation. Clin Infect Dis 2002;35(5):526–32.

126. Lindemans CA, Leen AM, Boelens JJ. How I treat adenovirus in hematopoietic stem cell transplant recipients. Blood 2010;116(25):5476–85.

127. Lion T, Kosulin K, Landlinger C, et al. Monitoring of adenovirus load in stool by real-time PCR permits early detection of impending invasive infection in patients after allogeneic stem cell transplantation. Leukemia 2010;24(4):706–14.

128. Ohrmalm L, Lindblom A, Omar H, et al. Evaluation of a surveillance strategy for early detection of adenovirus by PCR of peripheral blood in hematopoietic SCT recipients: incidence and outcome. Bone Marrow Transplant 2011;46(2):267–72.

129. Walls T, Hawrami K, Ushiro-Lumb I, et al. Adenovirus infection after pediatric bone marrow transplantation: is treatment always necessary? Clin Infect Dis 2005;40(9):1244–9.

130. Florescu DF, Pergam SA, Neely MN, et al. Safety and efficacy of CMX001 as salvage therapy for severe adenovirus infections in immunocompromised patients. Biol Blood Marrow Transplant 2012;18(5):731–8.

131. Hiwarkar P, Amrolia P, Sivaprakasam P, et al. Brincidofovir is highly efficacious in controlling adenoviremia in pediatric recipients of hematopoietic cell transplant. Blood 2017;129(14):2033–7.

132. Grimley MS, Chemaly RF, Englund JA, et al. Brincidofovir for asymptomatic adenovirus viremia in pediatric and adult allogeneic hematopoietic cell transplant recipients: a randomized placebo-controlled phase II trial. Biol Blood Marrow Transplant 2017;23(3):512–21.

133. Lankester AC, Heemskerk B, Claas EC, et al. Effect of ribavirin on the plasma viral DNA load in patients with disseminating adenovirus infection. Clin Infect Dis 2004;38(11):1521–5.

134. Heemskerk B, Lankester AC, van Vreeswijk T, et al. Immune reconstitution and clearance of human adenovirus viremia in pediatric stem-cell recipients. J Infect Dis 2005;191(4):520–30.

135. van den Hoogen BG, de Jong JC, Groen J, et al. A newly discovered human pneumovirus isolated from young children with respiratory tract disease. Nat Med 2001;7(6):719–24.

136. Wyde PR, Chetty SN, Jewell AM, et al. Comparison of the inhibition of human metapneumovirus and respiratory syncytial virus by ribavirin and immune serum globulin in vitro. Antiviral Res 2003;60(1):51–9.

137. Shahda S, Carlos WG, Kiel PJ, et al. The human metapneumovirus: a case series and review of the literature. Transpl Infect Dis 2011;13(3):324–8.

138. Hoppe BP, de Jongh E, Griffioen-Keijzer A, et al. Human metapneumovirus in haematopoietic stem cell transplantation recipients: a case series and review of the diagnostic and therapeutic approach. Neth J Med 2016;74(8):336–41.

139. El Chaer F, Shah DP, Kmeid J, et al. Burden of human metapneumovirus infections in patients with cancer: Risk factors and outcomes. Cancer 2017;123(12):2329–37.

140. Nitschinsk KM, Clarke DT, Idris A, et al. RNAi targeting of human metapneumovirus P and N genes inhibits viral growth. Intervirology 2018;61(3):149–54.

141. Allander T, Tammi MT, Eriksson M, et al. Cloning of a human parvovirus by molecular screening of respiratory tract samples. Proc Natl Acad Sci U S A 2005;102(36):12891–6.

142. Schenk T, Strahm B, Kontny U, et al. Disseminated bocavirus infection after stem cell transplant. Emerg Infect Dis 2007;13(9):1425–7.

143. Schildgen O, Muller A, Allander T, et al. Human bocavirus: passenger or pathogen in acute respiratory tract infections? Clin Microbiol Rev 2008;21(2): 291–304.

144. Hakki M, Rattray RM, Press RD. The clinical impact of coronavirus infection in patients with hematologic malignancies and hematopoietic stem cell transplant recipients. J Clin Virol 2015;68:1–5.

145. Pene F, Merlat A, Vabret A, et al. Coronavirus 229E-related pneumonia in immunocompromised patients. Clin Infect Dis 2003;37(7):929–32.

146. Oosterhof L, Christensen CB, Sengelov H. Fatal lower respiratory tract disease with human corona virus NL63 in an adult haematopoietic cell transplant recipient. Bone Marrow Transplant 2010;45(6):1115–6.

147. Ferguson PE, Gilroy NM, Faux CE, et al. Human rhinovirus C in adult haematopoietic stem cell transplant recipients with respiratory illness. J Clin Virol 2013; 56(3):255–9.

148. Ison MG, Hayden FG, Kaiser L, et al. Rhinovirus infections in hematopoietic stem cell transplant recipients with pneumonia. Clin Infect Dis 2003;36(9): 1139–43.

149. Ghosh S, Champlin R, Couch R, et al. Rhinovirus infections in myelosuppressed adult blood and marrow transplant recipients. Clin Infect Dis 1999;29(3):528–32.

Fungal Infections of the Stem Cell Transplant Recipient and Hematologic Malignancy Patients

Derek J. Bays, MD[a], George R. Thompson III, MD[b,c,*]

KEYWORDS

- Fungal infections • Candidiasis • Aspergillosis • Mucormycosis
- Hematologic malignancies • Hematopoietic stem cell transplant

KEY POINTS

- Investigate the risk factors and epidemiology of invasive fungal infections (IFIs) in the hematopoietic stem cell transplant (HSCT) and hematologic malignancy (HM) population.
- Discuss diagnostic strategies and challenges pertaining to IFIs.
- Examine clinical manifestations of different types of IFIs in the HSCT and HM population.
- Review treatment strategies and their efficacy for IFIs.

INTRODUCTION

Despite advances in chemotherapy options, morbidity and mortality remain high for patients with hematologic malignances (HMs). Those who require hematopoietic stem cell transplantation (HSCT) as a part of their therapy often experience significant immunosuppression and are subject to a variety of complications. These patients carry multiple risk factors for infectious complications, and are at high risk for development of invasive fungal infections (IFIs) when compared with the general population. Fluconazole prophylaxis among HSCT and neutropenic patients with HMs became standard of care after a landmark trial demonstrated its efficacy in preventing IFIs.[1] In 2007, Cornely and colleagues[2] showed improved outcomes in patients with

Disclosures: All authors no disclosures.
[a] Department of Internal Medicine, University of California Davis Medical Center, 4150 V Street, Suite 3100, Sacramento, CA 95817, USA; [b] Department of Internal Medicine, Division of Infectious Diseases, University of California Davis Medical Center, 4150 V Street, Suite G500, Sacramento, CA 96817, USA; [c] Department of Medical Microbiology and Immunology, University of California – Davis, One Shields Avenue, Tupper Hall, Davis, CA 95616, USA
* Corresponding author. Department of Medical Microbiology and Immunology, University of California – Davis, One Shields Avenue, Tupper Hall, Davis, CA 95616.
E-mail address: grthompson@ucdavis.edu

Infect Dis Clin N Am 33 (2019) 545–566
https://doi.org/10.1016/j.idc.2019.02.006
0891-5520/19/© 2019 Elsevier Inc. All rights reserved.

id.theclinics.com

posaconazole prophylaxis compared with fluconazole. However, there continue to be high rates of mortality associated with IFIs in these vulnerable populations.[3,4] We aim to discuss the epidemiology, clinical manifestations, diagnosis, and management in HSCT recipients and patients with HM.

CANDIDIASIS

Epidemiology of Candida spp Affecting Hematopoietic Stem Cell Transplantation Recipients

Before the adoption of antifungal prophylaxis in HSCT recipients, *Candida* spp were the primary etiology of IFIs and led to significant mortality.[5] The 1992 trial of Goodman and colleagues[1] demonstrated the efficacy of systemic antifungal prophylaxis with fluconazole in the HSCT population. Subsequent epidemiologic studies have demonstrated an increased incidence of molds, as the etiology of IFIs compared with *Candida* spp.[3,6] This trend may be explained by fluconazole's inferiority at preventing IFI from molds compared with triazoles such as posaconazole.[2]

The 3 most common species are *Candida glabrata, Candida albicans,* and *Candida parapsilosis* (in decreasing order of prevalence).[3] Whenever possible, the species should be identified given differences in susceptibilities (**Table 1**).[7] In addition, *Candida* species are notorious for forming biofilms on indwelling catheters,[9] which should prompt clinicians to be vigilant in removing these as part of treatment of all cases of candidemia.

Epidemiology of Candida spp Affecting Patients with Hematologic Malignancy

The incidence of candidemia in patients with HM and has been estimated 18.6 to 23.2 episodes per 100,000 inpatient days and remained stable from 2001 to 2006.[10] Previously, candidemia was most commonly caused by *C albicans.*[11] However, in the hematologic population, there have been increasing reports of a change in the causative organism with an increase in non–*C albicans* species.[10,12–14] Hachem and colleagues[14] demonstrated *C glabrata* as the leading cause of candidemia at a tertiary hospital in Texas followed closely by *Candida krusei.* During their 10-year surveillance, *C albicans* was the cause only 13.5% of the time, compared with 34.4% during the preceding 4 years before surveillance began. Hachem's group[14] also demonstrated that this shift may be explained by fluconazole prophylaxis, as this was an independent risk factor for development of *C glabrata* and *C krusei* candidemia, both of which having increased resistance compared with *C albicans.*[15] This trend has not been geographically isolated, with Zirkel and colleagues[13] also showing non–*C albicans* species being the most common in a retrospective study in Germany and Dewan and colleagues[12] showing *Candida tropicalis* as the etiology in 46% of patients in a tertiary-care hospital in India.

Clinical Manifestations of Local Mucocutaneous Candidiasis

Candida spp also can lead to noninvasive mucocutaneous infections in the oropharynx (thrush), esophagus (esophagitis), and vagina (vulvovaginitis). Oropharyngeal candidiasis, despite prophylaxis, remains a common entity occurring in approximately 10% of patients with HM[16] and approximately 17% of patients with HSCT.[17] In both esophageal and oropharyngeal candidiasis, the causative species is typically *C albicans.*[7] Symptoms and physical manifestations of oropharyngeal candidiasis range from painless white plaques along the buccal mucosa and oral cavity (pseudomembranous oral candidiasis) to painful erythematous lesions without plaques on the oral mucosa (atrophic oral candidiasis) and angle of the mouth (angular cheilitis).[18] The major symptoms of *Candida* esophagitis are odynophagia and dysphagia, and

Table 1
Susceptibility pattern of *Candida* spp

Candida spp	Susceptibility Patterns						
	Fluconazole	Voriconazole	Posaconazole	Itraconazole	Echinocandin	Amphotericin B	Flucytosine
C albicans	S	S	S	S	S	S	S
C glabrata	S-DD to R	S to S-DD?	S to S-DD?	S-DD to R	S to R[a]	S to I	S
C krusei	R	S to S-DD?	S to S-DD?	R	S	S to I	I to R
C lusitaniae	S	S	S	S	S	S to R	S
C parapsilosis	S	S	S	S	S to I	S	S
C tropicalis	S	S	S	S	S	S	S

Abbreviations: I, intermediate; R, resistant; S, susceptible; S-DD, susceptible-dose dependent.

[a] Echinocandin resistance in *C glabrata* is institution specific with some centers observing resistance rates up to 14%.[8]

Adapted from McCarty TP, Pappas PG. Invasive candidiasis. Infect Dis Clin North Am 2016;30(1):107; with permission.

in the HSCT and HM population these symptoms suggest disease regardless of the presence of concurrent oral candidiasis.

Clinical Manifestations of Invasive Candidiasis

Candidemia, defined as the presence of *Candida* spp in the blood, confers a high associated mortality. Risk factors for candidemia include both hematologic and solid organ malignancies, organ transplantation, neutropenia, immunosuppressive agents, renal failure with and without hemodialysis, intensive care unit stay with and without mechanical ventilation, indwelling catheters including urinary and central venous, high Acute Physiology and Chronic Health Evaluation (APACHE) II scores, broad-spectrum antimicrobials, immunosuppression, total parenteral nutrition, prior colonization of *Candida* spp, and surgical procedures (particularly those that transect the bowel wall lumen).[11] There are not specific symptoms for candidemia, and it should be considered in patients with HM and HSCT that have fever or hypotension, as these may be the only presenting symptoms.[19] Candidemia carries a high rate of mortality in this population, with mortality of 40% to 45% at 4 weeks,[10,20–22] further emphasizing the need for high clinical suspicion in this vulnerable population.

Once a patient is diagnosed with candidemia, disseminated complications need to be considered. All patients with candidemia should have a dilated eye examination by ophthalmology to evaluate for chorioretinitis and endophthalmitis.[7] Neutropenic patients frequently need repeated examination after count recovery.[7] In the immunocompromised, ocular candidiasis typically does not present with symptoms.[23] When symptoms are present, patients typically complain of blurred vision or new "floaters" consistent with vitritis.[23] Rarely, candidemia can be complicated by endocarditis. In the general population, *Candida* endocarditis typically carries a high mortality approaching 80% and often requires surgical involvement.[24]

Chronic disseminated candidiasis (also known as hepatosplenic candidiasis) occurs in 3% to 29% of patients of patients with HM.[25] However, the true incidence is thought to be lower (closer to 3%–6%), especially in the era of antifungal prophylaxis.[26] It typically occurs in patients who have been neutropenic for longer than 15 days; however, clinical symptoms and diagnosis often do not develop until neutropenia resolves and white blood cell count recovers.[25] The most common presentation is fever despite broad-spectrum antimicrobial agents, right upper quadrant pain, and elevated alkaline phosphatase.[25] Cultures of lesions are often negative, with pathology showing dead yeast. Because lesions may not typically develop until resolution of neutropenia, this manifestation argues for an immune reconstitution inflammatory syndrome phenomenon.[27] It often carries a high rate of mortality, ranging from 21% to 74%, but this appears to be largely be influenced by duration of neutropenia and underlying malignancy.[7,27]

Diagnosis of Candidiasis

The diagnosis of candidiasis depends on the presenting manifestation. Oropharyngeal and vaginal candidiasis are often diagnosed clinically, based on typical symptoms and physical examination appearance.[28] *Candida* esophagitis is confirmed via esophageal endoscopy with esophageal brushing and biopsy; however, it can be clinically diagnosed in patients with oropharyngeal candidiasis combined with symptoms of odynophagia and/or dysphagia.[29] If there is not clinical improvement over 3 to 4 days following empiric therapy, then endoscopy should be pursued to assess for coinfection or resistance.

Candidemia is diagnosed via growth on blood cultures; however, it often takes 2 to 3 days for *Candida* spp to grow in a blood culture and the sensitivity is poor, at approximately 50%.[30] In addition, different species have different rates of time to first positive blood culture, with *C glabrata* taking longer to grow compared with *C parapsilosis*.[30] This is thought to be related to the degree of fungemia burden, as *C glabrata* typically has fewer than 5 colony forming units (CFUs)/mL of blood compared with *C parapsilosis*, which typically has a high CFU/mL of blood.[31] Despite the poor sensitivity of blood cultures, this remains the gold standard given that the limit of detection for blood cultures is generally considered superior to polymerase chain reaction (PCR).[7]

Other non–culture-based methods have been the subject of recent investigation in an attempt to obtain the diagnosis earlier. T2Candida uses T2 magnetic resonance in a dedicated instrument to detect *Candida* directly in whole blood samples and is an effective adjunct to culture based methods.[30] $(1 \rightarrow 3)$-β-D-glucan, a cell wall component of multiple different fungi, including *Candida* spp, is also potentially useful in diagnosing invasive candidiasis.[7] In a pooled metanalysis for diagnosing invasive candidiasis with $(1 \rightarrow 3)$-β-D-glucan, the pooled sensitivity and specificity were 75% to 80% and 80%, respectively.[7] However, a number of conditions cause false positives, including infections caused by other fungi (eg, *Pneumocystis jirovecii*), hemodialysis, medical products containing glucan, and mucositis.[32–34]

The diagnosis of chronic disseminated candidiasis is challenging and requires a high clinical suspicion. In febrile patients with a history of prolonged neutropenia without other identifiable cause, this diagnosis should be considered. Concurrent abdominal pain and/or elevated alkaline phosphatase should prompt abdominal imaging by either computed tomography (CT) or MRI.[25] Ultrasound was originally used to describe the classic findings of chronic disseminated candidiasis: an echogenic core surrounded by a hypoechoic core (bull's eye lesion), which can also contain a central hypoechoic focus (wheel within a wheel).[35,36] CT and MRI show hypoattenuating lesions with hyperattenuating rims.[37] If imaging is consistent with chronic disseminated candidiasis, then percutaneous biopsy should be performed for culture and pathology.[25] Positive cultures for *Candida* spp or pathology demonstrating hyphae or pseudohyphae are considered proven chronic disseminated candidiasis, whereas negative pathology/culture is indicative of probable (in the setting of other mycologic support, such as positive $[1 \rightarrow 3]$-β-D glucan) or possible (no other mycologic support).[25]

Management of Local Mucocutaneous Candidiasis

The Infectious Disease Society of America published expert guidelines on candidiasis in 2015, which is the basis of our management recommendations.[7] Oropharyngeal candidiasis can typically be managed for 7 to 14 days with topical therapy, including clotrimazole troches, miconazole mucoadhesive tablets, and nystatin suspension when symptoms are mild.[7] More severe forms require systemic therapy with fluconazole for 7 to 14 days.[7] Empiric systemic therapy for 14 to 21 days with fluconazole for *Candida* esophagitis when clinical suspicion is high.[7] If dysphagia is severe enough that oral intake is prohibited, intravenous (IV) fluconazole or an echinocandin can be used.[7] *Candida* vulvovaginitis treatment in the HM/HSCT population is considered complicated.[28] Therefore, treatment should consist of 5 to 7 days of intravaginal azole (clotrimazole, miconazole, or econazole) or 3 to 5 days or oral fluconazole.[7]

Management of Invasive Candidiasis

Given the propensity for *C krusei* and *C glabrata* to be the etiology of candidemia in this population, as discussed earlier, the echinocandins (anidulafungin, caspofungin, or micafungin) are recommended as first-line therapy in the treatment of candidemia. Empiric therapy should be initiated in patients with risk factors and septic shock, as this improves mortality.[38] Given changing patterns of resistance (see **Table 1**), susceptibility testing should be performed.[7] In patients who rapidly clear their candidemia and have neutropenia resolution, duration of therapy can be 14 days with a step down to an oral triazole after clearance of candidemia (pending species identification and susceptibility testing). When neutropenia persists, suppressive therapy with an oral agent should be continued until engraftment.[7] If candidemia is complicated by endocarditis, then initial therapy should be either liposomal amphotericin B or high-dose echinocandin.[7]

Chorioretinitis management should be done in a collaborative effort with an ophthalmologist.[7] Management is partially dictated by involvement of the macula. Chorioretinitis alone requires fluconazole, voriconazole, or liposomal amphotericin B, pending susceptibilities.[7] If there is macular involvement, guidelines recommend additional intravitreal amphotericin B deoxycholate or voriconazole.[7] Duration of therapy should be 4 to 6 weeks.[7]

Chronic disseminated candidiasis management has a paucity of literature and treatment guidance is often anecdotal.[7] Therapy should be initiated with either liposomal amphotericin or an echinocandin followed by step down to fluconazole.[7] Ultimate duration is dictated by time for hepatosplenic lesions to resolve.[7] In cases in which symptoms persist despite antifungal therapy, adjunctive corticosteroids and nonsteroidal anti-inflammatories can be considered, but this is based on small studies.[7,39] Given that mortality appears to be driven by uncontrolled malignancy, management with chemotherapy and stem cell transplantation should not be withheld due to this diagnosis and can be considered following clinical improvement and control of the underlying infection.[7]

Rare Yeasts

Although occurring in only 0.6% of patients during the transplant-associated infection surveillance network (TRANSNET) study, the emergence of non-Candida, non-Cryptococcus yeast (also referred to as "cryptic yeast") warrant consideration in the HSCT and HM population.[3] The most common of these organisms are Trichosporon, Geotrichum capitatum (formerly Blastoschizomyces capitatum), Saccharomyces, Pichia, and Rhodotorula.[40] Despite their rareness, they should be considered given their high degree of mortality[41] and unfavorable susceptibility pattern.[40] Trichosporon spp are the most common of the cryptic yeast infections in patients with HMs, and is associated with fungemia and widespread disseminated disease due to hematogenous spread.[41] Because of resistance to amphotericin B and echinocandins, azoles have been the mainstay of therapy, including voriconazole and isavuconazole.[40]

INVASIVE MOLD INFECTIONS
Diagnosis for Invasive Mold Infections

The diagnosis of invasive mold infections (IMIs) is partially based on the European Organization for Research and Treatment of Cancer/Invasive Fungal Infections Cooperative Group and the Mycoses Study Group (EORTC/MSG).[42] The diagnostic criteria were revised in 2008 and categorize diagnosis as proven, probable, or possible.[42] For an IMI to be proven, it requires visualization of hyphae or melanized forms seen on histopathologic, cytopathologic, or direct microscopic evaluation from a sterile site obtained via needle aspiration or biopsy.[42] In addition, positive culture for a mold from a normally sterile site (including blood in the case of Fusarium and Scedosporium spp) obtained via a sterile procedure, such as biopsy, is considered proven.[42] Of note, this excludes cultures from bronchoalveolar lavage (BAL).[42] Probable infection is based on the presence of a host factor (neutropenia, allogeneic stem cell transplantation, use of corticosteroids for >3 weeks, use of T-cell immunosuppressants, or severe immunodeficiency), a clinical criterion (imaging findings suggestive of IMI, tracheobronchitis on bronchoscopy, sinonasal infection, central nervous system [CNS] infection), and a mycologic criterion (mold on a culture collected with nonsterile technique [ie, BAL]; galactomannan (GM) in blood, BAL fluid, or cerebrospinal fluid; and elevated β-D-glucan).[42] Possible infection is defined by host factors and clinical criteria *without* mycologic criteria.[42] Although these criteria are most commonly used for enrollment and analysis in clinical trials, they are helpful to the clinician in their description of the "certainty" of diagnosis.

With regard to noninvasive ways of investigating IMIs, the main serum markers are $(1 \rightarrow 3)$-β-D-glucan and GM. Aspergillus PCR is emerging as a viable method, and is now commercially available.[43] The goals of these assays are to have noninvasive ways to support diagnosis in a population that often has innate difficulties in obtaining invasive tissue specimens secondary to thrombocytopenia and neutropenia, putting them at increased risk of bleeding and infectious complications, respectively.[44] However, there has been significant heterogeneity in identifying the sensitivity and specificity of these assays for IMIs.[45]

In a meta-analysis from 2006, Pfeiffer and colleagues[45] demonstrated pooled sensitivity and specificity for GM in diagnosing proven invasive aspergillosis (IA) in patients with HM to be 70% and 92%, respectively. In addition, pooled sensitivity and specificity for GM in diagnosing proven IA in patients with HSCT was 65% for both.[45] However, the sensitivity and specificity improved to 79% and 86%, respectively, when the cutoff for a positive GM was greater than 0.5 optical density index (ODI).[45] These results were similar to a meta-analysis from 2015 from Leeflang and colleagues[46] in which they showed pooled sensitivity and specificity of 78% and 85% when the cutoff was greater than 0.5 ODI. Of note, Hachem and colleagues[32] showed that GM was more sensitive for non-*fumigatus Aspergillus* spp (49% compared with 6%), which further demonstrates the significant heterogeneity of the literature surrounding this assay. In a meta-analysis from 2012, Lamoth and colleagues[47] showed pooled sensitivity and specificity for β-D-glucan in IA in HM and HSCT patients was 57% and 97%, respectively. In a systematic review of the literature in 2015, it was shown that *Aspergillus* PCR had pooled sensitivity and specificity of 77% to 88% and 75% to 95%, which performed similarly to $(1 \rightarrow 3)$-β-D-glucan and GM.[43] The authors of this review proposed adding *Aspergillus* PCR to the next iteration of EORTC/MSG diagnostic guidelines.

With regard to other molds causing IMIs, $(1 \rightarrow 3)$-β-D-glucan and GM are not useful for diagnosing mucormycosis, as these serum markers are not present in the agents causing mucormycosis.[48] In the case of mucormycosis, there are molecular studies looking at PCR of BAL samples.[48] In addition, there are emerging serum and urine-based PCR diagnostics for mucormycosis that are promising.[49] However, these assays are not commercially available yet and not included in the most recent guidelines for mucormycosis diagnosis and treatment (although these guidelines are currently being updated). Therefore, diagnosis is dependent on direct microscopy of histopathology samples along with culture.[50]

Fusariosis and scedosporiosis, unlike other IMIs, are often diagnosed as fungemia using blood cultures.[51,52] Other methods of diagnosis are related to culture and/or biopsy of body sites of suspected infection.[51,52] In fusariosis, GM has been shown to have a sensitivity and specificity of 83% and 67%, respectively, in patients with HM[53]; however, this is based on a single study with small sample size. There are not sufficient patient data to support the use of $(1 \rightarrow 3)$-β-D-glucan in fusariosis.[54]

There are cases in the literature demonstrating positive GM in scedosporiosis,[55] as well as $(1\rightarrow3)$-β-D-glucan reactivity with *Scedosporium* spp[56]; however, there are insufficient data to comment on GM and $(1\rightarrow3)$-β-D-glucan levels in relation to scedosporiosis.

Invasive Aspergillosis

Epidemiology of invasive aspergillosis affecting hematopoietic stem cell transplantation recipients

The epidemiology of IA in HSCT was updated through the TRANSNET study.[3] This multisite study investigated 23 US transplant centers from 2000 to 2006 to investigate the incidence of IFIs. The overall incidence of IA at 6 and 12 months was 1.3% and 1.6%, respectively, with an overall incidence of 3.4% for all IFIs.[3] This study demonstrated that IA was the most common IFI among HSCT recipients (43% of IFIs).[3] *Aspergillus fumigatus* was the most common species in IA occurring in 44% to 45% of patients, with *Aspergillus niger* (9% of IA), *Aspergillus flavus* (7%–8% of IA), and *Aspergillus terreus* (5%–6% of IA) being the 3 most common non-*fumigatus Aspergillus* species.[3] Of note, identification to the species level was not accomplished in 23% to 26% of IA infections.[3] Median time to development of IA from HSCT was 99 days, compared with 61 for invasive candidiasis in the same population.[3] Most patients with HSCT with IA had grade III/IV graft versus host disease (GVHD) and neutropenia, and received allogeneic stem cell transplantation.[3]

Epidemiology of invasive aspergillosis affecting patients with hematologic malignancy

The SEIFEM study in 2004 was a multicenter retrospective cohort study across 18 hematology wards in Italy to better characterize IA in patents with HM, without HSCT.[4] The overall incidence of IFI was similar to HSCT at 4.6%, with IA having an incidence of 2.6.[4] Fifty-eight percent of IFIs were due to IA, with *A fumigatus* being the most common at 53%, but the breakdown of non-*fumigatus Aspergillus* spp was not available.[4] In a 10-site study in the Czech and Slovak Republics (FIND analysis), *A fumigatus* was the predominant cause of IA (79%), with *Aspergillus terreus, A niger*, and *A flavus* all occurring in 4.2% of IA.[57] Forty-three percent of the IA cases occurred during induction chemotherapy,[4] and 94% of cases occurred in patients with either acute myelocytic leukemia (AML) or acute lymphocytic leukemia (ALL).[4] A 2013 study showed that "cryptic" *Aspergillus* spp are common and are more likely to be resistant to first-line mold-active triazole agents.[58] With improvements in accurate identification of species, there will likely be improved characterization of these cryptic *Aspergillus* spp and their clinic outcomes.[59]

Clinical manifestations of invasive aspergillosis

IA has a wide variety of clinical manifestations, ranging from invasive pulmonary disease, invasive sinusitis, and disseminated disease, including CNS disease and cutaneous aspergillosis.[60] Invasive pulmonary aspergillosis (IPA) is the most common presenting syndrome, occurring in 86% to 94% of patients with HM with IA.[57,60] The most common symptom in IPA is fever, occurring in 77% to 97% of patients, and IPA should be considered in patients with prolonged fever despite broad-spectrum antibiotics.[60] Beyond fever, cough and dyspnea are predominant respiratory symptoms, occurring in 64% to 79% of patients.[57,60] Hemoptysis is a rare complication of IPA occurring only 1% to 8% of the time[57,61] compared with ~50% of patients with aspergillomas and without HM.[62]

Imaging findings in IPA for patients with HM vary and are influenced by the timing of disease and the degree of neutropenia.[63] Classically, a "halo" sign, which is a macronodule (≥1 cm in diameter) surrounded by a perimeter of ground-glass opacity, on lung CT imaging has been associated with IPA (**Fig. 1**), and has been reported to be sensitive and specific for IPA.[64] In a large study of 235 patients with IPA, only 61% of the patients had a halo sign.[63] Neutropenic patients were less likely to have a halo sign (47%) compared with non-neutropenic patients (62%), but the statistical significance of this is unclear.[63] This is potentially explained by the decreased inflammatory response in the neutropenic population, preventing the formation of the surrounding ground glass on CT imaging. The most likely abnormality in this study was a macro-nodule, which occurred in 95% of patients with IPA.[63] However, other studies have demonstrated nonspecific patterns to be the predominant abnormality, with the halo sign occurring in only 27% of patients.[57] High-resolution CT angiography is sensitive and specific in the diagnosis of invasive mold disease in the patients with hematologic malignancy.[65]

The incidence of invasive sinusitis secondary to molds was 6.1 of 100,000 patient days in a 10-year study at a large cancer center in Texas.[66] Mortality attributed to *Aspergillus* spp was 44% and 56% at 6 and 12 weeks of follow-up, respectively.[66] Symptoms typically included facial pain, swelling, nasal congestion, and erythema.[66] Sinus tenderness occurred in 31% of patients, and 54% patients who underwent a nasal endoscopic examination had a black eschar.[66] *Aspergillus* spp was the causative infection in 24% of evaluated patients.[66] Furthermore, in a study taking place in Taiwan, *A flavus* was the predominant species identified, and the investigators hypothesized that this may have been partially driven by differences in climate.[67]

CNS aspergillosis is a rare complication, accounting for 6% of IA in a single-site prospective study,[60] yet has a mortality approaching 100%.[68] In a small case series, fever was the most common symptom (57%), followed by focal neurologic deficit (36%), seizure (29%), altered level of consciousness (21%), and headache (14%).[68] There were nonspecific changes on CT/MRI, including ring-enhancing lesions and lesions expanding from the sinuses.[68]

Cutaneous aspergillosis can be either primary or secondary.[69] Primary cutaneous aspergillosis (PCA) occurs mostly in patients with large wounds, often from burns, and is typically caused by *A flavus*.[69,70] Secondary cutaneous aspergillosis (SCA) is a hallmark of disseminated aspergillosis and a harbinger of poor survival (30% 3-month survival).[69] Cutaneous aspergillosis typically presents with nodules/papules with erythema that evolves to a necrotic eschar (**Fig. 2**).[69] Any such lesions should

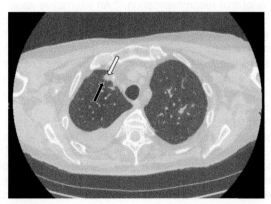

Fig. 1. CT chest demonstrating typical halo sign in a patient with chronic lymphocytic leukemia with IPA secondary to *A fumigatus*. White arrow: pulmonary nodule. Black arrow: Surrounding ground-glass opacity.

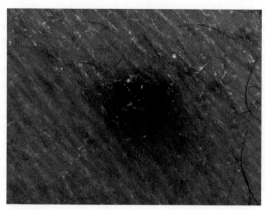

Fig. 2. Typical manifestation of disseminated mold infection to the skin: erythematous papules with central necrosis. Seen here in a patient with disseminated *S apiospermum*.

be biopsied in the HSCT and HM population, as they carry the highest risk for SCA and biopsy can aide in diagnosis.[69]

Management of invasive aspergillosis

Given the diagnostic challenges associated with IA, the role of empiric therapy must be considered. Febrile patients, who have been febrile for longer than 10 days, are at higher risk for IA.[71,72] However, it is generally recommended to wait to start empiric antifungals (liposomal amphotericin B, an echinocandin, or voriconazole) until after 96 hours of fever that persists despite empiric antibacterial antibiotics.[71] When considering empiric antifungals for IA, efforts should be made to diagnose a possible IFI definitively, particularly among those receiving antifungal prophylaxis, as recent evidence suggests a shift in IFI epidemiology with non-*Aspergillus* molds increasing in frequency.[73]

IPA should be treated initially with voriconazole or isavuconazole (unless in the setting of breakthrough infection while on azole prophylaxis).[71] A 2002 randomized clinical trial comparing voriconazole against amphotericin B deoxycholate demonstrated improved 12-week survival in the voriconazole treatment arm (71% vs 58%), which is the basis of this recommendation.[74] An alternative azole is isavuconazole, which was shown to be noninferior to voriconazole in a randomized clinical trial in 2016.[75] Liposomal amphotericin B, while having been subjected to less vigorous clinical trial assessment, can be used as an alternative initial therapy.[71] There are limited randomized clinical trials looking at combination therapy, but the consensus is to consider voriconazole and an echinocandin in combination for treatment of IPA in patients with severe disease and persistent, profound neutropenia, based on possible synergy between azoles and echinocandins.[71,76,77]

In cases in which there is breakthrough IPA despite prophylaxis, consensus is to change antifungal class while also monitoring drug levels if able and attempting to define definitive diagnosis to allow for antifungal susceptibilities.[71] The duration of treatment is not well established and largely dependent on the patient, especially considering immunosuppression and neutropenia. Expert consensus is to treat at least 6 to 12 weeks, but is dependent on severity, extent, and resolution of disease. Secondary prophylaxis is indicated on repeated or ongoing immunosuppression[71] Resolution is monitored by obtaining serial CT imaging of the chest, but with the understanding that lesions may worsen following initial neutropenia resolution.[71,78] Serial

GMs can be followed, as this appears in some studies to correlate with outcome on therapy.[71,79]

Invasive *Aspergillus* sinusitis often is treated with a combined surgical and systemic antifungal approach,[67,71] and patients often need repeated surgical debridement.[66] Treatment with a triazole as initial therapy may improve 6-week mortality.[66]

Treatment of cutaneous aspergillosis depends on if it is suspected primary cutaneous aspergillosis or SCA. Given that SCA often is a sign of disseminated aspergillosis, consensus guidelines recommend initiation of voriconazole while initiating a search for primary focus of infection.[71] PCA may be managed with a combined surgical and antifungal approach.[71]

As discussed earlier, CNS IA is a devastating disease that is almost uniformly fatal. Treatment focuses on reducing immunosuppressants and agents leading to neutropenia, while combining voriconazole with surgery (there are trends of improved mortality with this approach).[71,80] There may be benefits to combination antifungals with voriconazole and either liposomal amphotericin B or an echinocandin, but data are limited.[71]

Successful outcomes in IA are closely related to neutrophil count.[57] In the FIND analysis, there were only 21% successful outcomes in patients with an absolute neutrophil count (ANC) <100 at the end of treatment, compared with 81% in patients with an ANC greater than 1000.[57] Mortality at 3 months was 42% (predominantly contributed to by IA), compared with 57% at 12 months (predominantly contributed to by underlying conditions such as uncontrolled malignancy).[57] In the TRANSNET study, 1-year mortality was 75% in HSCT with IA, compared with 1-year all-cause mortality of 13% and 36% in autologous and allogeneic stem cell transplantation without IFIs, respectively.

MUCORMYCOSIS
Epidemiology of Mucormycosis Affecting Stem Cell Transplantation Recipients

Mucormycosis (formerly termed zygomycosis) is an invasive mold infection caused by the mucoromycetes: *Rhizopus*, *Mucor*, *Lichtheimia* (previously classified as *Absidia*), *Cunninghamella*, *Rhizomucor*, *Apophysomyces*, and *Saksenaea* with *Rhizopus* spp being the most common at 34%.[81] In the TRANSNET study, mucormycosis was the third most common IFI, accounting for 8% of cases.[3] The incidence ranged from 0.1% to 2.0% looking at 10 different series across 5 different global sites.[82] Median time to mucormycosis was 123 days.[3] GVHD and its subsequent therapy with corticosteroids have a strong association with mucormycosis.[83] This may be due to not only the immunosuppressive effects, but also the hyperglycemia caused by corticosteroids, which is an independent risk factor for mucormycosis and control of hyperglycemia improves survival.[84]

Epidemiology of Mucormycosis Affecting Patients with Hematologic Malignancy

In the SEIFEM study, the incidence of mucormycosis was 0.1% and had a similar incidence to fusariosis.[4] Mucormycosis occurred almost exclusively in patients with AML and ALL, with only 1 patient having non-Hodgkin lymphoma.[4] In a single-site analysis of mucormycosis in HM, 100% had neutropenia and 15% were on corticosteroids.[85] In a multisite analysis, 80% of patients had neutropenia and 49% of patients were on corticosteroids.[86]

Clinical Manifestations of Mucormycosis

The most common manifestations of mucormycosis in the HM and HSCT population are pulmonary (64%), sinus (25%), and CNS (19%) with gastrointestinal and cardiac disease rare (~2%) in a series of mucormycosis across 18 hospitals.[86] Pulmonary mucormycosis cannot be easily distinguished from IPA.[87] However, in cases in which there is an IMI with a negative GM, the suspicion for mucormycosis should be raised.[50] It carries a high rate of mortality, up to 76%.[87] Imaging findings are similar to aspergillosis,[87] with consolidations as the most frequent finding along with cavities in approximately 40%.[88] One distinguishing imaging finding from IPA is the reverse halo sign: an area of ground-glass opacification surrounded by consolidation, which occurs more frequently in pulmonary mucormycosis.[89]

Findings and symptoms of invasive sinusitis from mucormycosis are also similar to aspergillosis.[66] However, there is an increased predilection for mucormycosis to go to the sinuses, especially in the setting of hyperglycemia and corticosteroid use.[66] Given the angioinvasive nature of mucormycosis, sinusitis can progress to rhinocerebral mucormycosis (**Fig. 3**) and should be considered in any patient in this population who develops sinusitis with headache or neurologic deficits.[87] That being said, rhinocerebral mucormycosis was much more common in diabetic patients (33% of cases) compared with 4% of patients with malignancy.[90]

Cutaneous mucormycosis occurs less often in the HM population and HSCT, occurring in 12% and 9%, respectively.[90] Typically, cutaneous mucormycosis presents with a necrotic eschar with surrounding erythema and induration.[87]

Management of Mucormycosis

One of the biggest challenges in the management of mucormycosis is the aggressive nature of the disease that makes source control difficult combined with the difficulty in diagnosis. Delays in initiation of therapy lead to a twofold reduction in survival from 83% to 49% in a retrospective study of patients with HM.[91] First-line therapy for all forms of mucormycosis is liposomal amphotericin B with consideration of combination therapy with an echinocandin, which has shown improvements in mortality in a

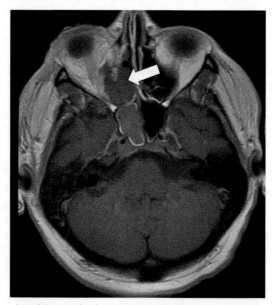

Fig. 3. MRI of invasive rhinocerebral mucormycosis (*Rhizopus* spp) in a patient receiving HSCT. *White arrow* showing rhino-orbital involvement.

retrospective study.[50,92] Unlike in aspergillosis, voriconazole is not active against mucormycosis and should be avoided.[93] However, isavuconazole appears to be effective treatment for mucormycosis in patients who cannot tolerate amphotericin B or who are being placed on an oral agent as part of suppressive management.[93,94] Given the angioinvasive nature of mucormycosis, adjunctive surgery is recommended whenever feasible.[50,82]

NON-*ASPERGILLUS* HYALINE MOLDS
Epidemiology of Non-Aspergillus Hyalohyphomycosis

Hyalohyphomycosis is a term that describes a fungal infection caused by molds whose basic tissue form is hyaline, light colored, and nonpigmented. It contains *Fusarium*, *Scedosporium*, *Lomentospora*, *Acremonium*, and *Paecilomyces* spp among others, and these infections are increasing in frequency among patients with HM and HSCT.[95–97] This review focuses on fusariosis and scedosporiosis, given the relative frequency of these infections. In the TRANSNET study, fusariosis occurred in 3% of patients with HSCT over the 6-year study.[3] In another multicenter trial of patients with HSCT, allogeneic HSCT carried the highest risk of fusariosis, with a fourfold increase in the incidence in HLA mismatched allogeneic stem cell transplantation (20.19 cases per 1000 in mismatched compared with 5 cases per 1000 in matched patients).[98] Fusariosis in the HM population was studied across 11 different sites and 56% of the cases were in acute leukemias, and prolonged neutropenia and corticosteroid use were the biggest risk factors for development of fusariosis.[99] The incidence of scedosporiosis in the HM and HSCT population increased from 0.82 cases per 100,000 patients to 1.33 cases per 100,000 patients when looking at 1993 to 1998 and 1995 to 2005, respectively.[100] As in fusariosis, the biggest risk factors for scedosporiosis are neutropenia and prior corticosteroid use.[100]

Clinical Manifestations of Fusariosis

Fusariosis differs in its presentation compared with other IMIs. It presents with fungemia in approximately half of patients with HSCT.[96,98] The most common symptom was fever, occurring in 92% of patients of a retrospective multisite study followed by skin lesions in 77% of patients.[99] Typical cutaneous manifestations are erythematous papules and nodules with and without central necrosis (similar to SCA).[99] Whereas IA and mucormycosis typically present with pulmonary symptoms and fungal sinusitis in the HM and HSCT population, fusariosis manifested only in the lungs or sinuses in 54% and 36% of cases, respectively.[99]

Clinical Manifestations of Scedosporiosis

Scedosporiosis is caused by *Scedosporium apiospermum* and *Lomentospora prolificans* (formerly *Scedosporium prolificans*). In the immunocompetent population, these organisms are known for infection following near-drowning experiences[101] or local cutaneous infections in agricultural workers following direct inoculation.[102] A comprehensive review of the literature from 2008 best characterizes its manifestations in the HSCT and HM population.[102] Pulmonary scedosporiosis is characterized by necrotizing pneumonia[102] and there is often concurrent pulmonary infection in disseminated scedosporiosis.[100] Fever was the most common symptom in sinopulmonary disease, occurring in 76% to 100% of patients.[102] As with fusariosis, there is a high propensity for dissemination, occurring in 64% of cases from a single-site retrospective study.[100] There was also a high rate of fungemia (44%)[100]; however, this seems to be more common in *L prolificans*.[102]

Management of Non-Aspergillus Hyalohyphomycosis

Management for fusariosis and scedosporiosis is challenging and both are associated with high mortality. Fusariosis has been shown to have a mortality of 67% in patients with HSCT and 65% of patients with HM,[51] although scedosporiosis has been shown to have even higher rates of mortality: ~70% with S apiospermum and ~100% in L prolificans for a total of 75%.[100]

First-line therapy for fusariosis is either liposomal amphotericin B or voriconazole.[103] Posaconazole can be used as salvage therapy. There are limited data regarding the combination of a polyene or a triazole with an echinocandin.[103] If there is significant cutaneous involvement, surgical debridement is recommended.[103] Reduction of immunosuppressive and myelosuppressive agents, if possible, is highly recommended, as persistent neutropenia or use of corticosteroids with concurrent fusariosis results in 100% mortality.[99]

Scedosporiosis management is dependent on the species involved. L prolificans has shown in vitro resistance to polyenes, azoles, and echinocandins,[104] which likely contributes to its significantly higher mortality compared with S apiospermum. S apiospermum is typically resistant to amphotericin B.[103] Guidelines recommend the use of voriconazole for S apiospermum with the use of surgical resection whenever possible (ie, cutaneous disease).[103,105] There are limited case reports/series showing the benefit of terbinafine in combination with voriconazole for both S apiospermum and L prolificans,[103] and combination therapy for all patients with HM and HSCT, given the high degree of mortality, is often recommended.

PNEUMOCYSTIS JIROVECII
Epidemiology of Pneumocystis jirovecii Affecting Stem Cell Transplantation Recipients

Before the use of prophylactic therapy, Pneumocystis jirovecii pneumonia (PJP) occurred in 5% to 16% of patients with allogeneic stem cell transplantation.[106] This has been reduced to fewer than 5% of patients since the widespread implementation of prophylactic antimicrobials starting in the early 1980s.[107] In the HSCT population, PJP can develop early (up to 6 months from HSCT) and late (after 6 months).[107] In a retrospective study of patients receiving HSCT at a single site, all of the early PJP infections occurred despite prophylaxis, in the setting of severe GVHD requiring high dose of immunosuppression.[107] The late PJP infections occurred 14.5 months from HSCT, on average, and none of the patients were receiving prophylaxis despite significant immunosuppression in all of the patients.[107] The incidence of PJP was 2.5%, which is greater than the incidence of less than 0.25% in the TRANSNET study. The median time to PJP infection was considerably less (~5 months) in the TRANSNET study.[3,107] Of note, both of these studies had only 13 patients with PJP, which could explain the large differences.

Epidemiology of Pneumocystis jirovecii Affecting Patients with Hematologic Malignancy

A retrospective study of PJP in patients with cancer was performed at MD Anderson Cancer Center from 1990 to 2003 to better characterize risk of PJP in HM.[108] The incidence in patients with HM was 187 per 100,000 patients compared with 16 and 386 for patients with solid malignancies and HSCT, respectively.[108] Forty-nine percent of the patients had leukemia and 45% had lymphoma[108]; 75% of the patients with HM had lymphopenia, with a median duration of 135 days and a median CD4+ T lymphocyte count of 55[108]; and 63% and 66% of patients were on corticosteroids and chemotherapy, respectively.[108]

Diagnosis of Pneumocystis jirovecii Pneumonia

The diagnosis of PJP should be considered in patients with risk factors, as described previously, who have symptoms of fever, dry cough, and dyspnea. Compared with PJP in adult patients with AIDS, there is a decreased burden of *P jirovecii* organisms in BAL fluid, which makes the diagnosis more difficult in patients who do not have AIDS.[109,110] Diagnosis is dependent on direct microscopic visualization of the organisms via direct fluorescent antibody (DFA) test or a variety of other stains[110] on either induced sputum or BAL. PCR for *P jirovecii* from BAL samples had a sensitivity of 87% and specificity of 92% when using DFA as the gold standard[111]; however, the positive predictive value was only 51% due to false positives in the setting of *P jirovecii* colonization; $(1 \rightarrow 3)$-β-D-glucan has also been found to be an effective screening tool for PJP with a pooled sensitivity of 96% in a meta-analysis from 2012.[112]

Clinical Manifestations of Pneumocystis jirovecii

Torres and colleagues[108] provided a 13-year retrospective study of patients with HM and found fever (86% of patients), dyspnea (75%), and dry cough (70%) were the predominant symptoms. Sixty percent of patients with HM had an arterial oxygen level less than 70 mm Hg compared with 35% of patients receiving HSCT.[108] Approximately 90% of patients present with bilateral infiltrates, ~70% patients had an interstitial pattern, and 13% of patients receiving HSCT had a spontaneous pneumothorax.[108] Mortality attributed to PJP was 29% in the patients with HM patients and 48% of the patients receiving HSCT.

Treatment of Pneumocystis jirovecii Pneumonia

Prophylaxis for PJP is indicated in patients with ALL, allogeneic HSCT, treatment with alemtuzumab, fludarabine/cyclophosphamide/rituximab combinations, or more than 4 weeks of treatment with corticosteroids (equivalent of $\geq$20 mg of prednisone per day).[113] Trimethoprim/sulfamethoxazole (TMP/SMX) is the first-line agent for prophylaxis with atovaquone, dapsone, and pentamidine as alternative agents.

Treatment of PJP is dependent on severity of disease (mild, moderate, or severe), which can be determined from oxygen saturation (SaO2) on room air and arterial oxygen level (Pao$_2$).[114] Pao$_2$ greater than 82.5 mm Hg and SaO2 greater than 96% is considered mild, Pao$_2$ 60.75 to 82.5 mm Hg and SaO2 91% to 96% is considered moderate, and Pao$_2$ less than 60% and SaO2 less than 91% is considered severe.[114] Mild disease can be treated with oral TMP/SMX for 2 to 3 weeks. Moderate-severe disease should be treated with IV TMP/SMX for 3 weeks.[114] The role of adjunctive glucocorticoids in patients not infected with human immunodeficiency virus has not been well defined and significant variability in practice patterns exists; they should be considered on an individual basis.[114]

SUMMARY

IFIs are a rare complication in the HM and HSCT population; however, they tend to be a devastating complication associated with high rates of mortality, approaching 100% in certain cases. Despite prophylaxis, we continue to see an incidence of IFIs of approximately 3.5%. In an age of novel chemotherapeutics and a growing immunosuppressed population, infectious complications remain problematic.[115] The incidence of breakthrough and newly described IFIs may increase as novel immunosuppressive agents are introduced. The scope of prophylaxis will need to be reevaluated to reflect new risk factors, and continued physician vigilance in the monitoring of patients in this population for the development of IFIs is needed.

ACKNOWLEDGMENTS

Support for this paper provided in part by the Burden Family Valley Fever Fund.

REFERENCES

1. Goodman JL, Winston DJ, Greenfield RA, et al. A controlled trial of fluconazole to prevent fungal infections in patients undergoing bone marrow transplantation. N Engl J Med 1992;326(13):845–51.
2. Cornely OA, Maertens J, Winston DJ, et al. Posaconazole vs. fluconazole or itraconazole prophylaxis in patients with neutropenia. N Engl J Med 2007;356(4): 348–59.
3. Kontoyiannis DP, Marr KA, Park BJ, et al. Prospective surveillance for invasive fungal infections in hematopoietic stem cell transplant recipients, 2001-2006: overview of the transplant-associated infection surveillance network (TRANSNET) database. Clin Infect Dis 2010;50(8):1091–100.
4. Pagano L, Caira M, Candoni A, et al. The epidemiology of fungal infections in patients with hematologic malignancies: the SEIFEM-2004 study. Haematologica 2006;91(8):1068–75.
5. Verfaillie C, Weisdorf D, Haake R, et al. Candida infections in bone marrow transplant recipients. Bone Marrow Transplant 1991;8(3):177–84.
6. Van Burik JA, Leisenring W, Myerson D, et al. The effect of prophylactic fluconazole on the clinical spectrum of fungal diseases in bone marrow transplant recipients with special attention to hepatic candidiasis: an autopsy study of 355 patients. Medicine 1998;77(4):246–54.
7. Pappas PG, Kauffman CA, Andes DR, et al. Clinical practice guideline for the management of candidiasis: 2016 update by the Infectious Diseases Society of America. Clin Infect Dis 2016;62(4):e1–50.
8. Alexander BD, Johnson MD, Pfeiffer CD, et al. Increasing echinocandin resistance in *Candida glabrata*: clinical failure correlates with presence of fks mutations and elevated minimum inhibitory concentrations. Clin Infect Dis 2013; 56(12):1724–32.
9. Branchini ML, Pfaller MA, Rhine-Chalberg J, et al. Genotypic variation and slime production among blood and catheter isolates of *Candida parapsilosis*. J Clin Microbiol 1994;32(2):452–6.
10. Sipsas NV, Lewis RE, Tarrand J, et al. Candidemia in patients with hematologic malignancies in the era of new antifungal agents (2001-2007): stable incidence but changing epidemiology of a still frequently lethal infection. Cancer 2009; 115(20):4745–52.
11. Yapar N. Epidemiology and risk factors for invasive candidiasis. Ther Clin Risk Manag 2014;10:95–105.
12. Dewan E, Biswas D, Kakati B, et al. Epidemiological and mycological characteristics of candidemia in patients with hematological malignancies attending a tertiary-care center in India. Hematol Oncol Stem Cell Ther 2015;8(3):99–105.
13. Zirkel J, Klinker H, Kuhn A, et al. Epidemiology of Candida blood stream infections in patients with hematological malignancies or solid tumors. Med Mycol 2012;50(1):50–5.
14. Hachem R, Hanna H, Kontoyiannis D, et al. The changing epidemiology of invasive candidiasis: *Candida glabrata* and *Candida krusei* as the leading causes of candidemia in hematologic malignancy. Cancer 2008;112(11):2493–9.
15. Lockhart SR, Iqbal N, Cleveland AA, et al. Species identification and antifungal susceptibility testing of Candida bloodstream isolates from population-based

surveillance studies in two U.S. cities from 2008 to 2011. J Clin Microbiol 2012; 50(11):3435–42.

16. Schelenz S, Abdallah S, Gray G, et al. Epidemiology of oral yeast colonization and infection in patients with hematological malignancies, head neck and solid tumors. J Oral Pathol Med 2011;40(1):83–9.

17. Epstein JB, Hancock PJ, Nantel S. Oral candidiasis in hematopoietic cell transplantation patients: an outcome-based analysis. Oral Surg Oral Med Oral Pathol Oral Radiol Endod 2003;96(2):154–63.

18. Thompson GR 3rd, Patel PK, Kirkpatrick WR, et al. Oropharyngeal candidiasis in the era of antiretroviral therapy. Oral Surg Oral Med Oral Pathol Oral Radiol Endod 2010;109(4):488–95.

19. Antinori S, Milazzo L, Sollima S, et al. Candidemia and invasive candidiasis in adults: a narrative review. Eur J Intern Med 2016;34:21–8.

20. Lortholary O, Renaudat C, Sitbon K, et al. The risk and clinical outcome of candidemia depending on underlying malignancy. Intensive Care Med 2017;43(5): 652–62.

21. Slavin MA, Sorrell TC, Marriott D, et al. Candidaemia in adult cancer patients: risks for fluconazole-resistant isolates and death. J Antimicrob Chemother 2010;65(5):1042–51.

22. Kullberg BJ, Viscoli C, Pappas PG, et al. Isavuconazole versus caspofungin in the treatment of candidemia and other invasive candida infections: the active trial. Clin Infect Dis 2018. [Epub ahead of print].

23. Shah CP, McKey J, Spirn MJ, et al. Ocular candidiasis: a review. Br J Ophthalmol 2008;92(4):466–8.

24. Baddley JW, Benjamin DK Jr, Patel M, et al. Candida infective endocarditis. Eur J Clin Microbiol Infect Dis 2008;27(7):519–29.

25. Rammaert B, Desjardins A, Lortholary O. New insights into hepatosplenic candidosis, a manifestation of chronic disseminated candidosis. Mycoses 2012; 55(3):e74–84.

26. Kontoyiannis DP, Luna MA, Samuels BI, et al. Hepatosplenic candidiasis. A manifestation of chronic disseminated candidiasis. Infect Dis Clin North Am 2000;14(3):721–39.

27. De Castro N, Mazoyer E, Porcher R, et al. Hepatosplenic candidiasis in the era of new antifungal drugs: a study in Paris 2000-2007. Clin Microbiol Infect 2012; 18(6):E185–7.

28. Sobel JD. Vulvovaginal candidosis. Lancet 2007;369(9577):1961–71.

29. Benson CA, Kaplan JE, Masur H, et al. Treating opportunistic infections among HIV-infected adults and adolescents: recommendations from CDC, the National Institutes of Health, and the HIV medicine association/Infectious Diseases Society of America. MMWR Recomm Rep 2004;53(RR-15):1–112.

30. Clancy CJ, Nguyen MH. Finding the "missing 50%" of invasive candidiasis: how nonculture diagnostics will improve understanding of disease spectrum and transform patient care. Clin Infect Dis 2013;56(9):1284–92.

31. Pfeiffer CD, Samsa GP, Schell WA, et al. Quantitation of Candida CFU in initial positive blood cultures. J Clin Microbiol 2011;49(8):2879–83.

32. Hachem RY, Kontoyiannis DP, Chemaly RF, et al. Utility of galactomannan enzyme immunoassay and (1,3) beta-d-glucan in diagnosis of invasive fungal infections: low sensitivity for *Aspergillus fumigatus* infection in hematologic malignancy patients. J Clin Microbiol 2009;47(1):129–33.

33. Pickering JW, Sant HW, Bowles CA, et al. Evaluation of a (1->3)-beta-d-glucan assay for diagnosis of invasive fungal infections. J Clin Microbiol 2005;43(12): 5957–62.

34. Mennink-Kersten MA, Warris A, Verweij PE. 1,3-beta-d-glucan in patients receiving intravenous amoxicillin-clavulanic acid. N Engl J Med 2006;354(26): 2834–5.

35. Pastakia B, Shawker TH, Thaler M, et al. Hepatosplenic candidiasis: wheels within wheels. Radiology 1988;166(2):417–21.

36. Lawrence PH, Holt SC, Levi CS, et al. Ultrasound case of the day. Hepatosplenic candidiasis. Radiographics 1994;14(5):1147–9.

37. Cornely OA, Bangard C, Jaspers NI. Hepatosplenic candidiasis. Clin Liver Dis 2015;6(2):47–50.

38. Kollef M, Micek S, Hampton N, et al. Septic shock attributed to candida infection: importance of empiric therapy and source control. Clin Infect Dis 2012; 54(12):1739–46.

39. Chaussade H, Bastides F, Lissandre S, et al. Usefulness of corticosteroid therapy during chronic disseminated candidiasis: case reports and literature review. J Antimicrob Chemother 2012;67(6):1493–5.

40. Thompson GR 3rd, Wiederhold NP, Sutton DA, et al. In vitro activity of isavuconazole against Trichosporon, Rhodotorula, Geotrichum, Saccharomyces and Pichia species. J Antimicrob Chemother 2009;64(1):79–83.

41. Pfaller MA, Diekema DJ. Rare and emerging opportunistic fungal pathogens: concern for resistance beyond Candida albicans and Aspergillus fumigatus. J Clin Microbiol 2004;42(10):4419–31.

42. De Pauw B, Walsh TJ, Donnelly JP, et al. Revised definitions of invasive fungal disease from the European Organization for Research and Treatment of Cancer/ Invasive Fungal Infections Cooperative Group and the National Institute of Allergy and Infectious Diseases Mycoses Study Group (EORTC/MSG) consensus group. Clin Infect Dis 2008;46(12):1813–21.

43. White PL, Wingard JR, Bretagne S, et al. Aspergillus polymerase chain reaction: systematic review of evidence for clinical use in comparison with antigen testing. Clin Infect Dis 2015;61(8):1293–303.

44. Masur H, Shelhamer J, Parrillo JE. The management of pneumonias in immunocompromised patients. JAMA 1985;253(12):1769–73.

45. Pfeiffer CD, Fine JP, Safdar N. Diagnosis of invasive aspergillosis using a galactomannan assay: a meta-analysis. Clin Infect Dis 2006;42(10):1417–27.

46. Leeflang MM, Debets-Ossenkopp YJ, Wang J, et al. Galactomannan detection for invasive aspergillosis in immunocompromised patients. Cochrane Database Syst Rev 2015;(12):CD007394.

47. Lamoth F, Cruciani M, Mengoli C, et al. Beta-glucan antigenemia assay for the diagnosis of invasive fungal infections in patients with hematological malignancies: a systematic review and meta-analysis of cohort studies from the Third European Conference on Infections in Leukemia (ECIL-3). Clin Infect Dis 2012; 54(5):633–43.

48. Lengerova M, Racil Z, Hrncirova K, et al. Rapid detection and identification of Mucormycetes in bronchoalveolar lavage samples from immunocompromised patients with pulmonary infiltrates by use of high-resolution melt analysis. J Clin Microbiol 2014;52(8):2824–8.

49. Baldin C, Soliman SSM, Jeon HH, et al. PCR-based approach targeting mucorales-specific gene family for diagnosis of mucormycosis. J Clin Microbiol 2018;56(10) [pii:e00746-18].

50. Cornely OA, Arikan-Akdagli S, Dannaoui E, et al. ESCMID and ECMM joint clinical guidelines for the diagnosis and management of mucormycosis 2013. Clin Microbiol Infect 2014;20(Suppl 3):5–26.
51. Campo M, Lewis RE, Kontoyiannis DP. Invasive fusariosis in patients with hematologic malignancies at a cancer center: 1998-2009. J Infect 2010;60(5):331–7.
52. Rodriguez-Tudela JL, Berenguer J, Guarro J, et al. Epidemiology and outcome of scedosporium prolificans infection, a review of 162 cases. Med Mycol 2009; 47(4):359–70.
53. Nucci M, Carlesse F, Cappellano P, et al. Earlier diagnosis of invasive fusariosis with aspergillus serum galactomannan testing. PLoS One 2014;9(1):e87784.
54. Ostrosky-Zeichner L, Alexander BD, Kett DH, et al. Multicenter clinical evaluation of the (1–>3) beta-d-glucan assay as an aid to diagnosis of fungal infections in humans. Clin Infect Dis 2005;41(5):654–9.
55. Grenouillet F, Botterel F, Crouzet J, et al. Scedosporium prolificans: an emerging pathogen in France? Med Mycol 2009;47(4):343–50.
56. Odabasi Z, Paetznick VL, Rodriguez JR, et al. Differences in beta-glucan levels in culture supernatants of a variety of fungi. Med Mycol 2006;44(3):267–72.
57. Racil Z, Weinbergerova B, Kocmanova I, et al. Invasive aspergillosis in patients with hematological malignancies in the Czech and Slovak republics: fungal infection database (FIND) analysis, 2005-2009. Int J Infect Dis 2013;17(2): e101–9.
58. Alastruey-Izquierdo A, Mellado E, Pelaez T, et al. Population-based survey of filamentous fungi and antifungal resistance in Spain (FILPOP study). Antimicrob Agents Chemother 2013;57(7):3380–7.
59. Negri CE, Goncalves SS, Xafranski H, et al. Cryptic and rare aspergillus species in Brazil: prevalence in clinical samples and in vitro susceptibility to triazoles. J Clin Microbiol 2014;52(10):3633–40.
60. Nicolle MC, Benet T, Thiebaut A, et al. Invasive aspergillosis in patients with hematologic malignancies: incidence and description of 127 cases enrolled in a single institution prospective survey from 2004 to 2009. Haematologica 2011; 96(11):1685–91.
61. Cornillet A, Camus C, Nimubona S, et al. Comparison of epidemiological, clinical, and biological features of invasive aspergillosis in neutropenic and nonneutropenic patients: a 6-year survey. Clin Infect Dis 2006;43(5):577–84.
62. Rafferty P, Biggs BA, Crompton GK, et al. What happens to patients with pulmonary aspergilloma? Analysis of 23 cases. Thorax 1983;38(8):579–83.
63. Greene RE, Schlamm HT, Oestmann JW, et al. Imaging findings in acute invasive pulmonary aspergillosis: clinical significance of the halo sign. Clin Infect Dis 2007;44(3):373–9.
64. Blum U, Windfuhr M, Buitrago-Tellez C, et al. Invasive pulmonary aspergillosis. MRI, CT, and plain radiographic findings and their contribution for early diagnosis. Chest 1994;106(4):1156–61.
65. Stanzani M, Sassi C, Lewis RE, et al. High resolution computed tomography angiography improves the radiographic diagnosis of invasive mold disease in patients with hematological malignancies. Clin Infect Dis 2015;60(11):1603–10.
66. Davoudi S, Kumar VA, Jiang Y, et al. Invasive mould sinusitis in patients with haematological malignancies: a 10 year single-centre study. J Antimicrob Chemother 2015;70(10):2899–905.
67. Chen CY, Sheng WH, Cheng A, et al. Invasive fungal sinusitis in patients with hematological malignancy: 15 years experience in a single university hospital in Taiwan. BMC Infect Dis 2011;11:250.

68. Kourkoumpetis TK, Desalermos A, Muhammed M, et al. Central nervous system aspergillosis: a series of 14 cases from a general hospital and review of 123 cases from the literature. Medicine (Baltimore) 2012;91(6):328–36.

69. Bernardeschi C, Foulet F, Ingen-Housz-Oro S, et al. Cutaneous invasive aspergillosis: retrospective multicenter study of the French invasive-aspergillosis registry and literature review. Medicine (Baltimore) 2015;94(26):e1018.

70. van Burik JA, Colven R, Spach DH. Cutaneous aspergillosis. J Clin Microbiol 1998;36(11):3115–21.

71. Patterson TF, Thompson GR 3rd, Denning DW, et al. Practice guidelines for the diagnosis and management of aspergillosis: 2016 update by the Infectious Diseases Society of America. Clin Infect Dis 2016;63(4):e1–60.

72. Caselli D, Cesaro S, Ziino O, et al. A prospective, randomized study of empirical antifungal therapy for the treatment of chemotherapy-induced febrile neutropenia in children. Br J Haematol 2012;158(2):249–55.

73. Lamoth F, Chung SJ, Damonti L, et al. Changing epidemiology of invasive mold infections in patients receiving azole prophylaxis. Clin Infect Dis 2017;64(11): 1619–21.

74. Herbrecht R, Denning DW, Patterson TF, et al. Voriconazole versus amphotericin b for primary therapy of invasive aspergillosis. N Engl J Med 2002;347(6): 408–15.

75. Maertens JA, Raad II, Marr KA, et al. Isavuconazole versus voriconazole for primary treatment of invasive mould disease caused by aspergillus and other filamentous fungi (secure): a phase 3, randomised-controlled, non-inferiority trial. Lancet 2016;387(10020):760–9.

76. Clemons KV, Stevens DA. Efficacy of micafungin alone or in combination against experimental pulmonary aspergillosis. Med Mycol 2006;44(1):69–73.

77. Kontoyiannis DP, Ratanatharathorn V, Young JA, et al. Micafungin alone or in combination with other systemic antifungal therapies in hematopoietic stem cell transplant recipients with invasive aspergillosis: short communication. Transpl Infect Dis 2009;11(1):89–93.

78. Caillot D, Couaillier JF, Bernard A, et al. Increasing volume and changing characteristics of invasive pulmonary aspergillosis on sequential thoracic computed tomography scans in patients with neutropenia. J Clin Oncol 2001;19(1):253–9.

79. Park SH, Choi SM, Lee DG, et al. Serum galactomannan strongly correlates with outcome of invasive aspergillosis in acute leukaemia patients. Mycoses 2011; 54(6):523–30.

80. Schwartz S, Ruhnke M, Ribaud P, et al. Improved outcome in central nervous system aspergillosis, using voriconazole treatment. Blood 2005;106(8):2641–5.

81. Skiada A, Pagano L, Groll A, et al. Zygomycosis in Europe: analysis of 230 cases accrued by the registry of the European Confederation of Medical Mycology (ECMM) working group on zygomycosis between 2005 and 2007. Clin Microbiol Infect 2011;17(12):1859–67.

82. Lanternier F, Sun HY, Ribaud P, et al. Mucormycosis in organ and stem cell transplant recipients. Clin Infect Dis 2012;54(11):1629–36.

83. Marr KA, Carter RA, Crippa F, et al. Epidemiology and outcome of mould infections in hematopoietic stem cell transplant recipients. Clin Infect Dis 2002;34(7): 909–17.

84. Yohai RA, Bullock JD, Aziz AA, et al. Survival factors in rhino-orbital-cerebral mucormycosis. Surv Ophthalmol 1994;39(1):3–22.

85. Nosari A, Oreste P, Montillo M, et al. Mucormycosis in hematologic malignancies: an emerging fungal infection. Haematologica 2000;85(10):1068–71.

86. Pagano L, Offidani M, Fianchi L, et al. Mucormycosis in hematologic patients. Haematologica 2004;89(2):207–14.
87. Petrikkos G, Skiada A, Lortholary O, et al. Epidemiology and clinical manifestations of mucormycosis. Clin Infect Dis 2012;54(Suppl 1):S23–34.
88. McAdams HP, Rosado de Christenson M, Strollo DC, et al. Pulmonary mucormycosis: radiologic findings in 32 cases. AJR Am J Roentgenol 1997;168(6): 1541–8.
89. Wahba H, Truong MT, Lei X, et al. Reversed halo sign in invasive pulmonary fungal infections. Clin Infect Dis 2008;46(11):1733–7.
90. Roden MM, Zaoutis TE, Buchanan WL, et al. Epidemiology and outcome of zygomycosis: a review of 929 reported cases. Clin Infect Dis 2005;41(5):634–53.
91. Chamilos G, Lewis RE, Kontoyiannis DP. Delaying amphotericin b-based frontline therapy significantly increases mortality among patients with hematologic malignancy who have zygomycosis. Clin Infect Dis 2008;47(4):503–9.
92. Reed C, Bryant R, Ibrahim AS, et al. Combination polyene-caspofungin treatment of rhino-orbital-cerebral mucormycosis. Clin Infect Dis 2008;47(3):364–71.
93. Guinea J, Pelaez T, Recio S, et al. In vitro antifungal activities of isavuconazole (BAL4815), voriconazole, and fluconazole against 1,007 isolates of zygomycete, *Candida, Aspergillus, Fusarium*, and *Scedosporium* species. Antimicrob Agents Chemother 2008;52(4):1396–400.
94. Marty FM, Ostrosky-Zeichner L, Cornely OA, et al. VITAL and FungiScope Mucormycosis Investigators. Isavuconazole treatment for mucormycosis: a single-arm open-label trial and case-control analysis. Lancet Infect Dis 2016; 16(7):828–37.
95. Nucci M, Anaissie E. Emerging fungi. Infect Dis Clin North Am 2006;20(3): 563–79.
96. Nucci M. Emerging moulds: *Fusarium, Scedosporium* and zygomycetes in transplant recipients. Curr Opin Infect Dis 2003;16(6):607–12.
97. Riches ML, Trifilio S, Chen M, et al. Risk factors and impact of non-*Aspergillus* mold infections following allogeneic HCT: a CIBMTR Infection & Immune Reconstitution analysis. Bone Marrow Transplant 2016;51(2):277–82. Corrigendum 51(3):322.
98. Nucci M, Marr KA, Queiroz-Telles F, et al. *Fusarium* infection in hematopoietic stem cell transplant recipients. Clin Infect Dis 2004;38(9):1237–42.
99. Nucci M, Anaissie EJ, Queiroz-Telles F, et al. Outcome predictors of 84 patients with hematologic malignancies and *Fusarium* infection. Cancer 2003;98(2): 315–9.
100. Lamaris GA, Chamilos G, Lewis RE, et al. *Scedosporium* infection in a tertiary care cancer center: a review of 25 cases from 1989-2006. Clin Infect Dis 2006;43(12):1580–4.
101. McCarthy M, Rosengart A, Schuetz AN, et al. Mold infections of the central nervous system. N Engl J Med 2014;371(2):150–60.
102. Cortez KJ, Roilides E, Quiroz-Telles F, et al. Infections caused by *Scedosporium* spp. Clin Microbiol Rev 2008;21(1):157–97.
103. Tortorano AM, Richardson M, Roilides E, et al. ESCMID and ECMM joint guidelines on diagnosis and management of hyalohyphomycosis: *Fusarium* spp., *Scedosporium* spp. and others. Clin Microbiol Infect 2014;20(Suppl 3):27–46.
104. Cuenca-Estrella M, Gomez-Lopez A, Mellado E, et al. Head-to-head comparison of the activities of currently available antifungal agents against 3,378 Spanish clinical isolates of yeasts and filamentous fungi. Antimicrob Agents Chemother 2006;50(3):917–21.

105. Troke P, Aquirrebengoa K, Arteaga C, et al. Treatment of scedosporiosis with voriconazole: clinical experience with 107 patients. Antimicrob Agents Chemother 2008;52(5):1743–50.

106. Meyers JD, Flournoy N, Thomas ED. Nonbacterial pneumonia after allogeneic marrow transplantation: a review of ten years' experience. Rev Infect Dis 1982;4(6):1119–32.

107. De Castro N, Neuville S, Sarfati C, et al. Occurrence of *Pneumocystis jirovecii* pneumonia after allogeneic stem cell transplantation: a 6-year retrospective study. Bone Marrow Transplant 2005;36(10):879–83.

108. Torres HA, Chemaly RF, Storey R, et al. Influence of type of cancer and hematopoietic stem cell transplantation on clinical presentation of *Pneumocystis jirovecii* pneumonia in cancer patients. Eur J Clin Microbiol Infect Dis 2006;25(6): 382–8.

109. Limper AH, Offord KP, Smith TF, et al. . *Pneumocystis carinii* pneumonia. Differences in lung parasite number and inflammation in patients with and without AIDS. Am Rev Respir Dis 1989;140(5):1204–9.

110. Thomas CF Jr, Limper AH. *Pneumocystis* pneumonia. N Engl J Med 2004; 350(24):2487–98.

111. Azoulay E, Bergeron A, Chevret S, et al. Polymerase chain reaction for diagnosing *Pneumocystis* pneumonia in non-HIV immunocompromised patients with pulmonary infiltrates. Chest 2009;135(3):655–61.

112. Onishi A, Sugiyama D, Kogata Y, et al. Diagnostic accuracy of serum 1,3-beta-d-glucan for *Pneumocystis jirovecii* pneumonia, invasive candidiasis, and invasive aspergillosis: systematic review and meta-analysis. J Clin Microbiol 2012; 50(1):7–15.

113. Maertens J, Cesaro S, Maschmeyer G, et al. ECIL guidelines for preventing *Pneumocystis jirovecii* pneumonia in patients with haematological malignancies and stem cell transplant recipients. J Antimicrob Chemother 2016;71(9): 2397–404.

114. Maschmeyer G, Helweg-Larsen J, Pagano L, et al. ECIL guidelines for treatment of *Pneumocystis jirovecii* pneumonia in non-HIV-infected haematology patients. J Antimicrob Chemother 2016;71(9):2405–13.

115. Morrison VA. Immunosuppression associated with novel chemotherapy agents and monoclonal antibodies. Clin Infect Dis 2014;59(Suppl 5):S360–4.

Parasitic Infections of the Stem Cell Transplant Recipient and the Hematologic Malignancy Patient, Including Toxoplasmosis and Strongyloidiasis

Driele Peixoto, MD[a],*, Daniel P. Prestes, MD[b,c]

KEYWORDS

- Parasitic infections • Hematopoietic stem cell transplantation • Immunosuppression
- Toxoplasmosis • Strongyloidiasis

KEY POINTS

- Parasitic infections are an emerging and potentially serious complication in HSCT.
- Diagnosis of toxoplasmosis can be challenging in the HSCT scenario, and it usually requires a high clinical suspicion as it may present with pleotropic symptoms.
- In the HSCT recipients and hematologic malignancy patients using immunosuppression may lead to severe forms of Strongyloides infection.
- In the setting of HSCT recipients and hematologic malignancy patients unusual parasitic infections such as leishmaniasis, chagas disease, malaria, schistosomiasis and other parasitic infections may occur.

INTRODUCTION

In the past decade, advances in the new antimicrobial agents, expanded immunosuppression protocols, and increased knowledge of immune reconstitution have led to changes in recommendations for prevention of infection in hematopoietic stem cell transplantation (HSCT) recipients. Despite these advances, infection is reported as the primary cause of death in up to 8% of autologous HSCT recipients and ranges from 17% to 20% of allogeneic (allo) HSCT patients.[1]

Disclosures: All authors report no conflict of interest.
[a] São Paulo State Cancer Institute (ICESP), Hospital das Clínicas, Av. Dr. Arnaldo, 251, São Paulo CEP: 01246-000, Brazil; [b] A. C. Camargo Cancer Center, Rua Professor Antonio Prudente, 211, Sao Paulo CEP: 01509-010, Brazil; [c] Emilio Ribas Infectious Diseases Institute, Av. Doutor Arnaldo, 165, Sao Paulo CEP: 01246-900, Brazil
* Corresponding author.
E-mail address: driele.peixoto@yahoo.com.br

Infect Dis Clin N Am 33 (2019) 567–591
https://doi.org/10.1016/j.idc.2019.02.009
0891-5520/19/© 2019 Elsevier Inc. All rights reserved.

id.theclinics.com

Nevertheless, the proportion of parasitic infections among HSCT patients seems to be lower than that of bacterial and viral infection, with an estimated frequency reported between 0.31% and 10%.[2] However, it is not known whether this small proportion is due to a small number of cases or if there is an underestimated reporting of cases, as parasitic diseases are often neglected and mainly occur in underdeveloped countries where the access to diagnostic methods is underresourced.

Therefore, in view of the increasing number of transplants performed worldwide and the severity of these diseases and their impact on public health, a better knowledge of parasitic infections would help to minimize their potentially fatal outcomes and improve patient care. This article reviews the key aspects of parasitic infections in individuals with hematologic malignancy and recipients of stem cell transplantations.

TOXOPLASMOSIS

Toxoplasma gondii is a ubiquitous intracellular protozoan parasite. Transmission to human host occurs by ingestion of raw or undercooked meat containing tissue cysts, by exposure to oocysts in soil contaminated with cat feces, or transplacentally (**Fig. 1**).

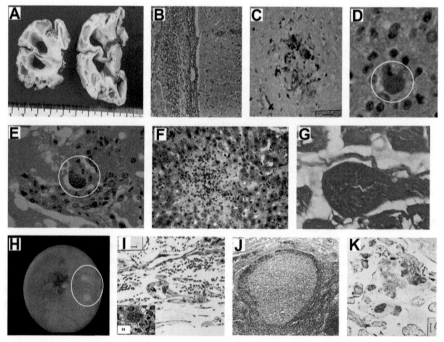

Fig. 1. Toxoplasmosis. (*A*) CNS congenital toxoplasmosis: dilated cerebral ventriculus and thinning of the cortex. (*B*) Histopathologic observation of a *Toxoplasma* meningoencephalitis with a mononuclear and polymorphonuclear infiltrate leading to a meningeal thickening. (*C*) *T gondii* immunohistochemical reaction in a microglial nodule. (*D*) *T cruzi* cyst within a microglial nodule. (*E*) Toxoplasmosis interstitial pneumonia with hemorrhage and a *T gondii* pseudocyst. (*F*) *T gondii* immunohistochemical reaction in the liver acinar cells. (*G*) *T gondii* pseudocyst in the myocardial cell. (*H*) Ocular toxoplasmosis showing whitish thickenings. (*I*) Toxoplasmosis retinitis immunohistochemical reaction showing *T gondii* antigens. (*I1*) Electron microscopy showing a *T gondii* pseudocysts in the retina. (*J*) Reactional lymph node with a lymphoid and germinative center hyperplasia. (*K*) *T gondii* antigens expressed in the placental villi. (*Courtesy of* Dr Maria Irma Seixas Duarte, MD, PhD, Sao Paulo, Brazil.)

Its prevalence varies geographically from less than 15% in the United States to 50% to 80% in Central Europe and some regions in Latin America (**Table 1**). In healthy individuals, primary infection is seldom asymptomatic; it usually manifests as fever and lymphadenopathy and is commonly diagnosed by serology.[3–5]

In immunocompromised patients such as HSCT recipients, toxoplasmosis is usually the result of a reactivation of a latent infection in seropositive patients rather than primary infection.[6] In this setting, *T gondii* presentation may include severe invasive organ disease as well as disseminated forms.[7] Most cases occur within the first 100 days following transplantation. The highest-risk patients are seropositive allo-HSCT recipients who have received cord blood transplant, unrelated donor graft, or T cell–depleted transplants, those with prior high-grade graft-versus-host disease (GVHD), and those who are unable to take trimethoprim-sulfamethoxazole (TMP/SMX) for *Pneumocystis jirovecii* prophylaxis.[8,9]

Several studies have reported an incidence of 0.3% to 8% in the first year after HSCT, depending on the seroprevalence of *T gondii* in the post-transplant toxoplasmosis studied population.[9] Additionally the prognosis of toxoplasmosis is poor, with reported mortality rates of up to 60%, including a considerable proportion of cases diagnosed post mortem, mostly in cases of disseminated disease.[10]

In immunocompromised patients, the clinical presentation may vary from constitutional symptoms such as fever, headache, and lymphadenopathy to symptoms of single-organ invasive disease, and to disseminated disease including myocarditis, pneumonitis, retinitis, and hepatitis (see **Fig. 1**).[7] In the immunosuppression scenario, the most commonly affected organ is the central nervous system (CNS), when clinical manifestations may include headache, altered mental status, peripheral nerve palsy, numbness, and visual changes.

The most common CNS toxoplasmosis neuroimaging findings on computed tomography or MRI studies are ring-enhanced lesions, usually localized in the basal ganglia, sometimes with perilesional edema.[6] Because these lesions are very characteristic, treatment should be started empirically whenever they are present. In general, a follow-up imaging study is recommended after 7 to 10 days to evaluate treatment response. In nonresponding cases brain biopsy should be considered, particularly to evaluate for other causes of similar lesions such as malignancies and other infections.[3] Because immunocompromised patients may lack the typical CNS lesion characteristics owing to immunosuppression,[11] the *T gondii* polymerase chain reaction (PCR) in the cerebrospinal fluid (CSF) can be a valuable confirmatory tool because of its high specificity (96% to 100%).[12]

Diagnosis of toxoplasmosis can be challenging in the HSCT scenario, and usually requires a high clinical suspicion index because it is a disease with pleiotropic symptoms at presentation. It is known that specific anti-*T gondii* antibodies are not a reliable diagnostic tool in the immunosuppression context and they can be absent in the early phase after HSCT.[7,9] Moreover, early diagnosis is of great importance because of its high mortality, particularly when treatment is delayed.[13,14] Thus, molecular techniques have been introduced as a pre-emptive strategy for those high-risk patients after HSCT, and some centers are developing pre-emptive protocols with weekly blood *T gondii* PCR monitoring. These protocols aim to help diagnose toxoplasmosis in an early phase and start treatment before the symptom onset. This might be a valuable option, particularly in high-burden areas, and recent publications have shown a favorable prognosis with a reduction in mortality.[8,15]

The treatment of choice for toxoplasmosis is based on the combination of pyrimethamine/sulfadiazine and folinic acid. Another alternative regimen that has been gaining popularity recently is the use of TMP/SMX, reported to have clinical efficacy similar to

Table 1
Main parasitic diseases in hematopoietic stem cell transplantation, and their distribution and transmission

Disease	Organism	Distribution/ Prevalence	Transmission
Toxoplasmosis	*Toxoplasma gondii*	Worldwide ~60% USA 11% of population (>6 years old)	Foodborne, zoonotic (cats), congenital, blood transfusion, organ transplant
Leishmaniasis NTD	*Leishmania* spp	90 countries in the tropics, subtropics, and southern Europe Cutaneous leishmaniasis 700,000–1.2 million/y Visceral leishmaniasis 100,000/y	Anthroponotic (bite of phlebotomine sand flies)
Chagas Disease NTD	*Trypanosoma cruzi*	Mexico Central America South America ~8 million infected persons	Infected triatomine Contaminated food Congenital Blood transfusion Organ transplant
Malaria	*Plasmodium falciparum* *Plasmodium vivax* *Plasmodium malariae* *Plasmodium ovale* *Plasmodium knowlesi*	Worldwide, tropical 216 million cases of malaria occurred in 2016	Mosquito-borne disease
Babesiosis	*Babesia microti* *Babesia divergens*	*B divergens* (Europe) *B microti* (USA)	Tick bites (*Ixodes scapularis*) Blood transfusion
Free-living amebae (acanthamebiasis)	*Naegleria fowleri* *Acanthamoeba* spp *Balamuthia mandrillaris*	Worldwide in the environment in water and soil	Nasal insufflation, contaminated water, swimming pools, soil Contact lenses
Schistosomiasis NTD	*Schistosoma mansoni* *Schistosoma japonica* *Schistosoma mekongi* *Schistosoma guineensis* *Schistosoma intercalatum*	200 million people infected worldwide	Skin comes in contact with contaminated freshwater (cercaria)
Strongyloidiasis	*Strongyloides stercoralis*	Tropical or subtropical climates 30–100 million infected persons	Skin penetration by contacting contaminated soil autoinfestation
Cryptosporidiosis	*Cryptosporidium hominis* *Cryptosporidium parvum*	Widespread	Fecal-oral route, person-to-person transmission, sexual partners and heath care works, animal to human in contact in farms

(continued on next page)

Table 1
(continued)

Disease	Organism	Distribution/ Prevalence	Transmission
Microsporidium	*Enterocytozoon bieneusi* *Encephalitozoon* spp	Widespread	Uncertain Water sources? Farm? Animals?
Amebiases	*Entamoeba histolytica*	Widespread	Ingestion of the infectious cyst, mainly through contact with contaminated hands, food, or water, but there is a new appreciation that exposure to fecal matter may occur during sexual contact
Giardiasis	*Giardia duodenalis* or synonymous *G lamblia*	Widespread	Infection is transmitted by ingestion of the cyst, which is found in contaminated water, food, or person to person
Blastocystosis	*Blastocystis* spp	Widespread	Eating food contaminated with feces from an infected human or animal

Abbreviation: NTD, neglected tropical diseases.
Adapted from www.cdc.gov/parasites/index.html. Accessed November 4, 2018.

that of the first-line therapy among AIDS patients with the advantage of a lower number of pills per day.[16] Alternative regimens are presented in **Table 2**. The treatment should be maintained for 4 to 6 weeks after resolution of symptoms; however, it may be continued longer depending on the degree of immunosuppression (**Table 2**).

Primary prophylaxis is recommended for all allogeneic recipients with a positive serology before transplant. In these cases, the first-line option is TMP/SMX (160/800 mg) 3 times per week starting after the engraftment[1] and maintained for at least 6 months. Moreover, prolonged prophylaxis courses may be needed if the recipient remains significantly immunocompromised (eg, the occurrence of GVHD requiring high-dose immunosuppressant). For high-risk patients who are intolerant to TMP/SMX, the first recommended alternative prophylactic regimen may include clindamycin plus pyrimethamine and folinic acid. Therefore, other options such as atovaquone, dapsone, clarithromycin, and azithromycin can be used although the evidence supporting their efficacy is limited.[17] Another alternative approach to prophylaxis is the use of a pre-emptive protocol based on weekly screening quantitative PCR in those high-risk recipients who are unable to take prophylaxis or combined with prophylaxis for high-risk patients requiring longer surveillance because of prolonged periods of immunosuppression.

Despite controversy on the need for widespread use of secondary prophylaxis in HSCT, most services agree on its need in individuals with a high risk of reactivation

Table 2
Recommended treatment of parasitic infections in hematopoietic stem cell transplantation recipients

Disease	Primary Treatment	Secondary Treatment
Toxoplasmosis	CNS disease: pyrimethamine 200 mg PO × 1 then 75 mg PO per day with sulfadiazine 1–1.5 g PO q6 h with folinic acid 10–25 mg per day for 4–6 wk then suppressive therapy or TMP/SMX 10/50 mg/kg per day PO IV divided q12 h × 6 wk then suppressive therapy	Pyrimethamine with folinic acid and clindamycin or clarithromycin or azithromycin or atovaquone for 4–6 wk then suppressive therapy
Leishmaniasis	Cutaneous and mucocutaneous: Sodium stibogluconate or meglumine antimonitate (Glucantime) at 20 mg/kg/d IV/IM × 28 days OR Liposomal amphotericin B 3 mg/kg IV daily with total dose of 20–60 mg/kg Visceral: Liposomal amphotericin B 3 mg/kg IV daily ON DAYS 1–5, 10, 17, 24, 31 and 38 (total of 40 mg/kg)	Fluconazole 200 mg PO daily × 6 wk (*L major* only); ketoconazole 600 mg PO daily for 30 d (*L mexicana, L panamensis, and L major*) Miltefosine 2,5 mg/kg/d (maximum of 150 mg/d) PO × 28 d
Chagas disease	Benznidazole 5–7 mg/kg/d PO bid, 60 d	Nifurtimox, 8–10 mg/kg/d PO divided 4×/d 90 d
Malaria	Uncomplicated (*P vivax, P malariae, P ovale, P knowlesi*) OR *P falciparum* (chloroquine sensitive): chloroquine phosphate 1 g (600 mg base) PO, then 0,5 g in 6 h, then 0,5 g daily × 2 d PLUS primaquine phosphate 52.6 mg PO once daily × 14 d (for *P vivax and P ovale*) Complicated (Artesunate 2.4 mg/kg IV at 0, 12, 24, 48 h Continue q24h if unable to take oral medication Follow parenteral therapy wiyh a complete oral course of one of: Atovaquone/proguanil × 3 days Artemether/lumefantrine × 3 days Doxycycline 100 mg q12h × 7 days * If severe P. vivax add Primaquine [see uncomplicated P. vivax])	Uncomplicated (*P vivax, P malariae, P ovale, P knowlesi*): none Uncomplicated (*P falciparum*): atovaquone-proguanil 4 adult tablets (100/400 mg) PO in a single dose daily × 3 d (with food) OR quinine sulfate 650 mg PO tid × 3 d PLUS doxycycline 100 mg PO bid
Babesiosis	Atovaquone 750 mg PO bid PLUS azithromycin 500–1000 PO on day 1, then 250–1000 mg/d PO for 7–10 d Treat 6 wk to include 2 wk after blood smear negative for severe cases	Clindamycin 600 mg PO tid PLUS Quinine 650 mg PO tid 7–10 d

Free-living amebae	Acanthamoeba sp: no proven therapy, can try: pentamidine + fluconazole + miltefosine 50 mg PO tid. May add TMP/SMX, metronidazole, and azithromycin Balamuthia mandrillaris: albendazole + fluconazole or itraconazole + miltefosine 50 mg PO tid + pentamidine. May add TMP/SMX Naegleria fowleri: amphotericin B deoxycholate + rifampin 10 mg/kg/d + fluconazole 10 mg/kg/d + miltefosine 50 mg PO tid + azithromycin 500 mg.
Schistosomiasis	Praziquantel: 20 mg/kg/dose PO bid × 1 d S mansoni, S hematobium, or S intercalatum 20 mg/kg PO tid × 1 d S japonicum or S mekongi	Oxamniquine and artemether (antimalarial) Oxamniquine (S mansoni)
Strongyloidiasis	For disseminated disease with larvae in stool and sputum, repeat treatment every 15 days while stools positive and then 1 more treatment cycle Ivermectin 200 μg/kg/d PO for 2 d (asymptomatic or intestinal disease) For hyperinfection or disseminated disease in immunocompromised patients: Ivermectin 200 μg/kg/d PO per day until stool and/or sputum exams are negative for 2 wk	Albendazole 400 mg PO bid × 7 d for asymptomatic or intestinal disease
Cryptosporidiosis	Nitazoxanide 500 mg PO bid, 14 d	Paromomycin or azithromycin
Microsporidium	Albendazole 400 mg PO bid, 2–4 wk	Fumagillin
Amebiasis Diarrhea	Metronidazole 500–750 mg PO tid, 5–10 d Followed by Paromomycin (25–35 mg/kg/d PO divided 3 doses × 7 d) or iodoquinol (650 mg PO tid × 20 d)	Tinidazole 2 g PO daily 3 d Followed Paromomycin (25–35 mg/kg/d PO divided 3 doses × 7 d) or iodoquinol (650 mg PO tid × 20 d)
Giardiasis	Tinidazole 2 g, 1 day	Nitazoxanide 500 mg PO bid × 3 d Metronidazole 500–750 mg PO tid × 5 d, paromomycin 500 mg PO qid × 10 d
Blastocystosis	Nitazoxanide, 500 mg PO bid for 3 d	Metronidazole 1.5 g × 1 daily for 10 d

Abbreviations: bid, twice daily; IV, intravenously; PO, orally; q, every; qid, every day; SMX, sulfamethoxazole; tid, 3 times daily; TMP, trimethoprim.
Adapted from Gilbert DN, Chambers HF, Eliopoulos GM, et al., editors. Sanford guide to antimicrobial therapy 2018, 48th edition. Sperryville (VA): Antimicrobial Therapy, Inc; 2018; with permission.

after therapy discontinuation. This population includes those with a history of chronic toxoplasmosis and previous infection, and those who develop recurrent GVHD.[14,18]

LEISHMANIASIS

Leishmaniasis is an anthropozoonotic infection caused by protozoans of the genus *Leishmania* (see **Table 1**). It is transmitted to humans by the bite of a mosquito from the genus *Phlebotomus* (New World) or *Lutzomya* (Old World).[19] However, other forms of transmission including donor-derived transmission and incidental transmission by blood transfusion or by needle sharing among intravenous drug users have also been reported.[19–21]

There are 3 major forms of leishmaniasis: visceral (VL), cutaneous (CL), and mucocutaneous. The disease is considered a public health issue because it affects some of the poorest regions of the world. Leishmaniasis is present in 4 continents and it is considered endemic in 88 countries, including 72 developing countries.[19]

In the HSCT setting, the derangement of host cellular immunity caused by the conditioning therapy or GVHD treatment could lead to leishmaniasis reactivation. However, post-HSCT leishmaniasis can also be a result of a primary infection, and the graft itself has been described as another potential source.[22]

The clinical presentation is variable and depends on the form of leishmaniasis as well as the degree of immunosuppression (**Fig. 2**). Among HSCT patients, VL is the form described in most cases, usually presenting with fever, hepatomegaly, splenomegaly, lymphadenopathy, and pancytopenia. Though less common, cutaneous disease has also been described in HSCT recipients and usually presents as single or multiple ulcerating papular lesions.[23] In addition, post-kala-azar dermal leishmaniasis is a cutaneous complication of VL characterized by a macular, maculopapular, and nodular rash, which should be considered in an HSCT patient who has recovered from a VL episode.[24]

Because symptoms of VL form are nonspecific, diagnostic delays are common. However, given mortality rates reaching 100% without specific treatment, clinicians should consider leishmaniasis a possible diagnosis in HSCT recipients from endemic areas who present with fever and pancytopenia.[25]

The proven diagnosis of leishmaniasis is the evidence of the parasite in tissue specimens such as the detection of amastigotes in the bone marrow. However, other methods can be used, including *Leishmania* PCR detection in the bone marrow or blood, which is a very sensitive and specific technique in the VL diagnosis. Among immunocompromised patients, it is also valuable for follow-up of treatment response.[26,27]

The serology tests for leishmaniasis include indirect fluorescent antibody test, enzyme-linked immunosorbent assay (ELISA), and direct agglutination. However, in the HSCT recipient a serology result should be carefully interpreted because there is impairment in the antibody production in these patients.[28] Skin test is considered a marker of previous exposure to *Leishmania* and it is not a valuable diagnostic tool for active infection, especially for patients from high-burden areas.[25]

The 2 most used drugs for treatment of leishmaniasis are pentavalent antimonials and amphotericin B.[25] According to the pharmacologic properties of these drugs, there are many variables that can affect their efficacy such as the *Leishmania* species, patient characteristics, drug availability, disease extent, and previous treatments.[29] Indeed, among HSCT patient data comparing both drugs are lacking and evidence relies mostly on case reports describing VL treatment with liposomal amphotericin B, with a good response.[22,28] Data from other immunocompromised

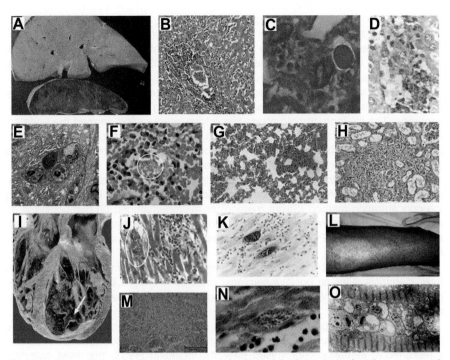

Fig. 2. Leishmaniasis and Chagas disease. (*A*) Visceral leishmaniasis showing a steatosis yellowish enlarged liver and an enlarged parasitized spleen with reticuloendothelial cell hyperplasia. (*B*) Histopathologic observation of a liver showing a mononuclear infiltrate of the portal space and hyperplasia of the Kupffer parasitized cells. (*C*) Kupffer cells cytoplasm containing amastigote parasites. (*D*) Immunohistochemical reaction revealing amastigotes parasitizing Kupffer cells. (*E*) Electronic microscopy illustrating amastigote forms in Kupffer cells' cytoplasm. (*F*) Spleen red pulp with macrophages containing amastigotes. (*G*) Leishmaniasis interstitial pneumonitis with mononuclear cells infiltrate. (*H*) Histopathologic observation of a leishmaniasis interstitial nephritis with mononuclear cells infiltrate. (*I*) Chagas enlarged heart with dilated cavities and a left ventricular thrombosis. (*J*) *T cruzi* amastigotes form parasitized heart myocardial cells with an interstitial mononuclear cells infiltrate. (*K*) Immunohistochemical reaction showing *T cruzi* antigens expressed in the myocardial cells cytoplasm. (*L*) Chagas skin lesions in a renal transplant patient. (*M*) Chronic Chagas myocarditis with an extensive inflammation and fibrosis. (*N*) Myocardial with *T cruzi* amastigotes. (*O*) Electron microscopy showing *T cruzi* amastigotes in the cardiac cell cytoplasm. (*Courtesy of* Dr Maria Irma Seixas Duarte, MD, PhD, Sao Paulo, Brazil.)

populations such as HIV and solid organ transplant patients show similar efficacy of both therapies when used to treat VL (see **Table 2**).[30] However, currently amphotericin B is considered the drug of choice for the treatment of VL according to international guidelines, owing to greater antimonial-related severe side effects when systemically administered, leading to treatment interruptions.[30] Also, the development of resistance of *Leishmania* to pentavalent antimonials is another drawback of these drugs.[31–33]

CHAGAS DISEASE

Chagas disease, also referred to as American trypanosomiasis, is caused by *Trypanosoma cruzi*, a protozoan parasite transmitted by infected triatomine bugs.

Transmission may also occur through oral transmission, contaminated blood transfusion, tissue/organ transplantation, or vertical transmission.[34] Chagas disease is a public health concern in endemic areas in South America, Mexico, and Central America, although more than 200,000 people live with *T cruzi* infection in the United States, mostly immigrants from endemic areas (see **Table 1**).[35]

The disease has acute and chronic phases. In the acute cases symptoms can vary from mild, nonspecific febrile illness to life-threatening myocarditis or meningoencephalitis. The life-long chronic phase has a long latent period, termed the undetermined phase. This phase may include cardiac complications such as heart rhythm abnormalities or dilated cardiomyopathy, and gastrointestinal tract complications such as megaesophagus and megacolon (see **Fig. 2**).[36]

Because a high number of parasites circulating in blood characterizes the acute phase, the diagnosis relies on: (1) direct methods of parasitologic identification using the concentration method (Strout method) or microhematocrit; (2) hemocultures as indirect methods of parasitologic identification; and (3) techniques based on nucleic acid detection such as PCR, which have high sensitivity even among immunocompromised patients.[37]

Chronic infection is characterized by intermittent and extremely low parasitemia; thus, diagnosis relies on positive serology, most commonly ELISA and immunofluorescent antibody test. When results are discordant, a third assay or repeat sampling may be required.[34]

Chagas disease reactivation is defined as an increase in parasitemia that can be detected by direct parasitologic and/or PCR methods, even in the absence of clinical symptoms. In immunocompromised patients, including HSCT, the most common presentation of Chagas disease is reactivation. Particularly for HSCT the risk of reactivation varies from 17% to 40% for autologous or allogeneic HSCT, respectively.[38] The most common presentation in reactivation is febrile illness, subcutaneous nodules (chagoma), panniculitis, myocarditis, meningitis, encephalitis, and stroke. In this clinical scenario, direct parasitologic tests and blood PCR are usually needed, although other specific tests may be performed on skin lesion biopsy samples or on CSF.[37] Additionally a rare presentation of Chagas reactivation with retinitis in HSCT transplant patients, with vitreous biopsy PCR positive for *T cruzi*, was published recently.[39]

Another peculiarity of Chagas management in the immunocompromised population is the need to investigate proactively high-risk individuals, even if asymptomatic, before the use of chemotherapy or conditioning regimens.[37] This higher-risk population includes individuals from endemic areas, those born to mothers from such areas, and those who receive blood transfusion in endemic countries. This investigation can be performed with serologic tests for antibody detection, although caution is needed when interpreting results because false negatives may occur.[40]

Among HSCT candidates, monitoring of possible reactivation during the chemotherapy phase before the transplant is recommended. The recommended follow-up schedule is based on directed parasitologic methods and PCR repeated weekly for 2 months, bimonthly between second and sixth months post transplant, and annually thereafter.[37] This protocol is of importance because early treatment has been shown to reduce the incidence of severe cases and fatal disease.[41]

The treatment of Chagas disease is based on benznidazole and nifurtimox. Because of its better tolerance, benznidazole is considered a first-line treatment.[36] In addition, antiparasitic treatment is indicated for all cases of reactivated Chagas disease (see **Table 2**).[34]

MALARIA

Malaria is an acute parasitic infection caused by 5 human plasmodia species: *Plasmodium falciparum*, *Plasmodium vivax*, *Plasmodium malariae*, *Plasmodium ovale*, and *Plasmodium knowlesi*.[42] It is transmitted to humans mostly by the mosquito bite of the female *Anopheles* (see **Table 1**), although it can be acquired through blood product transfusion or grafts in the HSCT scenario.[43,44]

Although successive exposures to malaria do not produce a protective immune response, some degree of tolerance and resistance is achieved through persistence of plasmodia in the liver, the microvasculature, and the bloodstream. This incomplete acquired immunity does not eradicate the infection but elucidates the lack of parasitemia and higher incidence of asymptomatic disease in adults from endemic regions, although it may also pose a problem for blood and organ donation.[45]

The disease has been described after solid organ transplantation, including in recipients of liver, kidney, and heart transplants.[45] Infection following HSCT is considered an unusual infectious complication of the transplant procedure, mainly described by case reports. In this population, fever is the main symptom reported and may be accompanied by pancytopenia.[46]

Classically, definitive diagnosis is made by direct microscopy of thick and thin blood smears by Giemsa or acridine orange stain (**Fig. 3**).[12] This method was most commonly used for diagnosis of febrile patients after HSCT. Nevertheless it is time consuming, has low sensitivity, and is not recommended for donor blood screening, as it is not suitable for detection of asymptomatic cases with low parasitemia. Molecular diagnostic methods, including DNA hybridization and PCR for DNA and mRNA amplification, are more sensitive than direct stains and can detect low levels of parasitemia earlier than examination of blood film.[42] Serology may be useful to investigate a potential donor; however, it might be negative in case of acute disease. Rapid diagnostic tests are available by using dipsticks, allowing the detection of specific plasmodia antigens, although they are not suitable for detecting submicroscopic parasitemia because of their low sensitivity.[12]

In endemic areas, previous episodes of malaria are not considered an exclusion criterion for donation; however, active surveillance is strongly recommended for recipients from these regions, those who had previous malaria infection, and recipients of donors from endemic areas. After a malaria episode the disease can persist for a long period, which can vary from 3 to 40 years depending on the *Plasmodium* species.[42] Therefore, in the transplant setting the parasitized red cells are a potential source of transmission and clinical malaria can emerge from a pre-existent subclinical infection in the donor, which is exacerbated during the immunosuppression period.[2]

The anti-*Plasmodium* treatment is based on the *Plasmodium* species, and takes into account the geographic distribution and sensitivity profile. Special attention is needed to the interaction between antimalarial drugs and immunosuppressive therapy. In brief, individuals in uncomplicated areas should be treated with chloroquine or artemisinin-based combination therapy (ACT). In areas with chloroquine-resistant infections, *P vivax*, *P ovale*, *P malariae*, or *P knowlesi* malaria should be treated with ACT. To prevent relapse, cases of *P vivax* and *P ovale* should have primaquine added to the primary treatment. Uncomplicated *P falciparum* malaria should be treated with one of the ACTs. For severe disease, intravenous treatment with artesunate is recommended (see **Table 2**).

BABESIOSIS

Babesiosis is an infectious disease caused by intraerythrocytic protozoal parasites of the genus *Babesia*. Transmission to humans occurs via ticks or blood transfusion (see

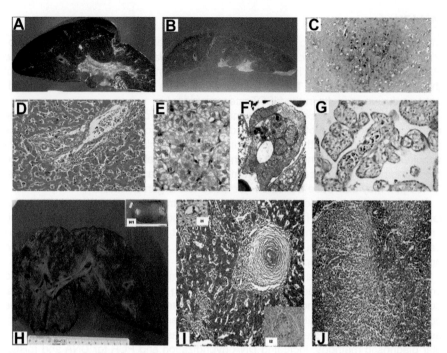

Fig. 3. Malaria and schistosomiasis. (*A*) Malaria enlarged liver with dark-brown color result-ing from hemosiderin and malaria pigment deposition. (*B*) Malaria splenomegaly with accentuation of red pulp. (*C*) Histopathologic observation of CNS malaria duck granuloma with mononuclear infiltrate and malaria pigment impregnation. (*D*) Histopathologic aspect of a malaria-affected liver with mononuclear infiltrate confined to the portal space and Kupffer cells hyperplasia. (*E*) Kupffer cells with a malaria-positive immunohistochemical re-action. (*F*) Electron microscopy of cerebral malaria showing *P falciparum* trophozoites clustered into a macrophage cytoplasm. (*G*) Placental villi red blood cells with malaria immu-nohistochemical positive reaction. (*H*) Enlarged liver showing portal spaces fibrosis. (*H1*) Congestive sclerosis splenomegaly. (*I*) Histopathologic observation of a liver with a granu-loma containing *S mansoni* ova. (*I1,I2*) Schistosomiasis granuloma with eggs and cells showing an *S mansoni*-positive antigen immunohistochemical reaction. (*J*) Liver biopsy showing hepatosplenic schistosomiasis and histiocytic lymphoma. (*Courtesy of* Dr Maria Irma Seixas Duarte, MD, PhD, Sao Paulo, Brazil.)

Table 1). A case reported in transplant recipients has been tracked back to pretrans-plant blood transfusion in an HSCT recipient.[47]

The incubation period is typically 1 to 9 weeks post exposure. *Babesia* infection can range from asymptomatic in healthy individuals to life-threatening disease in immuno-compromised patients. Symptoms may develop within a few weeks or months after exposure. Early symptoms may be fever and malaise, which can progress to severe hemolytic anemia, adult respiratory distress syndrome, multiorgan failure, and even death.[48] Risk factors for severe babesiosis include anatomic or functional asplenia, immunocompromised state, rituximab use, thrombocytopenia, parasitemia greater than 10%, and older age (>60 years).[49]

Reports of babesiosis in transplant recipients are few; nonetheless babesiosis can be a cause of anemia post HSCT,[50] and hemophagocytic lymphohistiocystosis has been described in immunocompetent patients and splenectomized renal transplant patients.

The babesiosis diagnostic involves the identification of intraerythrocytic parasites in blood smears, indirect immunofluorescence, or the PCR testing of blood for *Babesia* DNA.[51]

The treatment requires a combination of atovaquone plus azithromycin or clindamycin plus oral quinine for at least 7 to 10 days (see **Table 2**). However, in a series of 14 immunocompromised subjects, most with B cell lymphoma, asplenic, or treated with rituximab, the treatment was required for at least 6 weeks to achieve a cure. Three (21%) subjects died, highlighting the severity of disease in this population and the importance of blood smears for monitoring response to therapy and relapse after completion of treatment.[52]

For those patients with high-level parasitemia (>10%) or severely ill patients, exchange transfusion should be considered as part of the treatment. Though rare, resistance to the atovaquone/azithromycin regimen can occur, more commonly in immunocompromised hosts.[53]

FREE-LIVING AMEBAE

Acanthamoeba species are ubiquitous in the environment and infective forms can occur through the eye, the nasal passages to the lower respiratory tract, and ulcerated or broken skin (see **Table 1**). Systemic infection is increasingly reported in immunocompromised hosts,[54] except the *Acanthamoeba* keratitis that occurs in healthy individuals and is associated with contact lens use.[55]

A high index of suspicion is necessary to make this diagnosis, and recipients of autologous HSCT may be at increased risk for amebic reactivation.[54] *Acanthamoeba* spp and *Balamuthia mandrillaris* cause cutaneous infection and chronic granulomatous amebic encephalitis, whereas *Naegleria fowleri* causes an acute, fulminant primary amebic meningoencephalitis.[54,56] Despite the limited data of *Acanthamoeba* encephalitis among HSCT recipients, at least 1 case series of 10 individuals reported 100% lethality, even in adequately treated individuals.[57]

Diagnosis is usually made by the identification of cysts or trophozoites in infected tissue. Cutaneous lesions should be biopsied because early diagnosis is imperative to optimize the chance of survival. Brain computed tomography and MRI can also be helpful in the diagnostic investigation, although its results may be nonspecific, particularly in *Naegleria* cases. Direct examination of CSF should be performed.[58] In *Acanthamoeba* infections, a brain biopsy may be needed to investigate for trophozoites, specific tissue abnormalities, and immunofluorescence. Additionally an increasing number of PCR-based techniques for detection and identification of free-living amebic infections have been described.[59]

Optimal treatment regimens for free-living amebic infections remain unknown.[60] Thus, antimicrobial therapy must have wide spectrum and be aggressive. Related treatments with combinations of drugs have been used with inconsistent results (see **Table 2**).[58,61]

SCHISTOSOMIASIS

Schistosomiasis is a neglected tropical disease caused by trematode worms of the genus *Schistosoma*. The infection affects almost 240 million people worldwide, mostly in tropical and subtropical areas. Six species are responsible for human infection, with diverse geographic distributions: *Schistosoma mansoni* is prevalent in Africa, South America, and the Caribbean islands; *Schistosoma japonicum* in China and the Philippines; *Schistosoma mekongi* in Southeast Asia; *Schistosoma guineensis* and related *Schistosoma intercalatum* in central Africa; and *Schistosoma haematobium* (the species related to urogenital schistosomiasis) in Africa and the Middle East (see **Table 1**).[62]

Intestinal schistosomiasis has a nonspecific clinical presentation that includes abdominal pain, diarrhea, bloody stools, and liver enlargement in advanced cases, whereas urogenital schistosomiasis usually presents with hematuria (see **Fig. 3**).[62]

Schistosomiasis is rare in immunocompromised populations, particularly among hematologic malignancy or stem cell transplanted patients, and most publications are limited to few case reports.[63,64] Nevertheless, for patients coming from endemic areas, routine stool and urine examinations and serologic tests of schistosomiasis should be performed, and proper treatment of schistosomiasis at least 3 to 8 weeks before HSCT is recommended.[65]

Schistosomal periportal fibrosis may thus be added to the known risk factors predisposing to the development of veno-occlusive disease (VOD) in allogeneic transplant recipients, as shown among 89 allogeneic HSCT recipients in whom VOD of the liver was higher in those with schistosomal periportal fibrosis.[66]

In general, stool and/or urine examination for ova is the primary diagnostic method for suspected schistosome infections. The choice of sample to diagnose schistosomiasis depends on the parasite species likely to be causing the infection. Whereas *S haematobium* adult worms are found in the venous plexus of the lower urinary tract and eggs are shed in urine, the other species' eggs are shed in feces. The eggs are shed irregularly, so to increase the sensitivity of the examination multiple samples are needed, and a set of 3 serial samples is usually recommended. The clinical investigation of individuals undergoing chemotherapy is particularly challenging because its use might reduce the amount of excreted eggs, hampering the diagnosis in many cases.[64,67]

The first-line treatment of schistosomiasis is oral praziquantel, a safe drug efficacious against all adult worms' species,[68] infrequently associated with parasite resistance. Patients should be retreated if stool or urine examination remains positive at 4 weeks.[69] Although some other treatments are available, they are rarely needed (see **Table 2**).

STRONGYLOIDIASIS

Strongyloides stercoralis is an intestinal nematode endemic to tropical and subtropical areas and has also been reported in temperate regions of Europe and the southeastern United States (see **Table 1**). The parasite has an autoinfective cycle that allows it to cause long-term persistent infections. This characteristic can be explained by its ability to complete the life cycle either in the environment or in the human host.[45]

The perpetuation of infection by the filariform larvae is limited by the host immunity, especially the T-helper 2 cell–mediated immune response. Thus, in the immunocompromised patient such as the HSCT recipient, autoinfection is facilitated and can culminate in the so-called *Strongyloides* hyperinfection syndrome (SHS).

In the transplant setting, risk factors for SHS are those linked to the use of immunosuppressive drugs such as corticosteroids and T cell–depleting drugs, although cyclosporine-containing regimens have a crucial impact in reducing *Stongyloides* reactivation among the transplant population, as the drug also has an anti-helminthic effect.[70] Indeed, among the allogeneic HSCT population, the period of highest reactivation risk is not the immediate post-transplant period but when GVHD develops and steroids are started with cyclosporine discontinuation.[71]

The clinical presentation is variable and the disease can present as: acute infection; chronic infection with autoinfection; SHS with high parasite burden leading to exuberant clinical manifestations, restricted to pulmonary and gastrointestinal symptoms; and disseminated disease characterized by the spreading of the larvae to other organs (**Fig. 4**).[45,70] The main symptoms reported include fever, bacteremia, rash, gastrointestinal pain, diarrhea, hemoptysis, wheezing, and CNS

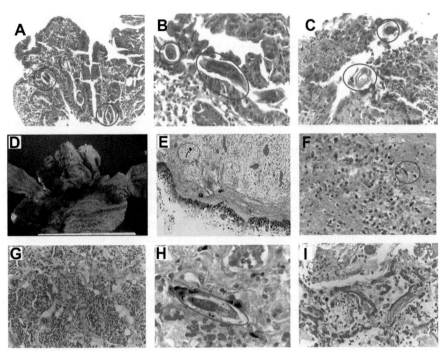

Fig. 4. Strongyloidiasis. (*A*) Duodenitis: histopathologic section with inflammatory infiltrate from *S stercoralis* rhabditoids and adult worms crypt invasion. (*B*) Small bowel with adult worms and eggs in the villi. (*C*) *S stercoralis* worms' transversal segment and eggs on an ulcerated gastric mucosa. (*D*) Hemorrhagic gastritis with edema and mucosal erosion. (*E*) Colonic mucosa showing edema and submucosal inflammation with *S stercoralis* worm. (*F*) CNS parenchymal inflammatory nodule with a filarioid worm. (*G*) *S stercoralis* hemorrhagic pneumonia. (*H*) Filarioid worm within the hemorrhagic area. (*I*) Hemorrhagic pneumonia with diffuse alveolar damage. (*Courtesy of* Dr Maria Irma Seixas Duarte, MD, PhD, Sao Paulo, Brazil.)

manifestations compatible with meningitis caused by gram-negative bacteria from intestinal flora.

The diagnosis of strongyloidiasis should be suspected when there is epidemiologic risk along with clinical signs and symptoms, eosinophilia, or suggestive serologic findings.[72] Eosinophilia is usually mild (5% to 15%); however, it is a nonspecific marker of disease, and patients with chronic infection, SHS, or disseminated disease may have normal or even low eosinophil counts.[73] Definitive diagnosis is made by identification of larvae on direct microscopy from clinical species mainly in stool and duodenal aspirate. In addition, if strongyloidiasis is clinically suspected in a seronegative patient or if serology tests are unavailable, a total of 3 or more stool examinations is recommended to increase the sensitivity of the test.[1]

Serology by ELISA is also available and may be used for diagnosis. It is highly sensitive (88%) and specific (90%) in an immunocompetent host,[72] although the sensitivity may be lower in the setting of immunosuppression.[74] In addition, the *Strongyloides* antibody test can cross-react with other helminth infections, which may result in a false-positive test.[72]

Ivermectin is considered the drug of choice for treatment of uncomplicated strongyloidiasis in the immunocompetent host.[45] Because the complete eradication of *Strongyloides* infection is difficult in immunocompromised patients, some experts recommend repeating the 2-day treatment 2 weeks later or even treating for longer until neutrophil counts recover.[75]

Albendazole is an alternative, and has been shown to clear stool of S stercoralis larvae in 38% to 45% of infected individuals and to normalize serology in chronic infected patients with a negative stool test.[70] Although thiabendazole was routinely used for the treatment of S stercoralis, the high rate of adverse events limits its use (see **Table 2**).[70]

The best treatment approach for SHS in immunocompromised patients is unclear, and clinical failure with ivermectin has been reported. Moreover, with high parasite burden it is recommended to continue treatment for a longer period, until the clinical syndrome resolves and larvae are no longer detectable. Also, for severe cases refractory to conventional treatment or for those patients who are unable to take oral ivermectin, there are some case reports advocating the use of subcutaneous ivermectin as a rescue treatment with good overall survival rates and microbiologic "cure."[76]

Strongyloidiasis is considered a devastating complication in the immunosuppression context, with mortality rates reported to range from 50% to 70% in SHS and disseminated infection, respectively. Because of this risk, adequate screening before transplantation is strongly recommended. The current recommendation for HSCT recipients is to screen those with unexplained eosinophilia who were exposed to/living in endemic areas.[1] Moreover, given the limitation of current diagnostics and considering the favorable tolerability of the drug, some authors suggest a pre-emptive therapy with ivermectin for high-risk patients regardless of serology result or eosinophilia.[75]

CRYPTOSPORIDIOSIS

Cryptosporidium is an intracellular protozoan parasite that has emerged as an important cause of diarrheal illness worldwide. Most infections worldwide have been attributed to *Cryptosporidium hominis* and *Cryptosporidium parvum* (see **Table 1**).[77]

Cryptosporidium infection in immunocompetent individuals is self-limited. However, the clinical presentation in immunocompromised patients is highly variable. The spectrum of its presentation may spread from asymptomatic individuals to life-threatening gastrointestinal and biliary tract disease, including cases of transient gastrointestinal symptoms and chronic diarrhea.[78] A Brazilian study of hematologic patients showed a significantly higher frequency of *Cryptosporidium* infection than in the control group with the same age and environmental exposition.[79]

Transmission is usually via the fecal-oral route, as well as person-to-person transmission particularly within households and nurseries, among sexual partners and heath care workers, and animal to human via contact in farms.[80]

Cryptosporidium infection has been reported with a variable prevalence following HSCT. In a study in southern India, its incidence was 4.61%,[81] whereas in a French study where a systematic screening was used, the cumulative incidence of digestive *Cryptosporidium* in allogeneic HSCT reached 9.6% in patients with diarrhea and 4% in all HSCT recipients.[82] In this population the entire gastrointestinal tract can be affected, and the infection may mimic intestinal GVHD.

Detection of *Cryptosporidium* infection is based on analysis of stool samples by use of microscopy with tinctorial and fluorescent stains or via antigen and nucleic acid detection. More sensitive, specialized tests available in reference facilities include PCR and, for maximum sensitivity in exceptional circumstances, immunomagnetic separation with immunofluorescence microscopy.[77] Serologic testing has a limited value for clinical diagnoses because it can remain elevated for more than a year after the infection.

The Food and Drug Administration–approved drug for treatment of *Cryptosporidium* is nitazoxanide,[83] a broad-spectrum antiparasitic with reported use as a deworming agent as well as a treatment of giardiasis and cryptosporidiosis in randomized trials (see **Table 2**).[69] An immunocompromised patient was successfully treated with a combination of azithromycin and nitazoxanide, aiming for a rapid combined action of drugs.[82]

MICROSPORIDIA

Microsporidia is a group of obligatory intracellular parasites currently considered to be related or belonging to the fungi kingdom. The commonest microsporidia in humans are *Enterocytozoon bieneusi* and *Encephalitozoon* spp. The routes of microsporidia infection are still uncertain, but the species that can infect humans have been identified in water sources as well as in farm, domestic, and wild animals (see **Table 1**).[84]

Although traditionally associated with diarrheal illness in patients with AIDS, extraintestinal infections involving various organs have been reported, particularly in immunocompromised hosts.[85] Clinical presentations may include enteropathy, keratoconjunctivitis, sinusitis, tracheobronchitis,[86] encephalitis, interstitial nephritis, hepatitis, cholecystitis, osteomyelitis, and myositis.[87]

Reports on the prevalence of *Microsporidium* in oncologic patients are limited. In a study of 320 patients with cancer, the prevalence of microsporidia infection has been reported to be as high as 11% using staining of the stool samples.[88] High-risk HSCT patients with gastrointestinal complaints should be evaluated for microsporidian pathogens regularly to improve their quality of life and decrease the problems during the treatment period.[89] In addition, microsporidia should be considered in the differential diagnosis of pulmonary infections in immunosuppressed patients.[90,91]

Albendazole is the first-line therapy for most species that infect humans (see **Table 2**).[69] Additionally the reduction of immunosuppression, whenever possible, is essential for clearing the infection. One alternative regimen is oral fumagillin, although its use is limited because of significant bone marrow toxicity.[85]

AMEBIASES

Intestinal amebiasis caused by *Entamoeba histolytica* is a leading cause of severe parasitic diarrhea worldwide, mostly in developing countries with poor sanitary conditions (see **Table 1**).[92]

The transmission of amebiasis occurs after the ingestion of the infectious cyst, mainly through contact with contaminated hands, food, or water, but there is a new appreciation that exposure to fecal matter may occur during sexual contact.[93]

Amebiasis presentation can range from asymptomatic infection, to invasive intestinal amebiasis (dysentery, colitis, appendicitis, toxic megacolon, amebomas), and to invasive extraintestinal amebiasis (liver abscess, peritonitis, pleuropulmonary abscess, cutaneous and genital amebic lesions).[94]

Amebiasis has rarely been reported in patients undergoing HSCT, although it is an extremely common infection worldwide.[95,96] More recently a study demonstrated that patients with either symptomatic or asymptomatic intestinal amebiasis treated with corticosteroid therapy were at higher risk of developing the potentially fatal complication of fulminant amebic colitis. Thus, patients from endemic areas with very high epidemiologic burden might benefit from screening before treatment with corticosteroids.[92]

Amebiasis can be diagnosed by stool examination, colonoscopy, and histologic examination. Antigen kits to detect *Entamoeba* require fresh (not formalin-preserved) stool for analysis, and stool PCR is a promising new technique. Serum antibodies are useful in a person from a nonendemic country.[97]

Amebic colitis should be treated with metronidazole followed by a luminal agent, such as paromomycin. Treatment with a luminal agent alone is sufficient for patients with asymptomatic intestinal amebiasis (see **Table 2**).[92] The luminal agent usually prescribed is either nitazoxanide or paromomycin, although an allogeneic bone marrow transplanted patient with diarrhea, intestinal amebiasis and acute GVHD was successfully treated with metronidazole in Japan.[98]

GIARDIASIS

Giardia lamblia is a flagellated protozoan and is a common cause of diarrheal disease throughout the world. Infection is transmitted by ingestion of the cyst, which is found in fecally contaminated water, food, or person-to-person transmission (see **Table 1**).[99]

Giardia infections can be asymptomatic, estimated in 5% to 15% of infected people, but typical symptoms include diarrhea flatulence, abdominal pain, and distension. Later the diarrhea becomes more intermittent, with periods of normal bowel function interspersed with diarrhea and malabsorption.

Immunosuppression in patients with *Giardia* can have serious effects, and it may be difficult to distinguish between infection and GVHD.[100–102] An Indian study including 29 renal, 2 liver, and 7 bone marrow transplant recipients documented a prevalence of *Giardia* of 11%,[103] and *Giardia* was a common cause of diarrhea in the Indian HSCT community.[104]

The diagnosis of giardiasis is generally made by the identification of cysts or trophozoites in fecal specimens. Shedding of cysts is somewhat intermittent, so a total of 3 fecal samples over a period of several days is generally recommended. Fecal coproantigen detection using enzyme immunoassays or immunochromatography detection and fluorescent antibody assays of fecal specimens are now used more frequently. Nucleic acid detection methods have also been studied extensively and include conventional and real-time PCR. Nucleic acid methods probably have greater sensitivity, although questions remain regarding their specificity.[99]

The most studied drugs to treat giardiasis are metronidazole, tinidazole, and albendazole (see **Table 2**). The efficacies of metronidazole and tinidazole have been uniformly excellent, whereas some studies of albendazole have shown inferiority to the nitroimidazoles.[99,105]

BLASTOCYSTOSIS

Blastocystis hominis is a protozoan parasite that inhabits the human gastrointestinal tract.[106] It has a worldwide distribution, although it is more frequent in developing countries. Fecal-oral route is the presumed route of transmission (see **Table 1**).[107,108]

The pathogenic role for *B hominis* is uncertain in the immunocompetent host, and in some communities prevalence is as high as 20% in asymptomatic individuals. However, infection has been reported in allogenic bone marrow transplantation with acute GVHD involving the gastrointestinal tract.[109]

In a Turkish study, 201 of 452 bone marrow transplant recipients (44%) experienced one or more episodes of diarrhea from the first day of the conditioning regimen to day 100 following transplantation. In this study, *B hominis* was found to be the only cause of diarrhea in 8 patients, although in 3 patients it was associated with other pathogens.[104]

Blastocystis is detected by standard clinical parasitologic techniques using preparations of fresh stool.[108] However, these methods have a low diagnostic sensitivity compared with molecular tools, such as PCR assays, and could greatly underestimate the real prevalence of the parasite.[110]

The clinical literature also offers no conclusive evidence as to what constitutes effective treatment for the eradication of *B hominis*. The main drugs that have been used are iodoquinol, metronidazole, and nitazoxanide (see **Table 2**).[108]

ACKNOWLEDGMENTS

The authors would like to thank Dr Maria Irma Seixas Duarte, MD, PhD, for providing all pathology images used in the article as a courtesy from her personal archives.

REFERENCES

1. Tomblyn M, Chiller T, Einsele H, et al. Guidelines for preventing infectious complications among hematopoietic cell transplantation recipients: a global perspective. Biol Blood Marrow Transplant 2009;15(10):1143–238.
2. Fabiani S, Fortunato S, Petrini M, et al. Allogeneic hematopoietic stem cell transplant recipients and parasitic diseases: a review of the literature of clinical cases and perspectives to screen and follow-up active and latent chronic infections. Transpl Infect Dis 2017;19(2). https://doi.org/10.1111/tid.12669.
3. Montoya JG, Liesenfeld O. Toxoplasmosis. Lancet 2004;363(9425):1965–76.
4. Derouin F, Pelloux H. Prevention of toxoplasmosis in transplant patients. Clin Microbiol Infect 2008;14(12):1089–101.
5. Prestes-Carneiro LE, Rubinsky-Elefant G, Ferreira AW, et al. Seroprevalence of toxoplasmosis, toxocariasis and cysticercosis in a rural settlement, Sao Paulo State, Brazil. Pathog Glob Health 2013;107(2):88–95.
6. Hakko E, Ozkan HA, Karaman K, et al. Analysis of cerebral toxoplasmosis in a series of 170 allogeneic hematopoietic stem cell transplant patients. Transpl Infect Dis 2013;15(6):575–80.
7. Busemann C, Ribback S, Zimmermann K, et al. Toxoplasmosis after allogeneic stem cell transplantation—a single centre experience. Ann Hematol 2012;91(7): 1081–9.
8. Martino R, Bretagne S, Einsele H, et al. Early detection of *Toxoplasma* infection by molecular monitoring of *Toxoplasma gondii* in peripheral blood samples after allogeneic stem cell transplantation. Clin Infect Dis 2005;40(1):67–78.
9. Fricker-Hidalgo H, Bulabois CE, Brenier-Pinchart MP, et al. Diagnosis of toxoplasmosis after allogeneic stem cell transplantation: results of DNA detection and serological techniques. Clin Infect Dis 2009;48(2):e9–15.
10. Mele A, Paterson PJ, Prentice HG, et al. Toxoplasmosis in bone marrow transplantation: a report of two cases and systematic review of the literature. Bone Marrow Transplant 2002;29(8):691–8.
11. Khalaf AM, Hashim MA, Alsharabati M, et al. Late-onset cerebral toxoplasmosis after allogeneic hematopoietic stem cell transplantation. Am J Case Rep 2017; 18:246–50.
12. Jarque I, Salavert M, Peman J. Parasitic infections in hematopoietic stem cell transplantation. Mediterr J Hematol Infect Dis 2016;8(1):e2016035.
13. Prestes DP, Mendes C, Batista MV, et al. A case-series of toxoplasmosis in hematopoietic stem cell transplantation: still a concern for endemic countries. Bone Marrow Transplant 2018;53(10):1336–9.
14. Martino R, Maertens J, Bretagne S, et al. Toxoplasmosis after hematopoietic stem cell transplantation. Clin Infect Dis 2000;31(5):1188–95.

15. Meers S, Lagrou K, Theunissen K, et al. Myeloablative conditioning predisposes patients for *Toxoplasma gondii* reactivation after allogeneic stem cell transplantation. Clin Infect Dis 2010;50(8):1127–34.

16. Torre D, Casari S, Speranza F, et al. Randomized trial of trimethoprim-sulfamethoxazole versus pyrimethamine-sulfadiazine for therapy of toxoplasmic encephalitis in patients with AIDS. Italian Collaborative Study Group. Antimicrob Agents Chemother 1998;42(6):1346–9.

17. Gajurel K, Dhakal R, Montoya JG. Toxoplasma prophylaxis in haematopoietic cell transplant recipients: a review of the literature and recommendations. Curr Opin Infect Dis 2015;28(4):283–92.

18. Brinkman K, Debast S, Sauerwein R, et al. Toxoplasma retinitis/encephalitis 9 months after allogeneic bone marrow transplantation. Bone Marrow Transplant 1998;21(6):635–6.

19. Machado CM, Martins TC, Colturato I, et al. Epidemiology of neglected tropical diseases in transplant recipients. Review of the literature and experience of a Brazilian HSCT center. Rev Inst Med Trop Sao Paulo 2009;51(6):309–24.

20. le Fichoux Y, Quaranta JF, Aufeuvre JP, et al. Occurrence of *Leishmania infantum* parasitemia in asymptomatic blood donors living in an area of endemicity in southern France. J Clin Microbiol 1999;37(6):1953–7.

21. Cruz I, Morales MA, Noguer I, et al. *Leishmania* in discarded syringes from intravenous drug users. Lancet 2002;359(9312):1124–5.

22. Sirvent-von Bueltzingsloewen A, Marty P, Rosenthal E, et al. Visceral leishmaniasis: a new opportunistic infection in hematopoietic stem-cell-transplanted patients. Bone Marrow Transplant 2004;33(6):667–8.

23. Komitopoulou A, Tzenou T, Baltadakis J, et al. Is leishmaniasis an "unusual suspect" of infection in allogeneic transplantation? Transpl Infect Dis 2014;16(6):1012–8.

24. Zijlstra EE, Musa AM, Khalil EA, et al. Post-kala-azar dermal leishmaniasis. Lancet Infect Dis 2003;3(2):87–98.

25. Gajurel K, Dhakal R, Deresinski S. Leishmaniasis in solid organ and hematopoietic stem cell transplant recipients. Clin Transplant 2017;31(1). https://doi.org/10.1111/ctr.12867.

26. Lachaud L, Dereure J, Chabbert E, et al. Optimized PCR using patient blood samples for diagnosis and follow-up of visceral leishmaniasis, with special reference to AIDS patients. J Clin Microbiol 2000;38(1):236–40.

27. Antinori S, Calattini S, Longhi E, et al. Clinical use of polymerase chain reaction performed on peripheral blood and bone marrow samples for the diagnosis and monitoring of visceral leishmaniasis in HIV-infected and HIV-uninfected patients: a single-center, 8-year experience in Italy and review of the literature. Clin Infect Dis 2007;44(12):1602–10.

28. Agteresch HJ, van 't Veer MB, Cornelissen JJ, et al. Visceral leishmaniasis after allogeneic hematopoietic stem cell transplantation. Bone Marrow Transplant 2007;40(4):391–3.

29. Sundar S, Chakravarty J. An update on pharmacotherapy for leishmaniasis. Expert Opin Pharmacother 2015;16(2):237–52.

30. Basset D, Faraut F, Marty P, et al. Visceral leishmaniasis in organ transplant recipients: 11 new cases and a review of the literature. Microbes Infect 2005;7(13):1370–5.

31. Clemente WT, Mourao PHO, Lopez-Medrano F, et al. Visceral and cutaneous leishmaniasis recommendations for solid organ transplant recipients and donors. Transplantation 2018;102(2S Suppl 2):S8–15.

32. Mitsuru M, Izumi N, Koichiro G. Strongyloidiasis and culture-negative suppurative meningitis, Japan, 1993-2015. Emerg Infect Dis J 2018;24(12):2378.
33. Aronson N, Herwaldt BL, Libman M, et al. Diagnosis and treatment of leishmaniasis: Clinical Practice Guidelines by the Infectious Diseases Society of America (IDSA) and the American Society of Tropical Medicine and Hygiene (ASTMH). Clin Infect Dis 2016;63(12):e202–64.
34. Dias JC, Ramos AN Jr, Gontijo ED, et al. 2nd Brazilian consensus on Chagas disease, 2015. Rev Soc Bras Med Trop 2016;49(Suppl 1):3–60.
35. Manne-Goehler J, Umeh CA, Montgomery SP, et al. Estimating the burden of Chagas disease in the United States. PLoS Negl Trop Dis 2016;10(11):e0005033.
36. Bern C, Montgomery SP, Herwaldt BL, et al. Evaluation and treatment of Chagas disease in the United States: a systematic review. JAMA 2007;298(18):2171–81.
37. Pinazo MJ, Miranda B, Rodriguez-Villar C, et al. Recommendations for management of Chagas disease in organ and hematopoietic tissue transplantation programs in nonendemic areas. Transplant Rev (Orlando) 2011;25(3):91–101.
38. Altclas J, Sinagra A, Dictar M, et al. Chagas disease in bone marrow transplantation: an approach to preemptive therapy. Bone Marrow Transplant 2005;36(2):123–9.
39. Conrady CD, Hanson KE, Mehra S, et al. The first case of *Trypanosoma cruzi*-associated retinitis in an immunocompromised host diagnosed with pan-organism polymerase chain reaction. Clin Infect Dis 2018;67(1):141–3.
40. Altclas J, Salgueira C, Riarte A. Reactivation of Chagas disease after a bone marrow transplant. Blood Trasfus 2014;12(Suppl 1):s380.
41. Guiang KM, Cantey P, Montgomery SP, et al. Reactivation of Chagas disease in a bone marrow transplant patient: case report and review of screening and management. Transpl Infect Dis 2013;15(6):E264–7.
42. Inoue J, Machado CM, Lima GF, et al. The monitoring of hematopoietic stem cell transplant donors and recipients from endemic areas for malaria. Rev Inst Med Trop Sao Paulo 2010;52(5):281–4.
43. O'Donnell J, Goldman JM, Wagner K, et al. Donor-derived *Plasmodium vivax* infection following volunteer unrelated bone marrow transplantation. Bone Marrow Transplant 1998;21(3):313–4.
44. Mejia R, Booth GS, Fedorko DP, et al. Peripheral blood stem cell transplant-related *Plasmodium falciparum* infection in a patient with sickle cell disease. Transfusion 2012;52(12):2677–82.
45. Kotton CN, Lattes R. Parasitic infections in solid organ transplant recipients. Am J Transplant 2009;9(Suppl 4):S234–51.
46. Raina V, Sharma A, Gujral S, et al. *Plasmodium vivax* causing pancytopenia after allogeneic blood stem cell transplantation in CML. Bone Marrow Transplant 1998;22(2):205–6.
47. Cirino CM, Leitman SF, Williams E, et al. Transfusion-associated babesiosis with an atypical time course after nonmyeloablative transplantation for sickle cell disease. Ann Intern Med 2008;148(10):794–5.
48. Akel T, Mobarakai N. Hematologic manifestations of babesiosis. Ann Clin Microbiol Antimicrob 2017;16(1):6.
49. Lubin AS, Snydman DR, Miller KB. Persistent babesiosis in a stem cell transplant recipient. Leuk Res 2011;35(6):e77–8.
50. Bade NA, Yared JA. Unexpected babesiosis in a patient with worsening anemia after allogeneic hematopoietic stem cell transplantation. Blood 2016;128(7):1019.
51. Vannier E, Krause PJ. Human babesiosis. N Engl J Med 2012;366(25):2397–407.

52. Krause PJ, Gewurz BE, Hill D, et al. Persistent and relapsing babesiosis in immunocompromised patients. Clin Infect Dis 2008;46(3):370–6.

53. Wormser GP, Prasad A, Neuhaus E, et al. Emergence of resistance to azithromycin-atovaquone in immunocompromised patients with *Babesia microti* infection. Clin Infect Dis 2010;50(3):381–6.

54. Feingold JM, Abraham J, Bilgrami S, et al. Acanthamoeba meningoencephalitis following autologous peripheral stem cell transplantation. Bone Marrow Transplant 1998;22(3):297–300.

55. Dos Santos DL, Kwitko S, Marinho DR, et al. *Acanthamoeba* keratitis in Porto Alegre (southern Brazil): 28 cases and risk factors. Parasitol Res 2018;117(3): 747–50.

56. Morrison AO, Morris R, Shannon A, et al. Disseminated *Acanthamoeba* infection presenting with cutaneous lesions in an immunocompromised patient: a case report, review of histomorphologic findings, and potential diagnostic pitfalls. Am J Clin Pathol 2016;145(2):266–70.

57. Coven SL, Song E, Steward S, et al. *Acanthamoeba* granulomatous amoebic encephalitis after pediatric hematopoietic stem cell transplant. Pediatr Transplant 2017;21(8). https://doi.org/10.1111/petr.13060.

58. Maritschnegg P, Sovinz P, Lackner H, et al. Granulomatous amebic encephalitis in a child with acute lymphoblastic leukemia successfully treated with multimodal antimicrobial therapy and hyperbaric oxygen. J Clin Microbiol 2011; 49(1):446–8.

59. Qvarnstrom Y, Visvesvara GS, Sriram R, et al. Multiplex real-time PCR assay for simultaneous detection of *Acanthamoeba* spp., *Balamuthia mandrillaris*, and *Naegleria fowleri*. J Clin Microbiol 2006;44(10):3589–95.

60. Slater CA, Sickel JZ, Visvesvara GS, et al. Brief report: successful treatment of disseminated acanthamoeba infection in an immunocompromised patient. N Engl J Med 1994;331(2):85–7.

61. Schuster FL, Visvesvara GS. Opportunistic amoebae: challenges in prophylaxis and treatment. Drug Resist Updat 2004;7(1):41–51.

62. Colley DG, Bustinduy AL, Secor WE, et al. Human schistosomiasis. Lancet 2014;383(9936):2253–64.

63. Ferraz AA, de Sa VC, Lopes EP, et al. Lymphoma in patients harboring hepatosplenic mansonic schistosomiasis. Arquivos de gastroenterologia 2006;43(2): 85–8 [in Portuguese].

64. Sanchez-Montalva A, Salvador F, Ruiz-Camps I, et al. Imported disease screening prior to chemotherapy and bone marrow transplantation for oncohematological malignancies. Am J Trop Med Hyg 2016;95(6):1463–8.

65. Yalcin A, Avcu F, Ural AU, et al. *Schistosoma mansoni* infection following allogeneic bone marrow transplantation. Turk J Haematol 1999;16(4):181–4.

66. Mahmoud HK. Schistosomiasis as a predisposing factor to veno-occlusive disease of the liver following allogeneic bone marrow transplantation. Bone Marrow Transplant 1996;17(3):401–3.

67. Montes M, White AC Jr, Kontoyiannis DP. Symptoms of intestinal schistosomiasis presenting during treatment of large B cell lymphoma. Am J Trop Med Hyg 2004;71(5):552–3.

68. Siqueira LDP, Fontes DAF, Aguilera CSB, et al. Schistosomiasis: drugs used and treatment strategies. Acta Trop 2017;176:179–87.

69. Schwartz BS, Mawhorter SD. Parasitic infections in solid organ transplantation. Am J Transplant 2013;13(Suppl 4):280–303.

70. Keiser PB, Nutman TB. *Strongyloides stercoralis* in the immunocompromised population. Clin Microbiol Rev 2004;17(1):208–17.
71. Orlent H, Crawley C, Cwynarski K, et al. Strongyloidiasis pre and post autologous peripheral blood stem cell transplantation. Bone Marrow Transplant 2003;32(1):115–7.
72. Siddiqui AA, Berk SL. Diagnosis of *Strongyloides stercoralis* infection. Clin Infect Dis 2001;33(7):1040–7.
73. Vadlamudi RS, Chi DS, Krishnaswamy G. Intestinal strongyloidiasis and hyperinfection syndrome. Clin Mol Allergy 2006;4:8.
74. Schaffel R, Nucci M, Carvalho E, et al. The value of an immunoenzymatic test (enzyme-linked immunosorbent assay) for the diagnosis of strongyloidiasis in patients immunosuppressed by hematologic malignancies. Am J Trop Med Hyg 2001;65(4):346–50.
75. Alpern JD, Arbefeville SS, Vercellotti G, et al. *Strongyloides* hyperinfection following hematopoietic stem cell transplant in a patient with HTLV-1-associated T-cell leukemia. Transpl Infect Dis 2016;19(1):e12638.
76. Barrett J, Broderick C, Soulsby H, et al. Subcutaneous ivermectin use in the treatment of severe *Strongyloides stercoralis* infection: two case reports and a discussion of the literature. J Antimicrob Chemother 2016;71(1):220–5.
77. Checkley W, White AC Jr, Jaganath D, et al. A review of the global burden, novel diagnostics, therapeutics, and vaccine targets for cryptosporidium. Lancet Infect Dis 2015;15(1):85–94.
78. Manivel C, Filipovich A, Snover DC. Cryptosporidiosis as a cause of diarrhea following bone marrow transplantation. Dis Colon Rectum 1985;28(10):741–2.
79. Chieffi PP, Paschoalotti MA, Vergueiro CS, et al. Infection by *Cryptosporidium* sp. in immunocompromised haematological patients. Rev Inst Med Trop Sao Paulo 2005;47(5):301–2.
80. Davies AP, Chalmers RM. Cryptosporidiosis. BMJ 2009;339:b4168.
81. Kang G, Srivastava A, Pulimood AB, et al. Etiology of diarrhea in patients undergoing allogeneic bone marrow transplantation in South India. Transplantation 2002;73(8):1247–51.
82. Legrand F, Grenouillet F, Larosa F, et al. Diagnosis and treatment of digestive cryptosporidiosis in allogeneic haematopoietic stem cell transplant recipients: a prospective single centre study. Bone Marrow Transplant 2011;46(6):858–62.
83. Sebastian E, Martin J, McDonald GB, et al. Cryptosporidium parvum infection vs GVHD after hematopoietic SCT: diagnosis by PCR with resolution of symptoms. Bone Marrow Transplant 2011;46(4):612–4.
84. Tabatabaie F, Abrehdari Tafreshi Z, Shahmohammad N, et al. Molecular detection of microsporidiosis in various samples of Iranian immunocompromised patients. J Parasit Dis 2015;39(4):634–8.
85. Ramanan P, Pritt BS. Extraintestinal microsporidiosis. J Clin Microbiol 2014; 52(11):3839–44.
86. Orenstein JM, Russo P, Didier ES, et al. Fatal pulmonary microsporidiosis due to encephalitozoon cuniculi following allogeneic bone marrow transplantation for acute myelogenous leukemia. Ultrastruct Pathol 2005;29(3–4):269–76.
87. Kelkar R, Sastry PS, Kulkarni SS, et al. Pulmonary microsporidial infection in a patient with CML undergoing allogeneic marrow transplant. Bone Marrow Transplant 1997;19(2):179–82.
88. Karaman U, Atambay M, Daldal N, et al. The prevalence of microsporidium among patients given a diagnosis of cancer. Turkiye Parazitol Derg 2008; 32(2):109–12 [in Turkish].

89. Cetinkaya U, Hamamci B, Kaynar L, et al. Investigation of the presence of *Encephalitozoon intestinalis* and *Enterocytozoon bieneusi* in bone marrow transplant patients by IFA-MAbs method. Mikrobiyol Bul 2015;49(3):432–8 [in Turkish].

90. Teachey DT, Russo P, Orenstein JM, et al. Pulmonary infection with microsporidia after allogeneic bone marrow transplantation. Bone Marrow Transplant 2004; 33(3):299–302.

91. Ozkoc S, Bayram Delibas S, Akisu C. Evaluation of pulmonary microsporidiosis in iatrogenically immunosuppressed patients. Tuberk Toraks 2016;64(1):9–16.

92. Shirley DA, Moonah S. Fulminant amebic colitis after corticosteroid therapy: a systematic review. PLoS Negl Trop Dis 2016;10(7):e0004879.

93. Salit IE, Khairnar K, Gough K, et al. A possible cluster of sexually transmitted *Entamoeba histolytica*: genetic analysis of a highly virulent strain. Clin Infect Dis 2009;49(3):346–53.

94. Shirley DT, Farr L, Watanabe K, et al. A review of the global burden, new diagnostics, and current therapeutics for amebiasis. Open Forum Infect Dis 2018; 5(7):ofy161.

95. Bavaro P, Di Girolamo G, Di Bartolomeo P, et al. Amebiasis after bone marrow transplantation. Bone Marrow Transplant 1994;13(2):213–4.

96. Perret C, Harris PR, Rivera M, et al. Refractory enteric amebiasis in pediatric patients with acute graft-versus-host disease after allogeneic bone marrow transplantation. J Pediatr Gastroenterol Nutr 2000;31(1):86–90.

97. Haque R, Ali IK, Akther S, et al. Comparison of PCR, isoenzyme analysis, and antigen detection for diagnosis of *Entamoeba histolytica* infection. J Clin Microbiol 1998;36(2):449–52.

98. Numata A, Itabashi M, Kishimoto K, et al. Intestinal amoebiasis in a patient with acute graft-versus-host disease after allogeneic bone marrow transplantation successfully treated by metronidazole. Transpl Infect Dis 2015;17(6):886–9.

99. Minetti C, Chalmers RM, Beeching NJ, et al. Giardiasis. BMJ 2016;355:i5369.

100. Ajumobi AB, Daniels JA, Sostre CF, et al. Giardiasis in a hematopoietic stem cell transplant patient. Transpl Infect Dis 2014;16(6):984–7.

101. Rubin RH. Gastrointestinal infectious disease complications following transplantation and their differentiation from immunosuppressant-induced gastrointestinal toxicities. Clin Transplant 2001;15(Suppl 4):11–22.

102. Bromiker R, Korman SH, Or R, et al. Severe giardiasis in two patients undergoing bone marrow transplantation. Bone Marrow Transplant 1989;4(6):701–3.

103. Yadav P, Khalil S, Mirdha BR. Molecular appraisal of intestinal parasitic infection in transplant recipients. Indian J Med Res 2016;144(2):258–63.

104. Pala C, Kaynar L, Buyukoglan R, et al. Diarrhea in peripheral stem cell transplant recipients: a developing country's experience. J Infect Dev Ctries 2014;8(5): 635–41.

105. Cernikova L, Faso C, Hehl AB. Five facts about *Giardia lamblia*. PLoS Pathog 2018;14(9):e1007250.

106. Zierdt CH. *Blastocystis hominis*—past and future. Clin Microbiol Rev 1991;4(1): 61–79.

107. Leelayoova S, Rangsin R, Taamasri P, et al. Evidence of waterborne transmission of *Blastocystis hominis*. Am J Trop Med Hyg 2004;70(6):658–62.

108. Coyle CM, Varughese J, Weiss LM, et al. Blastocystis: to treat or not to treat. Clin Infect Dis 2012;54(1):105–10.

109. Ghosh K, Ayyaril M, Nirmala V. Acute GVHD involving the gastrointestinal tract and infestation with *Blastocystis hominis* in a patient with chronic myeloid

leukaemia following allogeneic bone marrow transplantation. Bone Marrow Transplant 1998;22(11):1115–7.

110. El Safadi D, Cian A, Nourrisson C, et al. Prevalence, risk factors for infection and subtype distribution of the intestinal parasite *Blastocystis* sp. from a large-scale multi-center study in France. BMC Infect Dis 2016;16(1):451.

Vaccination of the Stem Cell Transplant Recipient and the Hematologic Malignancy Patient

Mini Kamboj, MD[a],*, Monika K. Shah, MD[b]

KEYWORDS

- Vaccines • Stem cell transplant • Hematologic • Cancer

KEY POINTS

- Patients with hematologic malignancy are at increased risk of morbidity and mortality from certain vaccine-preventable illnesses, such as influenza, pneumococcal disease, and zoster.
- Stem cell transplantation (SCT) recipients lose their preexisting immunity over time following SCT and require primary reimmunization strategies once T- and B-cell immunities have sufficiently recovered.
- Newer vaccines appear to be more immunogenic and show promise in terms of clinical efficacy in these vulnerable patient populations.
- Special vaccination considerations are required for household contacts of immunocompromised individuals as well as immunocompromised travelers.

INTRODUCTION

Due to advances in cancer treatment and earlier cancer detection, coupled with the aging and overall growth of the population, the number of cancer survivors in the United States is predicted to reach more than 20 million by 2026.[1] A five-fold increase in number of hematopoietic stem cell transplantation (SCT) survivors is expected in the United States between 2009 and 2030.[2] The Centers for Disease Control and Prevention (CDC) Advisory Committee on Immunization Practices (ACIP) recommends certain vaccines for routine use in all persons, stratified by age and clinical indication.[3]

Patients with malignancies affecting the bone marrow or lymphatic system and SCT recipients are considered severely immunocompromised (high risk) when it comes to

The authors have no relevant disclosures. This article was supported in part through the NIH/NCI Cancer Center Support Grant P30 CA008748.

[a] Infectious Disease Service, Department of Medicine, Memorial Sloan Kettering Cancer Center, Weill Cornell Medical College, 1275 York Avenue, Box 9, New York, NY 10065, USA; [b] Infectious Disease Service, Department of Medicine, Weill Cornell Medical College, 275 York Avenue, Box 420, New York, NY 10065, USA

* Corresponding author.

E-mail address: kambojm@mskcc.org

evaluation for travel vaccination.[4] Antibody titers to vaccine-preventable illnesses decline following SCT, so primary reimmunization is required when the immune system has sufficiently reconstituted. Three major societies and consensus groups have published guidelines for SCT recipients: Infectious Disease Society of America (IDSA), American Society of Blood and Bone Marrow Transplantation (ASBMT), and the European Group of Blood and Marrow Transplantation.[5–7] These recommendations, coupled with ACIP recommendations and newly available published data, serve as the basis of this review.

VACCINE TYPES AND TIMING

Inactivated vaccines are typically protein or polysaccharide based. Polysaccharide vaccines are less immunogenic and can be conjugated to proteins to enhance the immune response. Recombinant vaccines consist of genetically engineered antigens and are typically inactivated but can occasionally be live attenuated (LAV). Some vaccines contain adjuvants to enhance immunogenicity.[8] LAV uses a weakened but replication-competent organism. High-risk patients should not receive LAV until at least 2 years have elapsed since transplant, no evidence of systemic graft-versus-host disease (GVHD), and cessation of all immunosuppressive medication.[6] For patients undergoing elective splenectomy as a part of cancer treatment, indicated vaccines should be administered at least 2 weeks before the operation.[9]

Inactivated vaccines should be administered at least 2 weeks before initiation of cytotoxic therapy and/or a pretransplant conditioning regimen when needed. Consensus guidelines on post-SCT immunization protocols stipulate introduction of immunization with inactivated vaccines at 3 to 12 months following transplantation and acknowledge the lack of available prospective data to support more specific practices, including assessment of immune parameters before vaccination.[5–7] The recommended immunization schedule after SCT is presented in **Fig. 1**. SCT type, presence of GVHD, and ongoing immunosuppressive therapy may necessitate a delay in vaccine initiation.[10]

Special Consideration

Anti-CD20 therapy
Patients receiving monoclonal anti-CD20 antibody (Rituximab) or other B-cell–depleting therapies may not develop adequate antibody response to vaccines. An interval of at least 6 months is recommended between the last rituximab dose and vaccination.

Intravenous immunoglobulin
Intravenous immunoglobulin (IVIG) does not interfere with antibody response to inactivated vaccines. Administration of vaccines at different anatomic sites is permissible. Simultaneous or close administration of antibody-containing products and live vaccines can have a neutralizing effect with reduction in vaccine efficacy (serologic response). IVIG should therefore not be administered for 8 to 11 months before, and for at least 2 weeks after, measles, mumps, and rubella (MMR) and varicella vaccination (see sections on zoster and MMR in later discussion).

Chimeric antigen receptor T-cell therapy
In 2017, chimeric antigen receptor (CAR) T-cell therapies were approved by the US Food and Drug Administration (FDA) for treatment of refractory acute lymphoblastic leukemia in children and advanced B-cell lymphomas.[11] Using a genetic engineering technology, T cells gain the ability to recognize and destroy specific antigens on tumor cells. The most developed CAR T-cell therapy is targeted toward CD19, an antigen

VACCINES			Mo since transplant												
			1	2	3	4	5	6	7	8	9	10	11	12	24 mo
Inactivated influenza[a]	I	●				i					1 dose				
Pneumococcal conjugate[b]	I	●	3 doses										i		
Tetanus, diphtheria, pertussis[c]	I	●									3 doses				
Haemophilus influenzae B (Hib)	I	●									3 doses				
Inactivated Polio	I	●									3 doses				
Recombinant hepatitis B[d]	I	●									3 doses				
Mumps,measles, rubella[e]	L	●													2 doses
Varicella[f]	L	●													2 doses
Meningococcal[g] conjugate (MCV-4)	I	O									2 doses				
Human papilloma (HPV)[h]	I	O									3 doses				

I, inactivated; L, live.
● Recommended for all
O Age/ risk based

Fig. 1. Immunization schedule for SCT recipients. [a] Inactivated influenza vaccines: For children <9 years of age, 2 doses of inactivated influenza vaccines (IIV) 1 month apart. In elderly patients (≥65 years of age), consider the following if readily available: High-dose (HD-IIV3; Fluzone) or adjuvanted (aIIV3; Fluad). [b] PCV. [c] Tetanus, diphtheria, acellular pertussis vaccination: Various combinations and doses of vaccines exist, including DTaP, DT, Tdap, and Td. Capital letters indicate higher toxoid or antigen amounts. Give DTaP × 3 doses to all children ≤7 years; can consider for all patients irrespective of age, although DTaP is only licensed in children <7 years of age. Alternatively, can give 3 doses of Tdap, or 1 dose of Tdap, followed by 2 doses of Td. Among Tdap vaccines, *Boostrix* contains higher pertussis antigen than *Adacel*. *Boostrix* is preferred in adults ≥65 years. [d] Recombinant hepatitis B: Check serology after 3 doses; if negative anti-Hbs titer, revaccinate with 3-dose series; alternative, 1 dose booster of either high-antigen dose vaccine or standard dose and recheck anti-Hbs titer. If vaccinating with combined hepatitis A and B vaccine product, must still check anti-Hbs titer and revaccinate with hepatitis B vaccine if negative. [e] MMR: If measles antibody negative, vaccinate with 2 doses at least 1 month apart. [f] Recommended for use in VZV-seronegative patients. See text for data on recombinant zoster vaccine (Shingrix) in autotransplant recipients. [g] MCV-4: Recommended for persons aged 11 to 18 years, with a booster at 16–18 years. Meningococcal B vaccines should additionally be administered to SCT recipients aged 10-25 years with at-risk conditions (asplenia, terminal complement deficiency, laboratory worker, travel, outbreak). [h] HPV: Now available as 9-valent vaccine. Vaccinate in patients 9-26 years of age; FDA has recently expanded indicated age range to up to 45 years. [i] May administer vaccine at 4 months if widespread influenza in community. [j] Give fourth dose of PCV-13 if GVHD requiring immunosuppression. For all others, PPSV-23 booster (23 valent polysaccharide vaccine) is given at 1 year.

expressed on B cells. Once administered, CD19-directed CAR T cells destroy not only tumor cells that express CD19 but also normal B cells. Consequently, B-cell aplasia and hypogammaglobulinemia occur. The duration and degree of these effects after CAR-T are highly variable, and many individuals require IVIG replenishment. No studies have examined serologic response to the inactivated vaccines in patients treated with CAR T-cell therapy but lack reliable responses is not entirely unexpected.[11]

VACCINES
Inactivated Influenza Vaccine

Patients with hematologic malignancy and SCT recipients are at an elevated risk for influenza-related complications.[12–15] A third of SCT recipients with influenza develop lower airway disease. Overall mortality ranges from 6% to 15%, increasing to 28% to

45% when infection has progressed to include lower respiratory tract involvement.[14–23] Response to seasonal influenza immunization is mediated by the generation of neutralizing antibodies against viral antigens and $CD4^+$- and $CD8^+$- specific cytotoxic responses.[24]

Clinical effectiveness of the inactivated influenza vaccine in the SCT population is not rigorously studied. Routine strategies may not offer an optimal level of protection, especially early after SCT.[14] Several observational reports suggest reduced risk of lower respiratory tract infection and hospitalization among vaccinated SCT patients.[25–30]

Newer Food and Drug Administration–Approved Influenza Vaccines and Other Novel Strategies

To overcome the limitations of standard dose (SD) inactivated influenza vaccine, several strategies have been evaluated to see if they enhance protection from influenza following SCT.

A high-dose (HD) vaccine contains 4 times the amount of antigen compared with SD. An early phase randomized study comparing HD versus SD **(Table 1)** demonstrated superior immunogenicity with HD only for the A/H3N2 component. Local reactions were common with HD (67% vs 31% for SD), although most of these were mild.[31] Administration of HD vaccine in patients less than 65 years is not recommended.[32] In small-randomized studies, a second vaccine dose within the same season did not substantially improve immune response after SCT.[33,34]

Among the adjuvanted vaccines, AS03-[35] and MF59-[36] containing vaccines have been evaluated. MF59-containing vaccine, FLUAD (Seqirus), is the only adjuvanted influenza vaccine approved in the United States for elderly patients.[37] Specifically, in SCT, a single randomized trial failed to show superior seroconversion rates with FLUAD compared with SD-inactivated influenza vaccine (see **Table 1**).[36] Patients immunized greater than 6 months after transplant had higher seroconversion rates, indicating a potential benefit by waiting at least 6 months following SCT.

Pretransplant donor vaccination is without benefit, but vaccination of the SCT recipient may offer protection, although corroboration by additional studies is desired (see **Table 1**).[38]

Granulocyte macrophage colony stimulating factor has no role in improving vaccine effectiveness after SCT.[39]

Among recently approved vaccines, recombinant (egg free) and cell-based vaccines are promising new advancements. Recombinant vaccine (RIV4; Flublok)[40] retains genetic fidelity to circulating viruses, offering broader protection with a quadrivalent formulation and containing a high amount of antigen (3 times higher compared with SD). These vaccines are now licensed for use in adults over the age of 18.[41]

Despite data on clinical superiority in the general population of HD compared with SD inactivated influenza vaccines, no existing studies have compared the recombinant, HD, and adjuvanted vaccines among SCT patients. These vaccines are among the ACIP recommended options for adults ≥65 years, plausibly rendering better clinical protection for older transplant recipients. No conclusions can be drawn on the preferential use of 1 formulation over the other.

Recommendations

There is consensus across existing guidelines recommending seasonal influenza vaccination regardless of transplant type.[6,29] The key recommendations are as follows:

- Administer greater than 6 months after transplant but may begin at 4 months if influenza activity has begun. Influenza activity in United States peaks between December and February in 8 out of every 10 seasons.

Table 1
Key randomized studies of inactivated influenza vaccines in allogeneic stem cell transplant recipients

Study	Study Population and Season	Outcomes Assessed	Median Time to Vaccination	Findings
Halasa et al,[31] 2016 Phase 1 randomized safety study SD vs HD; n = 15 vs 29	Adult allogeneic SCT recipients 2010–11 2011–12	Safety (primary) Immunogenicity (secondary)	8.5 mo (HD) and 7.1 mo (SD)	• Higher local site reactions with HD (67% vs 31%) • HD had significantly higher seroprotection for A/H3N2 compared with the SD group; 81% vs 36% • No significant difference in seroprotection or seroconversion for A/H1N1 or B viruses
Karras et al,[34] 2013 Randomized open label Two doses of trivalent inactivated influenza vaccine (TIV) 4 wk apart vs single dose (33 vs 32)	Adult allogeneic SCT recipients 2010–2011	Immune response Viral-specific T-cell responses; seroprotection; seroconversion	0.9 (2 doses) and 0.7 (single)	• No significant difference in seroprotection or seroconversion for H3 or H1 N1 • Time from transplant >1 y associated with better seroprotection • CD+19 correlated with antibody response
Natori et al,[36] 2017 Randomized pilot trial Adjuvanted (Ad) vs SD TIV (35 vs 32)	Adult allogeneic SCT recipients 2015–2016	Serologic response	19 mo (Ad) and 10 mo (SD)	• No significant difference in immunogenicity • Seroconversion to at least 1 antigen 62.9 (Ad) vs 53.1% (SD) (highest for A/H3N2) • Trend toward higher immunogenicity with Ad among those >6 mo post-SCT
Ambati et al,[38] 2015 Open randomized prospective study of pre-SCT vaccination No vaccine (n = 38), donor (n = 44), recipient (n = 40),	Adult and pediatric allogeneic SCT recipients 2007–2010	Seroprotection rate at day 180 after transplant	Pretransplant and day +180	• Antibody titers against H1 and H3 were highest in the pretransplant recipient vaccination group through day 180 after transplantation • No beneficial effect of donor vaccination before transplant

- Two doses administered 1 month apart for children less than 9 years of age.
- Live-attenuated influenza vaccine is contraindicated.

Inactivated Influenza Vaccination in Patients with Hematologic Malignancy

Despite reduced effectiveness when compared with the general population, annual vaccination of patients with hematologic malignancy is an important preventive strategy.[6,30] Clinical studies in persons with hematologic malignancy show only marginal benefit with second doses.[42,43] Efficacy of inactivated influenza vaccine with certain malignancy treatment agents is specifically addressed in each of the following 2 paragraphs:

Rituximab

Antibody responses to adjuvanted influenza vaccine (AS03) were entirely subdued in a cohort of 67 patients vaccinated within 6 months after rituximab (71% on cyclophosphamide, doxorubicin, vincristine, and prednisone plus the monoclonal antibody rituximab).[44] A second vaccine is not helpful in boosting the immune response.

Ibrutinib

Ibrutinib is an immunomodulatory drug currently being used in the treatment of chronic lymphocytic leukemia (CLL), B-cell lymphomas, and Waldenström macroglobulinemia. It acts by inhibition of Bruton tyrosine kinase (BTK). Disruption in B-cell signaling, maturation, and immunoglobulin synthesis following BTK inhibition cause agammaglobulinemia.[45] Two studies on serologic response after inactivated influenza vaccine in ibrutinib-treated patients showed mixed results.[46,47] There are currently inadequate data to determine if inactivated influenza vaccination is ineffective in a certain subset of patients on treatment with this agent.

Pneumococcal Conjugate Vaccine -13 and Pneumococcal Polysaccharide Vaccine-23

Patients with hematologic malignancy and SCT recipients are at a 45 to 55 times higher risk (annual incidence 217–266/100,000 persons) of developing invasive pneumococcal disease (IPD) than the general population, primarily because of acquired hypogammaglobulinemia.[48,49] Multiple myeloma carries the greatest risk of IPD.

Conjugated vaccines induce early T-cell–dependent responses after SCT and elicit long-term immune memory. Since the introduction of conjugate vaccines for universal immunization, IPD rates have declined in high-risk patients.[49,50] The FDA approved conjugated pneumococcal vaccines starting in early 2000s with the 7-valent pneumococcal conjugate vaccine-7 (PCV-7), followed by expanded coverage to 13 serotypes with FDA-approval of PCV-13 in 2010, including the virulent serotype 19A.[51]

Prospective studies established the superior immunogenicity of conjugated pneumococcal vaccines when given 6 to 12 months after SCT[52]; 74.4% of pediatric recipients achieve seroprotection.[53] Vaccine response as early as 3 months after SCT was first shown in a randomized study with PCV-7 (3 months vs 9 months; 79% vs 82%). Notable findings in early vaccinees (vaccinated at 3 months following SCT) were a trend toward lower antibody concentration at 2 years as well as inferior priming for pneumococcal polysaccharide vaccine-23 (PPSV-23) when compared with PCV-7.[54] In a long-term follow-up study[55] of 30 surviving patients, persistent antibody response at 8 to 11 years from SCT was assessed; 10/17 in the late versus 2/13 in early group had PCV-7 antibodies $\geq$50 μg/mL (P = .03). PPSV-23 booster after the initial series was without any additional benefit. Collectively, these findings suggest that PCV administered at 3 months has the probable benefit of clinical protection against *Streptococcus pneumoniae* earlier after SCT, but durable responses may be compromised.

In 2009, ASBMT guidelines were updated to include PCV-7 at 3 to 6 months after SCT, with consideration for a fourth dose in patients with chronic GVHD, as a substitute to PPSV-23 (although graded as weak evidence). In other guidelines, PPSV-23 is recommended at 1 year.[5,56] Experience with PCV-13 in SCT recipients was reported in 2015 from a multicenter study, when 251 patients were immunized with a 4-dose PCV-13 series at 3 to 6 months following SCT. The fourth dose (booster) was administered at a 6-month interval, and 1 month before PPSV-23. Significant increase in geometric mean fold increase was observed after the fourth dose, but comparisons with PPSV-23 boost only were not conducted. The fourth dose of PCV-13 was associated with an increased local and systemic reaction.[57]

Recommendations
Current guidelines[6] recommend 3 doses of PCV-13 starting at 3 to 12 months after SCT, and 1 dose of PPSV-23 at 12 months in patients without GVHD (with an additional fourth dose of PCV-13 instead in those with GVHD). Although common practice, the optimal interval for post–vaccine serologic monitoring, and the benefit of booster doses beyond the first year, are not known.

Pneumococcal Vaccination in Patients with Hematologic Malignancy

PCV-13 is immunogenic in patients undergoing treatment of hematologic malignancy; duration of response can vary with the type of cancer and type of treatment. Patients with myeloma, especially those receiving lenalidomide,[58] can mount an immune response. PCVs[59] are superior to PPSV-23 among splenectomized patients with treated Hodgkin disease. PCV also performs better than PPSV-23 among patients treated with rituximab within the previous year. ACIP recommends starting with PCV-13, followed by PPSV-23 8 weeks later.[6,51,60]

Varicella and Zoster Vaccines

Adult patients with cancer have a higher overall incidence of herpes zoster compared with age-matched persons without cancer, particularly those with hematological malignancies.[61] Elderly patients with hematologic malignancy have a 2-fold higher rate of zoster compared with those with solid tumors (31.0 vs 14.9 per 1000 patient-years).[62]

Currently, 1 varicella vaccine and 2 zoster vaccines are licensed for use in adults.

The varicella vaccine, Varivax (Merck), and the older zoster vaccine, Zostavax (Merck), both contain the live-attenuated Oka strain virus and therefore have limited use in high-risk immunocompromised patients. Death following live zoster virus vaccination to a patient with CLL has been reported.[63]

The new recombinant subunit (non-live) vaccine, Shingrix (GlaxoSmithKline), is clinically superior to Zostavax. Shingrix was approved by the FDA on October 20, 2017. The vaccine is a 2-dose series licensed for adults aged greater than 50 years, including those with a previous episode of zoster or who previously received Zostavax. Shingrix is the preferred zoster vaccine as stated by ACIP.[64]

Studies demonstrate that Shingrix is highly effective in preventing zoster and postherpetic neuralgia (PHN) in all age groups without immunocompromising conditions, including the elderly (91% in adults $\geq$70 years old, 97% in adults 50–69 years old).[65,66] There is a lack of efficacy data among immunocompromised patients, although clinical trials are ongoing.[67,68] No current recommendations from ACIP exist for Shingrix use in patients with an active hematologic malignancy.[3]

Vaccination Against Varicella and Herpes Zoster in Stem Cell Transplant Recipients

Varicella zoster virus (VZV) reactivation after SCT is reported to be as high as 20% to 53%.[69] Breakthrough and late reactivations occur despite use of antiviral prophylaxis.[70]

Live vaccine (Varivax and Zostavax)

The 2009 consensus[7] and 2013 IDSA[6] guidelines recommend initiating Varivax immunization in seronegative recipients who are at least 24 months post-SCT, without systemic GVHD or active immune compromise.[6,7] Because of possible interference by neutralizing antibodies, patients should also be without receipt of IVIG within the preceding 8 to 11 months.[6] VZV-specific T-cell immunity does not adequately reconstitute in all situations following SCT,[71] so preventive strategies that include vaccination of individuals irrespective of serostatus are required.[72] A single retrospective study assessed the impact of Varivax administration at 24 months after allogenic SCT, in most seropositive recipients, and after antiviral prophylaxis was discontinued.[72] At 5 years, the overall rate of zoster and PHN was significantly lower in the Varivax versus nonvaccinated group (zoster, 17% vs 33%; PHN, 0% vs 8%). Several single-center observational studies have demonstrated short-term safety of Zostavax following SCT.[73–75] The vaccine, which contains 14 times the dose of virus compared with Varivax, remains largely contraindicated in this patient population.[64]

Inactivated varicella zoster vaccines (Shingrix and other)

Two recent major clinical trials that evaluated inactivated zoster vaccines are summarized in **Table 2**. De la Serna and colleagues[67] found significant efficacy of Shingrix when given as early as 50 to 70 days after autotransplant: 68% and 89% effective in preventing zoster and PHN, respectively. Another phase 3 trial assessed an investigational heat-inactivated vaccine among autologous SCT recipients, with the first dose given before SCT and 3 additional doses given within the first 3 months after SCT. Incidence of zoster was 32.9/1000 person-years in the vaccine group versus 91.9/1000 person-years in the placebo group, translating to an efficacy of 63.8%.[68]

Recommendations

For seronegative patients, Varivax can be given at 24 months post-SCT. The inactive subunit vaccine (Shingrix) is the preferred zoster vaccine for immunocompetent adults ≥50 years; patients who are no longer considered severely immunocompromised from their hematologic malignancy and/or SCT should be vaccinated. Insufficient data exist to recommend varicella vaccination earlier after transplant, although clinical trials with inactivated varicella vaccine are ongoing.

Tetanus, Diphtheria, Pertussis Vaccines

Various combinations and doses of vaccines exist, including Diphtheria-Tetanus-acellular Pertussis (DTaP), Diphtheria-Tetanus (DT), Tetanus-Diphtheria-acellular pertussis (Tdap), and Tetanus-diphtheria (Td). Capital letters indicate higher toxoid or antigen amounts. DTaP should be administered to all children ≤7 years of age. For patients aged ≥7 years of age, the 2013 IDSA guidelines stipulate that DTaP should be considered, or alternatively, 1 dose of Tdap vaccine should be administered followed by 2 doses of DT or Td (see **Fig. 1**).[6] Among the available Tdap vaccinations in the United States, Boostrix (GlaxoSmithKline) contains 8 μg of pertussis toxoid in comparison to Adacel (Sanofi Pasteur), which contains 2.5 μg.[76] There are scant data to recommend one over the other.[77]

Recommendations

SCT recipients should be immunized with 3 doses of tetanus, diphtheria, pertussis-containing vaccines at 6 months post-SCT. Patients with hematologic malignancy should receive a dose of Tdap if not previously given in adulthood.

Table 2
Randomized studies of inactivated zoster vaccines in autologous stem cell transplant recipients

Study	Study Population	Outcomes Assessed	Dosing Schedule (Days in Relation to SCT)	Findings
de la Serna et al,[67] 2018 Recombinant subunit (RZV) Phase 3 observer-blind, placebo controlled, randomized 1:1 Modified cohort: RZV (n = 870) Placebo (n = 851) Median follow-up = 21 mo	Adult autologous SCT recipients	Clinical efficacy (primary) Safety (primary)	2 doses 1. +50 to +70 2. +80 to +130 (or 30–60 d after dose 1)	Incident disease (per person, vaccine vs placebo) • HZ: 49 vs 135 (68.2% efficacy) • PHN: 1 vs 9 (89.3% efficacy)
Winston et al,[68] 2018 Heat-inactivated VZV vaccine (investigational) Phase 3 double-blind, placebo-controlled, randomized 5:1:5 Vaccine lot (n = 560) High antigen lot (n = 164) Placebo (n = 564) Mean follow-up = 2.4 y	Adult autologous SCT recipients 2010–2013 135 centers	Clinical efficacy (primary) Safety (primary-high lot group) Immunogenicity (secondary)	4 doses 1. −5 to −60 2. +30 3. +60 4. +90	Incident disease (per 1000 person-years, vaccine lot vs placebo): • HZ: 32.9/vs 91.9 (63.9% efficacy) • PHN: 2.3 vs 14.6 (83.7% efficacy) VZV-specific responses higher in vaccine group; T-cell responses sustained at 3 y; B-cell responses plateau after 1 y

Abbreviation: HZ, herpes zoster.

Hepatitis B

Hepatitis B vaccine is administered starting as early as 6 months following SCT. If administered earlier than 1 year following SCT, vaccine hepatitis B surface antibody titers should be checked, and if negative, the patient should be reimmunized with a second 3-dose series. Higher-antigen-dose hepatitis B vaccine[6] is available, and although it is primarily for use in patients on hemodialysis, it can also be used for booster dosing in this setting. Although not discussed in the 2013 guidelines, hepatitis B vaccine is also available as a coformulated vaccine with hepatitis A (Twinrix; GlaxoSmithKline). Twinrix has been given as a 3-dose series following SCT. This option offers the ability to achieve concurrent hepatitis A seroprotection.

Measles, Mumps, and Rubella Vaccine

MMR vaccination is only available as a trivalent formulation in the United States. It is an LAV and thus is contraindicated in high-risk patients. Vaccine titers to MMR decline in the years following SCT.[78,79] After SCT, the vaccine is given as a 2-dose series (often to measles-seronegative SCT recipients, although there is transplant center variability and some centers may administer to any recipient eligible for live virus vaccination).[6] The vaccine can be considered after 24 months following SCT (among those without GVHD, as well as 8–11 months after last receipt of IVIG products). Epidemic measles and mumps cases have reemerged worldwide,[80] and vaccine should be administered irrespective of last IVIG use in an outbreak situation.

Other Vaccines

Haemophilus influenza B conjugate and inactivated polio vaccines should be given to all SCT recipients, starting as early as 6 months. *Human papillomavirus vaccine* should be offered to all immunocompromised adults through 26 years of age if they have not previously received the series. The FDA recently approved the vaccine for expanded use in adults aged 27 to 45 years. *Conjugate meningococcal vaccines* should be given to SCT recipients according to age or at-risk condition. Two doses of quadrivalent meningococcal conjugate vaccine (MCV 4) (serotypes A, C, W-135, and Y) should be administered 6 to 12 months after SCT to persons aged 11 to 18 years, with a booster at 16 to 18 years. Meningococcal B vaccines should additionally be administered to SCT recipients aged 10 to 25 years with at risk conditions.[81] ACIP recommends either a 3-dose series of MenB-FHbp (Trumenba, Pfizer) or a 2-dose series of MenB-4C (Bexsero, GSK).[81]

OTHER VACCINATION CONSIDERATIONS
Donor Vaccination

Pretransplant donor immunization may enhance early expansion of humoral immunity in the recipient for some but not all vaccines.[38,82] This approach raises unique ethical and practical challenges and is not endorsed by existing guidelines.

Before International Travel

International travel is common among patients with cancer and SCT recipients.[83,84] Routine vaccinations should be up-to-date before travel. Some additional vaccines (**Table 3**) are specifically considered based on specific epidemiologic- and destination-based risk.[85,86]

Table 3
Vaccination in immunocompromised travelers[a]

Safe to Give[b]	Unsafe-Contraindicated
Hepatitis A[c]	Yellow fever (YFV)[e,f]
Intramuscular typhoid[d]	Oral typhoid
Inactivated polio (IPV)[e]	Oral polio (OPV)[g]
Hepatitis B	Oral cholera
Meningitis (MCV-4)[e]	
Rabies[d]	
Japanese encephalitis[d]	

[a] Country- and indication-specific vaccine recommendations available through the CDC.[85]
[b] Vaccines are injections unless otherwise indicated.
[c] Can also consider hepatitis A–specific immunoglobulin for short-term preexposure prophylaxis if unlikely to mount immune response to vaccination.
[d] Immunogenicity not known in immunocompromised recipients.
[e] Proof of vaccine receipt may be required for entry to certain destinations. If YFV cannot safely be given, a waiver letter can be granted from certified YFV providers. Risks of disease at destination versus benefits of travel should be discussed.
[f] Many clinicians remain reluctant to vaccinate with YFV after hematopoietic stem cell transplantation (SCT) regardless of immune status and time elapsed. One recent study demonstrated immunogenicity and safety in a cohort of 21 allogeneic HSCT recipients who were immunized with YFV, a median of 33 months after HSCT.[86]
[g] Not available in United States; give IPV.

Vaccination of Household Contacts (Including Children) and Health Care Workers

All household members of patients with hematologic malignancy or following SCT should receive age-appropriate vaccinations as recommended by the ACIP, including all inactivated vaccines as well as most LAVs (**Table 4**).

Table 4
Safety of live vaccines in household contacts of patients with high-risk immunocompromising conditions

Vaccine	Transmission in High-Risk Household Contacts	Recommendation	Special Precautions/ Comments
MMR	—	Safe	
Varicella	Mild/subclinical disease	Safe	If skin lesions develop, 1. Cover with dressing until scabbed 2. Avoid direct contact
LAIV	—	Do not administer	For patients requiring protective isolation, contacts should receive inactivated vaccine
Rotavirus	Persistent shedding	Safe	Avoid handling diapers for 4 wk
Oral polio (outside United States)		Do not administer	Use inactivated polio vaccine
Oral typhoid		Safe	
Yellow fever		Safe	

Abbreviation: LAIV, live-attenuated influenza vaccine.
   Data from Kamboj M, Sepkowitz KA. Risk of transmission associated with live attenuated vaccines given to healthy persons caring for or residing with an immunocompromised patient. Infect Control Hosp Epidemiol 2007;28(6):702–7.

REFERENCES

1. Miller KD, Siegel RL, Lin CC, et al. Cancer treatment and survivorship statistics, 2016. CA Cancer J Clin 2016;66(4):271–89.
2. Majhail NS, Tao L, Bredeson C, et al. Prevalence of hematopoietic cell transplant survivors in the United States. Biol Blood Marrow Transplant 2013;19(10): 1498–501.
3. Kim DK, Riley LE, Harriman KH, et al. Advisory committee on immunization practices recommended immunization schedule for adults aged 19 years or older - United States, 2017. MMWR Morb Mortal Wkly Rep 2017;66(5):136–8.
4. Kotton CN, Kroger AT, Freedman DO. Chapter 8: immunocompromised travelers. In: Centers for Disease Control and Prevention, editor. The CDC health information for international travel (The Yellow Book). 2018. Available at: https://wwwnc.cdc.gov/travel/yellowbook/2018/advising-travelers-with-specific-needs/immunocompromised-travelers. Accessed October 24, 2018.
5. Tomblyn M, Chiller T, Einsele H, et al. Guidelines for preventing infectious complications among hematopoietic cell transplantation recipients: a global perspective. Biol Blood Marrow Transplant 2009;15(10):1143–238.
6. Rubin LG, Levin MJ, Ljungman P, et al. 2013 IDSA clinical practice guideline for vaccination of the immunocompromised host. Clin Infect Dis 2014;58(3):309–18.
7. Ljungman P, Cordonnier C, Einsele H, et al. Vaccination of hematopoietic cell transplant recipients. Bone Marrow Transplant 2009;44(8):521–6.
8. Centers for Disease Control and Prevention. Epidemiology and prevention of vaccine-preventable diseases. In: Hamborsky J, Kroger A, Wolfe S, editors. 13th edition. Washington, DC: Public Health Foundation; 2015. Available at: https://www.cdc.gov/vaccines/pubs/pinkbook/genrec.html. Accessed October 24, 2018.
9. Bonanni P, Grazzini M, Niccolai G, et al. Recommended vaccinations for asplenic and hyposplenic adult patients. Hum Vaccin Immunother 2017;13(2):359–68.
10. Carpenter PA, Englund JA. How I vaccinate blood and marrow transplant recipients. Blood 2016;127(23):2824–32.
11. June CH, Sadelain M. Chimeric antigen receptor therapy. N Engl J Med 2018; 379(1):64–73.
12. Campbell AP, Guthrie KA, Englund JA, et al. Clinical outcomes associated with respiratory virus detection before allogeneic hematopoietic stem cell transplant. Clin Infect Dis 2015;61(2):192–202.
13. Legoff J, Zucman N, Lemiale V, et al. Clinical significance of upper airway virus detection in critically ill hematology patients. Am J Respir Crit Care Med 2019; 199(4):518–28.
14. Nichols WG, Guthrie KA, Corey L, et al. Influenza infections after hematopoietic stem cell transplantation: risk factors, mortality, and the effect of antiviral therapy. Clin Infect Dis 2004;39(9):1300–6.
15. Martino R, Porras RP, Rabella N, et al. Prospective study of the incidence, clinical features, and outcome of symptomatic upper and lower respiratory tract infections by respiratory viruses in adult recipients of hematopoietic stem cell transplants for hematologic malignancies. Biol Blood Marrow Transplant 2005; 11(10):781–96.
16. Ljungman P, de la Camara R, Perez-Bercoff L, et al. Outcome of pandemic H1N1 infections in hematopoietic stem cell transplant recipients. Haematologica 2011; 96(8):1231–5.
17. Ljungman P, Ward KN, Crooks BN, et al. Respiratory virus infections after stem cell transplantation: a prospective study from the Infectious Diseases Working

Party of the European Group for blood and marrow transplantation. Bone Marrow Transplant 2001;28(5):479–84.

18. Wei JY, Chen FF, Jin J, et al. Novel influenza A (H1N1) in patients with hematologic disease. Leuk Lymphoma 2010;51(11):2079–83.

19. George B, Ferguson P, Kerridge I, et al. The clinical impact of infection with swine flu (H1N109) strain of influenza virus in hematopoietic stem cell transplant recipients. Biol Blood Marrow Transplant 2011;17(1):147–53.

20. Espinosa-Aguilar L, Green JS, Forrest GN, et al. Novel H1N1 influenza in hematopoietic stem cell transplantation recipients: two centers' experiences. Biol Blood Marrow Transplant 2011;17(4):566–73.

21. Redelman-Sidi G, Sepkowitz KA, Huang CK, et al. 2009 H1N1 influenza infection in cancer patients and hematopoietic stem cell transplant recipients. J Infect 2010;60(4):257–63.

22. Kmeid J, Vanichanan J, Shah DP, et al. Outcomes of influenza infections in hematopoietic cell transplant recipients: application of an immunodeficiency scoring index. Biol Blood Marrow Transplant 2016;22(3):542–8.

23. Protheroe RE, Kirkland KE, Pearce RM, et al. The clinical features and outcome of 2009 H1N1 influenza infection in allo-SCT patients: a British Society of Blood and Marrow Transplantation study. Bone Marrow Transplant 2012;47(1):88–94.

24. Avetisyan G, Aschan J, Hassan M, et al. Evaluation of immune responses to seasonal influenza vaccination in healthy volunteers and in patients after stem cell transplantation. Transplantation 2008;86(2):257–63.

25. Kumar D, Ferreira VH, Blumberg E, et al. A 5-year prospective multicenter evaluation of influenza infection in transplant recipients. Clin Infect Dis 2018;67(9): 1322–9.

26. Pinana JL, Perez A, Montoro J, et al. Clinical effectiveness of influenza vaccination after allogeneic hematopoietic stem cell transplantation: a cross-sectional prospective observational study. Clin Infect Dis 2018. [Epub ahead of print].

27. Machado CM, Cardoso MR, da Rocha IF, et al. The benefit of influenza vaccination after bone marrow transplantation. Bone Marrow Transplant 2005;36(10): 897–900.

28. Engelhard D, Mohty B, de la Camara R, et al. European guidelines for prevention and management of influenza in hematopoietic stem cell transplantation and leukemia patients: summary of ECIL-4 (2011), on behalf of ECIL, a joint venture of EBMT, EORTC, ICHS, and ELN. Transpl Infect Dis 2013;15(3):219–32.

29. Tomblyn M, Chiller T, Einsele H, et al. Guidelines for preventing infectious complications among hematopoietic cell transplant recipients: a global perspective. Preface. Bone Marrow Transplant 2009;44(8):453–5.

30. Beck CR, McKenzie BC, Hashim AB, et al. Influenza vaccination for immunocompromised patients: summary of a systematic review and meta-analysis. Influenza Other Respir Viruses 2013;7(Suppl 2):72–5.

31. Halasa NB, Savani BN, Asokan I, et al. Randomized double-blind study of the safety and immunogenicity of standard-dose trivalent inactivated influenza vaccine versus high-dose trivalent inactivated influenza vaccine in adult hematopoietic stem cell transplantation patients. Biol Blood Marrow Transplant 2016;22(3): 528–35.

32. DiazGranados CA, Dunning AJ, Kimmel M, et al. Efficacy of high-dose versus standard-dose influenza vaccine in older adults. N Engl J Med 2014;371(7): 635–45.

33. Engelhard D, Nagler A, Hardan I, et al. Antibody response to a two-dose regimen of influenza vaccine in allogeneic T cell-depleted and autologous BMT recipients. Bone Marrow Transplant 1993;11(1):1–5.

34. Karras NA, Weeres M, Sessions W, et al. A randomized trial of one versus two doses of influenza vaccine after allogeneic transplantation. Biol Blood Marrow Transplant 2013;19(1):109–16.

35. Mohty B, Bel M, Vukicevic M, et al. Graft-versus-host disease is the major determinant of humoral responses to the AS03-adjuvanted influenza A/09/H1N1 vaccine in allogeneic hematopoietic stem cell transplant recipients. Haematologica 2011;96(6):896–904.

36. Natori Y, Humar A, Lipton J, et al. A pilot randomized trial of adjuvanted influenza vaccine in adult allogeneic hematopoietic stem cell transplant recipients. Bone Marrow Transplant 2017;52(7):1016–21.

37. Grohskopf LA, Sokolow LZ, Broder KR, et al. Prevention and control of seasonal influenza with vaccines: recommendations of the advisory committee on immunization practices-United States, 2018-19 Influenza Season. MMWR Recomm Rep 2018;67(3):1–20.

38. Ambati A, Boas LS, Ljungman P, et al. Evaluation of pretransplant influenza vaccination in hematopoietic SCT: a randomized prospective study. Bone Marrow Transplant 2015;50(6):858–64.

39. Pauksen K, Linde A, Hammarstrom V, et al. Granulocyte-macrophage colony-stimulating factor as immunomodulating factor together with influenza vaccination in stem cell transplant patients. Clin Infect Dis 2000;30(2):342–8.

40. Dunkle LM, Izikson R, Patriarca P, et al. Efficacy of recombinant influenza vaccine in adults 50 years of age or older. N Engl J Med 2017;376(25):2427–36.

41. Grohskopf LA, Sokolow LZ, Broder KR, et al. Prevention and control of seasonal influenza with vaccines: recommendations of the advisory committee on immunization practices - United States, 2017-18 influenza season. MMWR Recomm Rep 2017;66(2):1–20.

42. Sanada Y, Yakushijin K, Nomura T, et al. A prospective study on the efficacy of two-dose influenza vaccinations in cancer patients receiving chemotherapy. Jpn J Clin Oncol 2016;46(5):448–52.

43. Ljungman P, Nahi H, Linde A. Vaccination of patients with haematological malignancies with one or two doses of influenza vaccine: a randomised study. Br J Haematol 2005;130(1):96–8.

44. Yri OE, Torfoss D, Hungnes O, et al. Rituximab blocks protective serologic response to influenza A (H1N1) 2009 vaccination in lymphoma patients during or within 6 months after treatment. Blood 2011;118(26):6769–71.

45. Varughese T, Taur Y, Cohen N, et al. Serious infections in patients receiving ibrutinib for treatment of lymphoid cancer. Clin Infect Dis 2018;67(5):687–92.

46. Douglas AP, Trubiano JA, Barr I, et al. Ibrutinib may impair serological responses to influenza vaccination. Haematologica 2017;102(10):e397–9.

47. Sun C, Gao J, Couzens L, et al. Seasonal influenza vaccination in patients with chronic lymphocytic leukemia treated with ibrutinib. JAMA Oncol 2016;2(12):1656–7.

48. Cowan J, Do TL, Desjardins S, et al. Prevalence of Hypogammaglobulinemia in Adult Invasive Pneumococcal Disease. Clin Infect Dis 2018;66(4):564–9.

49. Shigayeva A, Rudnick W, Green K, et al. Invasive pneumococcal disease among immunocompromised persons: implications for vaccination programs. Clin Infect Dis 2016;62(2):139–47.

50. Lee YJ, Huang YT, Kim SJ, et al. Trends in invasive pneumococcal disease in cancer patients after the introduction of 7-valent pneumococcal conjugate vaccine: a 20-year longitudinal study at a major urban cancer center. Clin Infect Dis 2018;66(2):244–53.
51. Bonten MJ, Huijts SM, Bolkenbaas M, et al. Polysaccharide conjugate vaccine against pneumococcal pneumonia in adults. N Engl J Med 2015;372(12): 1114–25.
52. Kumar D, Chen MH, Welsh B, et al. A randomized, double-blind trial of pneumococcal vaccination in adult allogeneic stem cell transplant donors and recipients. Clin Infect Dis 2007;45(12):1576–82.
53. Meisel R, Kuypers L, Dirksen U, et al. Pneumococcal conjugate vaccine provides early protective antibody responses in children after related and unrelated allogeneic hematopoietic stem cell transplantation. Blood 2007;109(6):2322–6.
54. Cordonnier C, Labopin M, Chesnel V, et al. Randomized study of early versus late immunization with pneumococcal conjugate vaccine after allogeneic stem cell transplantation. Clin Infect Dis 2009;48(10):1392–401.
55. Cordonnier C, Labopin M, Robin C, et al. Long-term persistence of the immune response to antipneumococcal vaccines after Allo-SCT: 10-year follow-up of the EBMT-IDWP01 trial. Bone Marrow Transplant 2015;50(7):978–83.
56. Ljungman P, Engelhard D, de la Camara R, et al. Vaccination of stem cell transplant recipients: recommendations of the Infectious Diseases Working Party of the EBMT. Bone Marrow Transplant 2005;35(8):737–46.
57. Cordonnier C, Ljungman P, Juergens C, et al. Immunogenicity, safety, and tolerability of 13-valent pneumococcal conjugate vaccine followed by 23-valent pneumococcal polysaccharide vaccine in recipients of allogeneic hematopoietic stem cell transplant aged >/=2 years: an open-label study. Clin Infect Dis 2015;61(3): 313–23.
58. Noonan K, Rudraraju L, Ferguson A, et al. Lenalidomide-induced immunomodulation in multiple myeloma: impact on vaccines and antitumor responses. Clin Cancer Res 2012;18(5):1426–34.
59. Chan CY, Molrine DC, George S, et al. Pneumococcal conjugate vaccine primes for antibody responses to polysaccharide pneumococcal vaccine after treatment of Hodgkin's disease. J Infect Dis 1996;173(1):256–8.
60. Tomczyk S, Bennett NM, Stoecker C, et al. Use of 13-valent pneumococcal conjugate vaccine and 23-valent pneumococcal polysaccharide vaccine among adults aged ≥65 years: recommendations of the Advisory Committee on Immunization Practices (ACIP). MMWR Morb Mortal Wkly Rep 2014;63(37):822–5.
61. Hansson E, Forbes HJ, Langan SM, et al. Herpes zoster risk after 21 specific cancers: population-based case-control study. Br J Cancer 2017;116(12):1643–51.
62. Yenikomshian MA, Guignard AP, Haguinet F, et al. The epidemiology of herpes zoster and its complications in Medicare cancer patients. BMC Infect Dis 2015; 15:106.
63. Alexander KE, Tong PL, Macartney K, et al. Live zoster vaccination in an immunocompromised patient leading to death secondary to disseminated varicella zoster virus infection. Vaccine 2018;36(27):3890–3.
64. Dooling KL, Guo A, Patel M, et al. Recommendations of the Advisory Committee on immunization practices for use of herpes zoster vaccines. MMWR Morb Mortal Wkly Rep 2018;67(3):103–8.
65. Lal H, Cunningham AL, Godeaux O, et al. Efficacy of an adjuvanted herpes zoster subunit vaccine in older adults. N Engl J Med 2015;372(22):2087–96.

66. Cunningham AL, Lal H, Kovac M, et al. Efficacy of the herpes zoster subunit vaccine in adults 70 years of age or older. N Engl J Med 2016;375(11):1019–32.

67. de la Serna J, Campora L, Chandrasekar P, et al. Efficacy and safety of an adjuvanted herpes zoster subunit vaccine in autologous hematopoietic stem cell transplant recipients 18 years of age or older: first results of the phase 3 randomized, placebo-controlled ZOE-HSCT clinical trial. Abstract presented at the BMT Tandem Meeting. Salt Lake City, UT, February 25, 2018..

68. Winston DJ, Mullane KM, Cornely OA, et al. Inactivated varicella zoster vaccine in autologous haemopoietic stem-cell transplant recipients: an international, multicentre, randomised, double-blind, placebo-controlled trial. Lancet 2018; 391(10135):2116–27.

69. Lee CJ, Savani BN, Ljungman P. Varicella zoster virus reactivation in adult survivors of hematopoietic cell transplantation: how do we best protect our patients? Biol Blood Marrow Transplant 2018;24(9):1783–7.

70. Sahoo F, Hill JA, Xie H, et al. Herpes zoster in autologous hematopoietic cell transplant recipients in the era of acyclovir or valacyclovir prophylaxis and novel treatment and maintenance therapies. Biol Blood Marrow Transplant 2017;23(3): 505–11.

71. Distler E, Schnurer E, Wagner E, et al. Recovery of varicella-zoster virus-specific T cell immunity after T cell-depleted allogeneic transplantation requires symptomatic virus reactivation. Biol Blood Marrow Transplant 2008;14(12):1417–24.

72. Jamani K, MacDonald J, Lavoie M, et al. Zoster prophylaxis after allogeneic hematopoietic cell transplantation using acyclovir/valacyclovir followed by vaccination. Blood Adv 2016;1(2):152–9.

73. Issa NC, Marty FM, Leblebjian H, et al. Live attenuated varicella-zoster vaccine in hematopoietic stem cell transplantation recipients. Biol Blood Marrow Transplant 2014;20(2):285–7.

74. Naidus E, Damon L, Schwartz BS, et al. Experience with use of Zostavax((R)) in patients with hematologic malignancy and hematopoietic cell transplant recipients. Am J Hematol 2012;87(1):123–5.

75. Pandit A, Leblebjian H, Hammond SP, et al. Safety of live-attenuated measles-mumps-rubella and herpes zoster vaccination in multiple myeloma patients on maintenance lenalidomide or bortezomib after autologous hematopoietic cell transplantation. Bone Marrow Transplant 2018;53(7):942–5.

76. Liang JL, Tiwari T, Moro P, et al. Prevention of pertussis, tetanus, and diphtheria with vaccines in the United States: Recommendations of the Advisory Committee on Immunization Practices (ACIP). MMWR Recomm Rep 2018;67(2):1–44.

77. Small TN, Zelenetz AD, Noy A, et al. Pertussis immunity and response to tetanus-reduced diphtheria-reduced pertussis vaccine (Tdap) after autologous peripheral blood stem cell transplantation. Biol Blood Marrow Transplant 2009;15(12): 1538–42.

78. Forlenza CJ, Small TN. Live (vaccines) from New York. Bone Marrow Transplant 2012;48:749.

79. Kawamura K, Yamazaki R, Akahoshi Y, et al. Evaluation of the immune status against measles, mumps, and rubella in adult allogeneic hematopoietic stem cell transplantation recipients. Hematology 2015;20(2):77–82.

80. Whitaker JA, Poland GA. Measles and mumps outbreaks in the United States: Think globally, vaccinate locally. Vaccine 2014;32(37):4703–4.

81. Patton ME, Stephens D, Moore K, et al. Updated recommendations for use of MenB-FHbp serogroup B meningococcal vaccine - advisory committee on immunization practices, 2016. MMWR Morb Mortal Wkly Rep 2017;66(19):509–13.

82. Molrine DC, Antin JH, Guinan EC, et al. Donor immunization with pneumococcal conjugate vaccine and early protective antibody responses following allogeneic hematopoietic cell transplantation. Blood 2003;101(3):831–6.
83. Mikati T, Taur Y, Seo SK, et al. International travel patterns and travel risks of patients diagnosed with cancer. J Travel Med 2013;20(2):71–7.
84. Mikati T, Griffin K, Lane D, et al. International travel patterns and travel risks for stem cell transplant recipients. J Travel Med 2015;22(1):39–47.
85. CDC. Travelers health. Available at: Healthhttps://wwwnc.cdc.gov/travel/. Accessed: October 28, 2018.
86. Sicre de Fontbrune F, Arnaud C, Cheminant M, et al. Immunogenicity and Safety of Yellow Fever Vaccine in Allogeneic Hematopoietic Stem Cell Transplant Recipients After Withdrawal of Immunosuppressive Therapy. J Infect Dis 2018;217(3): 494–7.

Moving?

Make sure your subscription moves with you!

To notify us of your new address, find your **Clinics Account Number** (located on your mailing label above your name), and contact customer service at:

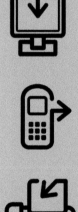

Email: journalscustomerservice-usa@elsevier.com

800-654-2452 (subscribers in the U.S. & Canada)
314-447-8871 (subscribers outside of the U.S. & Canada)

Fax number: 314-447-8029

Elsevier Health Sciences Division
Subscription Customer Service
3251 Riverport Lane
Maryland Heights, MO 63043

*To ensure uninterrupted delivery of your subscription, please notify us at least 4 weeks in advance of move.